PATIENT ASSESSMENT IN PSYCH. ... NURSING

Patient Assessment in Psychiatric Nursing

Philip J. Barker

Clinical Nurse Consultant in Behaviour Therapy

Tayside Area Clinical
Psychology Department
Royal Dundee Liff Hospital
Dundee DD2 5NF

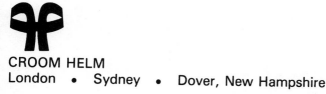

CROOM HELM
London • Sydney • Dover, New Hampshire

© Copyright 1985 Philip J. Barker
Croom Helm Ltd, Provident House, Burrell Row,
Beckenham, Kent BR3 1AT
Croom Helm Australia Pty Ltd, First Floor, 139 King Street,
Sydney NSW 2001, Australia
Croom Helm, 51 Washington Street, Dover, New Hampshire 03820, USA

British Library Cataloguing in Publication Data

Barker, Philip J.
  Patient assessment in psychiatric nursing.
  1. Psychiatric nursing
  I. Title
  610.73'68   RC440
  ISBN 0-7099-3254-5

Library of Congress Cataloging in Publication Data applied for.

Phototypeset in English Times by
Pat and Anne Murphy, 10 Bracken Way, Walkford, Christchurch,
Dorset, England

Printed and bound in Great Britain by
Biddles Ltd, Guildford and King's Lynn

CONTENTS

This book is for the old conjuror — for helping me to see; for Mr Eddy — for helping me to feel; for R. for helping me to think; and the significant others for teaching me that luck really does matter.

PREFACE

If my memory serves me right, I learned little about assessment when I was a student. At least not the kind of assessment I want to discuss here. We were encouraged to use our senses, in an effort to collect observations about the patient's 'state'. These observations tended to lend support to the doctor's diagnosis. On some occasions they served a real function, however limited, as a guide to the management of the patient. However, nurses did not talk readily about their 'assessment' of the patient. Nursing 'assessment' was a scaled-down version of the psychiatric diagnosis. Having learned all the major diagnostic criteria, we waited for patients who had been labelled in a particular way, to behave in a particular way. It was the nurse's task to monitor the patient's *condition*. The idea that patients were people did not have the philosophical credibility it has today. For this reason, nurses paid scant attention to studying the person who was sheltered by his towering label.

Assessment is the most important thing that any nurse can do in her interactions with patients. Historically speaking, it is the thing she does least well. In my own experience, nursing has no real tradition of assessment: the nursing textbooks seem to support this unfortunate conclusion. However, nurses are now trying to get some kind of assessment act together — especially through the medium of the 'nursing process'. However, there is a difference between 'doing' assessment, and doing it properly. Observing people through their behaviour; forming hypotheses about what it means; collecting data on its strength, weakness, severity, etc. are things which — in principle — anyone can do. This is much the same as saying that anyone can give massage or draw a house. What we are hoping for is sophisticated assessment, something which does justice to the problem under review. To continue my analogy, we want an assessment which is more like the sensitive manipulation of a physiotherapist, or the precise accuracy of a draughtsman.

I am under no illusions about the scope and potential of this book. It will *not* show you how to achieve the symbolic peak of reliable, sensitive, clinical judgement. I hope to introduce you to some of the principles and practices of assessment. It is not intended as a manual of assessment. I have spent a decade trying to learn about assessment and have had the good fortune to have worked with some very good 'tutors'. Still, as I write, I often find the enormity of the task overwhelming. I guess that I wrote this book for myself: a lifelong doubter of my own ability to judge. In this book I shall share with you my own ideas about assessment, as well as a few observations on the subject from some of the great thinkers. I shall also discuss the main methods briefly and shall finish by describing the use of several of these methods in the exploration of one or two of the more outstanding 'populations' in psychiatry: I refrain from saying the most outstanding *patients*.

Many of the assessment methods that I discuss in this book are influenced strongly by psychological research and practice. It has been my good fortune to have spent more time working closely with psychologists than I have with psychiatrists. This has allowed me the opportunity to see how the knowledge base of clinical psychology can be a stimulus for the practice of psychiatric nursing. I am aware that many nurses may feel uneasy about using some of the tools recommended here. Their anxiety may be fuelled by the common misconception that only 'psychologists should use psychological measures'. This is like arguing that only mathematicians should use pocket calculators, or even measuring tapes. The work of many a gifted psychologist has given the world a body of knowledge about the study of the human condition that it would be foolish to reject out of hand. There are many facets of psychiatric assessment which can only be undertaken by a suitably qualified psychologist. There are many other aspects of the lives of psychiatric patients which can only be seriously studied if nurses involve themselves in the business of *sophisticated* assessment. Let us not forget that traditional nursing 'assessment' methods — such as the temperature, pulse and respiration recording — are drawn from medical science. Does this mean that only doctors should use them?

I intend this book to be stimulating and informative. I hope that it will give the reader an idea about the kind of assessment methods which my colleagues and I have practised, with great satisfaction, for more than a decade. I do not know whether these methods have made us better 'carers' or not, but we have enjoyed the reassurance these methods gave us. I want to interest the reader in the philosophy of assessment — as distinct from diagnosis. I want to illustrate *which* kind of methods might be helpful in exploring *which* kinds of problems. I also want to communicate something of the thinking which needs to lie behind the selection of these methods. I have resisted the temptation to publish a catalogue of assessment methods, and hope that the reader will consult the original sources as we have done, to find out how to use the standardised methods in the correct manner. I have also tried to suggest how nurses might construct their own simple methods of assessment using principles which are very much 'tried and tested'. All the patients illustrated in the book are real. The methods discussed are examples of the kind of approaches we have adopted to try to understand the person called 'patient'.

Patient assessment in psychiatric nursing is a very wide remit. Such a range of problems and people are embraced by the term 'psychiatric' that I can do justice to some of these areas only by the exclusion of others. In the first four chapters I have tried to look at assessment in its most general sense and consider which principles or actual methods have widespread applicability. The remaining chapters look at specific problem areas which are of common concern to psychiatric nurses, whether working in hospital or community settings.

I have tried to ignore discussing psychiatric disorders as such. Instead, I have favoured looking at problems of living which are common to a variety of disorders. I have dealt exclusively with adult patients. Children, and the more elderly patient are missing from my coverage. Although both groups are important facets of the psychiatric scene I have excluded them for a number of good reasons. Children present with very special problems — whether they are physically or psychologically disturbed. They are not simply immature adults. The world of the child is a special place which demands special consideration. Children do not think like adults: as a result their behaviour, although similar in appearance, does not always follow the same rules as that of adults. Although many of the principles of assessment covered in the book can be adapted to suit children, I did not think that I could do this group justice within the space of a short chapter or even two. Given the pressure on space I thought that it would be more realistic to omit them altogether in the hope that the reader would be stimulated to pursue the subject of assessment in a specialist childhood text. My views on the elderly are similar. Although aspects of the assessment of the elderly are touched upon in Chapters 4 and 5, they are not dealt with in any detail. People who are changing, both physically and mentally, present special problems. I hope that by omitting any detailed consideration of this group I have conveyed — albeit obliquely — my feeling that the elderly are a very special case. They cannot, indeed should not, be seen as just another sub-group of the psychiatric scene.

In a similar vein I have excluded completely from consideration patients with an unambiguous *organic* disorder. I think that this omission is justified on the grounds that nurses have been well prepared to assess aspects of organic disorder: detecting and gauging muscular weakness, tremors, dyskenesia, paresis and paralysis, etc. I do not wish to suggest by my omission that these organic problems have no place in psychiatric nursing assessment. However, they may represent a group of problems which involve the presentation of mental symptoms based upon underlying physical disorder. In many senses they are qualitatively, and quantitatively different from the disorders reviewed here, where the problem is largely a psychological one, with no obvious underlying physical explanation. Despite these exclusions I am confident that many of the general principles of assessment covered in the early chapters, and some of the background issues which thread their way through the remaining chapters will be of some relevance to all three patient groups. In the sense that all are people first and patients second, this book was written with all patients in mind, whether they are specifically dealt with or not.

Throughout the book I have retained the use of the female gender (she) for the role of the nurse, and the male (he) for the patients. I have done so partly to reverse the unfortunate tradition in many texts where the active 'helper' or professional is usually a man, and the unfortunate passive individual on the receiving end is invariably a woman. In the final chapter I have alluded to the effect which sexism has had within the field of psychiatry. In attempting to give women their place in the text I hope that I have made a small contribution to the demise of the male chauvinist.

I should like to extend my heartfelt thanks to my colleagues who have shared my enthusiasm for 'care' in its broadest sense. To Mary Tosh, Sheena Greig, Jim McGlynn, Stan Phillips and my many students — thanks for putting up with me. To Doug Fraser and his many psychology colleagues — I say thanks for your generosity.

I am not sufficiently sure of my own identity to argue that what follows is undeniably 'nursing'. What I do is *assessment*. Why I do it is to understand the patient. I am not sure where my title 'nurse' fits in. I hope one day to establish this more clearly.

Phil Barker
Newport-on-Tay

1 PAINTING BY NUMBERS: AN OVERVIEW OF THE ASSESSMENT PROCESS

> Men are not be judged by their looks, habits and appearances; but by the character of their lives and conversations and by their works. It is better to be praised by one's own works than by the words of another. — L'Estrange

Looking to the Future

As I write the Scottish winter bites hard for the first time this year. Overnight, my neighbours and I seem to have become keen meteorologists. We discuss at length today's conditions, and make various predictions about the likelihood of further snow or the chance of a thaw. In a few short months our present concern will be transformed into an equally anxious search for signs of 'good weather' for our summer vacation. And so it goes throughout the seasons. Each day, men and women everywhere *assess* the weather, each one judging the role it might play in the fabric of their lives.

Although my neighbours and I do not talk about 'assessing' the weather, clearly this is what we are doing, day in and day out. Our 'weather assessment' differs little from the way we *judge* the value of a second-hand car; or how we *review* our social calendar; or how we *evaluate* our children's performance at school. In each case we are required to collect some information about the situation. We are then in a position to comment upon what we have observed. We can make judgements or pronouncements. Is the car worth the asking price? Are we going to be busy in the months ahead? How is Johnny progressing with his maths? Each of these everyday examples shares an important feature of all assessments: they are rarely, if ever, done for their own sake. Assessments are usually undertaken with a view to taking some action in the future. My assessment of the weather is done to help me to decide whether I should take an umbrella or sunglasses. The assessment of Johnny's school report may help us decide whether or not to give him some extra help with his homework. A very small proportion of assessments are done mainly for statistical purposes: to count how many depressed patients pass through a hospital service in one year, for instance. However, even here some action may result and there may be some change in the nature or organisation of the service. When

1

we turn our attention to the concept of *nursing assessment* we can safely assume that the aims are similar to the various simple examples I have quoted. In a small number of cases we collect information on patients to help to study the service offered to them. However, in the majority of cases assessment is undertaken with a view to *planning* and then *evaluating* some specific pattern of nursing care.

In this chapter I am going to try to discuss the meaning of the term *assessment*. I shall try to say what its role is in the care of psychiatric patients, and why it should be an integral part of the nurse's function. I shall take the line that you can't really help people unless you are first able to assess their problems. I am, however, well aware of the fact that many nurses would claim that they 'have no time for assessment' or that nurses have 'always assessed their patients'. With these views in mind I shall try to illustrate that assessment method can, on occasions, save time; and shall try to distinguish between 'intuitive' (or informal) assessments and those which are more structured or standardised. In this latter sense I shall try to plead a case for scientific assessment, if such a thing is possible within the 'art of nursing'. In this opening chapter I shall bear in mind that nurses have no real tradition of using assessment, in anything other than a casual or informal manner. In this sense we are quite unlike our psychology colleagues who are brimming over with the skills and knowledge of assessment, and also the doubts and uncertainties regarding their use in clinical practice. I have little interest in the tradition from which we have come. I am looking to the future of the art of nursing — a future which has already dawned in many areas as nurses gradually extend their natural abilities, becoming more methodical, systematic and effective as a result. This book was written with tomorrow in mind. Who know, by the time you come to read it, it may be today or even yesterday.

What is Assessment?

If you look to your dictionary for a definition of *assessment* you may find it to be fairly restrictive. Most dictionaries refer to assessment in relation to taxation: where an 'assessor' fixes the value of something. This seems to be the traditional meaning of the word. More recently we have come to understand the term as having something to do with *estimating the character of something or someone*. This definition seems to be more relevant to psychiatric nursing, where we are interested in estimating our patients in terms of 'who and what they are'. This meaning was first popularised by psychologists who believed that assessment should be concerned with the *worth* of a person.[1] This view was in stark contrast to traditional medical *diagnosis* which tried to identify the nature of the patient's pathology: looking for what was *wrong* with him. Recently, nurses have started to take a similar viewpoint, moving away from the strict use of a 'diagnostic model' in favour of an assessment of the worth of the individual. The voice of the nursing process movement[2] urges all nurses to show concern for the person behind the patient label, reminding us to look for 'worth' amidst what might seem like insurmountable problems. Although nurses are a long way from achieving this ideal there are many indications that each day brings us closer to dealing with the 'whole person', rather than simply the sum of his parts. Nurses are gradually beginning to appreciate that *assessment* involves looking at the patient from the broadest possible viewpoint. By implication, this will mean studying his *strengths* as well as his *weaknesses*.

Traditional forms of assessment in psychiatric nursing involve derivations of the diagnostic methods used by psychiatrists. In common with the practice of physical medicine, 'psychological medicine' also emphasises the search for a class of disorder. Unfortunately, experience has shown that 'real patients' often do not fit the rather tidy definitions of disorder covered by the diagnostic system.[3] Some psychiatrists have even suggested that psychiatric disorder should perhaps be seen as 'states' where different kinds of problems may be evident to varying degrees in the same patient, rather than assuming that the patient can have only 'one kind of psychiatric disease' that excludes the possibility of any other kind of psychological disorder.[4] In the United States especially this sort of philosophy has led to a broadening of traditional diagnostic categories. Consequently clinicians are acknowledging that there can be a wide range of (e.g.) psychotic disorder, rather than the restricted number of narrow definitions to which we have grown accustomed.[5]

Psychologists in particular have seriously questioned the value of 'pigeon-holing' patients in different diagnostic categories. Some psychologists have instead favoured looking at patients as people who have certain problems of living — which can range from the severely disabling to mild inconvenience. Such people also have strengths or assets, which might play a part in helping them to resolve these problems of living. This approach distinguishes traditional diagnosis from the emerging tradition of *assessment*.

Formal and Informal Methods

The *aim* of most assessments is the same. The process by which the assessment is conducted can vary enormously. These differences are highly significant. They can influence greatly the value of the information that is produced. The way that an assessment is carried out can make the exercise very worth while or largely a waste of time.

The main differences between assessment methods relate to the manner in which the information is collected. In general, this means that the process can be 'formal' or 'informal'. In a *formal* assessment some kind of structure is used. Usually, this is one which has been planned and studied carefully. Probably it will also have been found to be useful. In an *informal* assessment the information is collected by less structured, perhaps even haphazard, methods. Although formal and informal methods appear to have much in common, this similarity is often only superficial. For instance, an interview can be formal or informal, structured or unstructured. In both cases the patient is asked questions and his replies are noted. However, in a formal interview the questions will be worked out carefully in advance. They may even be worded in a particular way. The informal interview lacks this structure. The nurse simply asks the questions she thinks are important at that time and words them in the way she thinks appropriate.

Although *both* kinds of assessment are in common use, we should be aware that any formal system has important advantages over less structured ways of looking at patients. The rules, guidelines and specific procedures which are established in a formal system may help us to study different patients in more or less the same way. As a result, our own prejudices and idiosyncrasies are reduced, if not cancelled out entirely. The outcome of the assessment should be the same, irrespective of who completes it. The same cannot be said of more informal methods. Here our biases, opinions and other kinds of 'value judgement' influence how the assessment is conducted. Such factors can have a big influence on the kind of information collected.

We should emphasise the distinction between formal and informal methods when considering how nurses plan nursing care. In general, a nursing assessment calls for information about the nature and scale of the patient's problems. What is his problem, and how big is it? These questions should be as detailed and unambiguous as possible, especially where we hope to evaluate the effects of different forms of care or treatment. However, the way such information is collected often depends on the problem involved, and can even be influenced by the personality of the patient himself.

Traditionally, nurses have concentrated on assessing the patient's biophysical state. Here the nurse uses highly formalised methods of assessment. Even routine measures — such as taking a pulse or temperature, or testing the reaction of pupils to light — require the use of a precise, controlled procedure. Nurses are taught this 'assessment' procedure in a systematic manner. They are expected to use it with the minimum of adaptions, in an equally systematic manner. The reason for this is simple. Information about the patient's biophysical state needs to be as accurate as possible. The method used to collect this information reflects the need for reliability and precision. It must not be influenced by the attitudes or mood of the person carrying out the assessment. When we consider the nurse's assessment of the patient's non-physical state — his psychological or social functioning — the picture is quite different. The procedures a nurse uses to gauge the patient's core temperature or the various functions of his heart are orderly and fairly unreliable. The assessment of the patient's relationship with himself or the world around him, however, appears almost casual by comparison. Without doubt such 'psychosocial' targets are less clearly defined, and as such are more difficult to assess. However, if we want to understand this aspect of the patient we must strive to use equally formal methods of assessment — methods which will help clear away some of the mist of confusion and mystery which surrounds the patient's psychosocial state. In some situations the choice between formal and informal methods is determined by the patient himself. Where patients are talkative, intelligent and anxious to communicate, the nurse may get most of her information from open-ended conversations. Where the patient is less articulate or rarely speaks, the assessment is likely to favour more specific measures of his behaviour. This might involve the use of standardised rating scales, rather than casual interviewing, and will be more formal as a result. There appears to be a strong tradition in nursing for use of formal methods when studying the patient's physical state and more informal methods when studying him 'psychosocially'. We must ask ourselves whether it is time to discontinue this tradition.

What do we Need to Assess?

So far I have talked about studying the patient's functioning. I have also said that we can do this in a formal, or structured, manner; or can we be unstructured — even haphazard — about it. But what do I mean by the term 'the patient's functioning'? What do we look at or listen to when we say we are trying to study the 'whole person'?

Levels of Living

All of us funtion, or live, on a number of levels (see Figure 1.1). We live on a *basic physical* level. Although we are hardly sensitive to this level, our microscopic functioning — such as our biochemistry — is of crucial importance to the stability of our lives. The molecular or biochemical level of functioning is clearly the most basic level of our lives. At a level slightly removed from this lies our *biological* functioning. All the time our various organs are working to maintain the outward appearance of 'life' supported by our complex muscular and skeletal system, of which we have only the crudest awareness. At another level removed lies our *psychological* life. Here we experience thoughts and emotions, each varying from one day to the next or from one situation to another. At this level also lies our behaviour: how we deploy our thoughts, feelings and various perceptions to produce our own distinctive patterns of action. At another stage removed lies our *social* life: our relationships with the many people who make up our world. Some are close to us, such as family and friends. Others are simply the rest of 'humanity'. Finally, we have a level which can only be called our *spiritual* life. Here we live in the world of our hopes and our beliefs. Here we experience views of ourselves and our world that are often obscure, symbolic and ill-defined. For most of us this level is just beyond our reach. It is a bit like our molecular or biochemical 'life': it is important to our overall functioning; we know that it is there; but we do not fully understand what it does or indeed how it functions.

I have tried to distinguish between these levels of life to show that our life experience is not one thing. Rather, it is a complex interaction of different things: some which we can name and understand; others which are a total mystery to us. Most of us are only aware of how we live on a psychological and social level. Even

Figure 1.1: Levels of Living

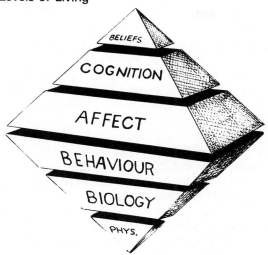

then, we are often confused about these 'open' aspects of our lives. It should be apparent that each of us lives on all these levels of experience all the time, whether we are aware of it or not. Often we only become aware of these levels when we begin to 'malfunction': when some aspect of out chemistry, biology, thoughts, emotions, habits, relationships or our symbolic view of 'ourselves' goes awry. This is also true of the patient. He needs help because some aspect of his functioning is 'dysfunctional'. However, it may well be that the patient experiences 'problems' on a number of levels, due to the interaction of his different life experiences. Although we can study how the patient functions, one level at a time, there may be disadvantages in such an approach. We should be aware of how one problem area — such as disturbed biochemistry — can influence how the patient thinks and feels. We should also be aware that such influences might also operate in the opposite direction.

How Long is a Piece of String?

Every time we set out to find out something, we embark upon an assessment. Each time we ask about what is happening *now*, what happened in the *past* or what might happen in the *future*, we are involved in the curious business of assessment. I say *curious*, for we are inquisitive and anxious to learn. Also the way we go about finding out can often appear strange or in some way extraordinary.

As I said at the start of this chapter, looking out of the window just now, making mental notes on cloud formation, the colour of the sky, how the wind bends the trees; these are all aspects of the assessment process. How can I describe today's weather to you, or make a prediction about tomorrow's, if I do not make some observation of the 'elements': how they appear and how they behave? Assessment of psychiatric patients differs only in *kind* from assessments of the weather, of educational progress or the worth of a painting or piece of pottery. They all share the same principle: that a reliable judgement can be made only if reliable information is available. If we do not scrutinise the painting carefully, we may judge it to be more valuable than it really is. The same is true of people. If we do not look at them carefully, methodically and with the minimum of bias, how can we reliably judge their 'worth'?

Presentation and Performance

There is a difference between a nursing assessment and judgements we might make about the weather, cars or objects. The judgement of the person that results from our assessment will, in most cases, be of crucial importance. In some cases a nursing assessment, combined with other forms of medical or psychological assessment, might make the difference between life and death. This could be said of the depressed patient who is a suicide risk, or the disturbed or disoriented patient who, unwittingly, might be a danger to himself. Having said that, we cannot afford to be glib about the potential value of assessment information. Neither should we complain too much about the work required to collect such information.

It is difficult to say anything concrete about psychiatric nursing assessment except to say that it is in its infancy, and is often gravely misunderstood. I opened this chapter from a rather oblique angle. I tried to show how assessment is a part of everyday life. It becomes *assessment* — the professional tool — only when we standardise or make more formal the things we do each day; and which we take very much for granted. It is very important that we grasp the idea that assessment is *not* 'something which psychologists do'. Certainly there are psychological forms of assessment. Certainly psychologists do carry out assessments. However, that does not mean that *only* psychologists can judge the worth of a person. Neither does it mean that someone who carries out such an assessment becomes, as if by magic, a psychologist. We must accept that the term 'assessment' is a word with a broad range of meanings, depending very much upon who defines it. I am aware that here I am simply adding my own interpretation of the word. However, each definition of assessment, including my own, emphasises the *collection of information* with the intention of *making a judgement*. These two actions are the very heart of assessment.

Nurses can assess patients in much the same way as mechanics might diagnose faults in a car engine. The mechanic is not diagnosing in the same way that a doctor would. Yet there are similarities. He is monitoring the functions of the engine, and he compares these with some ideal — what he would call normal engine running. When a doctor studies a patient's cardiovascular system and diagnoses some malfunction he uses the self-same process. I make this analogy merely to reinforce the point that nurses can embrace the idea of assessment in much the same way that a mechanic embraces diagnosis. The fact that these concepts have, by tradition, been associated with other professions is unimportant. If these concepts can help us fulfil our role, we should not hesitate in adopting them. It could be said that without the concept of assessment (or diagnosis) we cannot get on with the business of repairing, be it people or cars.

It is strange, however, that so little attention has been paid to assessment in psychiatric nursing textbooks. My own library shelf is packed with various directions about the kind of procedures to use, or suggestions about general processes to use in caring for patients. By comparison with this wealth of advice virtually nothing has been written about how we should go about identifying *what* should be done in the name of nursing care. As I noted earlier, in most areas of the patient's functioning the nursing assessment is a highly haphazard affair, governed by 'rules of thumb'. We need to translate these informal approaches into more systematic forms of assessment. Dare I say that we need to adopt more *scientific* ways of studying the patient?

Assessment involves looking at patients with a view to gaining a picture that will help us see them as unique human beings. This process involves developing a working model of the person. This model should show, in a simplified manner, how he funtions in relation to himself and the world around him. But before we set this process in motion we must decide what we are going to look at.

Any assessment involves collecting information about *performance* and *presentation*. If I were to ask you to assess a teapot or a car, you would make various notes on their appearance: size, colour, shape, etc. You would then try to relate these to the way in which they work: does the teapot pour easily? Is the handle easy to grip? What is the car's top speed? What is its average fuel consumption? Answers to these questions will give us *data* — or information — about presentation and performance. The appearance and the performance of things are not always related. The colour of a teapot has no relationship with how it pours. However, the *shape* of the spout or the contours of the car will have a relationship with 'pouring' or 'fuel consumption'. In this analogy I am trying to illustrate how the 'design' of something is related to its function: how it works in practice. We are often required to look for similar kinds of 'connections' — between presentation and performance — in our patients. The blushing (presentation) of a young man's cheeks and the stammering (performance) of his voice may have a relationship, one to the other. In assessment, we collect information about the appearance of the patient (his presentation) and how he behaves (his performance); and then try to see if we can understand him better by combining these two viewpoints.

Fishing for Clues

An assessment can be as broad or as narrow as we like. However, some kinds of assessment are concerned only with a narrow focus. These are usually called 'diagnostic assessments'. Some confusion seems to exist between the terms 'diagnosis' and 'assessment'. Before going any further perhaps we should clarify the difference between the two. These differences can best be illustrated by studying Figure 1.2. Here I have tried to describe the difference between assessment and diagnostic functions in a symbolic manner.

In a diagnosis the 'assessor' sets out to identify the presence of certain problems, dysfunctions or abnormalities. If these are *not* found the patient is given 'a clean bill of health'. Indeed, whether we are looking at a person's heart or a car engine, a diagnosis usually involves the detection of faults. The diagnostician rarely, if ever, looks for things which are right with the person, or are in good working order. A diagnostic report describes only those aspects of functioning which are abnormal. This is true of a doctor's diagnosis of a patient; a mechanic's diagnosis of a car; or an engineer's diagnosis of the structure of a bridge. The common denominator is the search for, and ultimate detection of, *problems*. This concept is illustrated on the left side of the figure. Here the

Figure 1.2

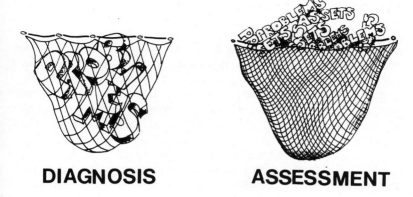

DIAGNOSIS　　　　**ASSESSMENT**

'net' which is cast is designed to catch only a certain size and shape of problem. All other aspects of the persons's functioning will pass through this net. This is the symbolic representation of the 'screening' or diagnostic process.

Assessment, in its purest sense, involves looking at people, or situations, in a more general sense. It tries to gain an overall picture, one which describes positive characteristics as well as problems. A full assessment describes the skills, assets and other positive features of a person. On the flip side of the coin can be seen his list of handicaps, disabilities or other dysfunctions. We often talk about cricketers 'assessing' the field of play. On the positive side the batsman studies the positioning of the fielders and tries to judge where to direct the ball to score maximum runs. On the negative side, he looks for possible problems: how he might be caught out. The assessment net shown on the right side of the illustration is designed to screen as many aspects of the person as possible. The weave of the net, which represents the format of the assessment, is much finer. As a result the person is subjected to a much finer-grained analysis. Aspects of the person's performance and presentation, which might be ignored or overlooked in a diagnosis, will be 'caught' under this broader form of assessment.

Objectivity and the Search for Meaning

So far I have discussed the concept of assessment by describing *what* we should look at and how we might organise our study of the patient. This is usually called the assessment *process*: suggesting that the activities involved in assessment can be isolated and defined. I have tried to show how some of our observations are objective where we use standardised methods. In other cases they are highly subjective, such as when we interview the patient casually. I have emphasised that there is a need to be as objective as possible. The importance of our assessment can never be over-stated. Can we ever afford to make casual observations, or snap judgements, when the quality of people's lives is at stake?

Although we try to collect information on the patient objec-tively, in the final analysis we must judge the significance of the information. Asking ourselves the question 'What does this mean?' requires some subjectivity. Critics of the trend towards a more scientific approach to care and treatment in psychiatry have said that 'dealing with human problems' and 'trying to be scientific' do not mix. Certainly, this would be true if we tried to assess people in exactly the same way that we studied atoms or chemical elements. If our aim was to make the assessment of people exactly the same as assessment in the physical sciences, then clearly this would not be appropriate. It goes without saying that it would hardly be possible either. However, that does not mean that we cannot try to abide by the spirit of the scientific approach, by weeding out our biases and prejudices. If we can do that we can make our observations more objective.

Judgements

Instead of comparing the assessment of people with traditional scientific methods it may be more appropriate to compare it with the *judicial* system. The courts use an assessment system which is not all that far removed from the assessment process of psychiatric nursing. Evidence is collected, presented and reviewed, so that a judgement can be made. This judgement is often made by someone in a 'learned' position: a person of high status whose impartiality is taken for granted. Where the judge is instructed by the jury, these laypersons are required to make an impartial judgement of the facts. Obviously, their judgement will rely on their own subjective viewpoint. However, they try to prevent their own prejudices and opinions from influencing their final decision.

Judgements of this sort are found in almost all forms of patient care. They are, however, more in evidence in some than in others. Even where we use highly objective means of recording or measuring the patient's state — as in temperature readings or electrocardiogram print-outs — we end up using our own subjective judgements. What does the height of mercury tell us about the patient? What do these traces on the ECG paper mean? Most often we ask, 'is this normal or abnormal?' We can ask this question about every level of the patient's life. Are these ESR levels normal? Is his heart rate normal? Is this level of anxiety normal? Is this kind of behaviour normal? Are these beliefs normal? These are rarely the straightforward questions which they seem. Do we mean 'average' or 'pathological'? Do we mean normal by comparison with ourselves; by comparison with most people in this hospital, in this town, this country or the whole world? Or are we talking about normality as it relates to this one individual? We shall return to a discussion of this concept later.

Even if the patient's problems are abnormal by most standards we must still judge whether or not they represent a serious threat to the patient or those around him. Virtually everyone, ourselves included, has some problem which others might consider in need of resolution. A key aspect of our assessment involves deciding whether or not the patient 'needs' help or treatment. A high temperature or an irregular heartbeat signifies a biological or physiological problem for most of us. The 'life problems' of the psychiatric patient are rarely so clear-cut. The range of so-called 'normal behaviour' is so wide that what is seen as disturbed by one person may be an acceptable way of life to another. The axiom that 'one man's meat is another man's poison' appears to extend to behavioural conventions also.

So how do we judge the seriousness of a patient's problems? If we accept that we have a right or duty to make such a judgement, it is apparent that we need some help to arrive at such an important decision. We often take for granted the biological knowledge that helps us decide that a certain temperature reading may indicate an infection, or that an irregular pulse may signify heart disease. In such cases the patient may even look ill. This 'fact' may even be evident to the layperson. However, we always take our 'layperson's hunch' a stage further, by applying more rigorous forms of assessment. As professionals, we make our diagnosis only after certain formal examinations have been made. In principle, the assessment of the patient's psychosocial problems should be no different. The patient may complain of certain problems — such as anxiety or hearing voices which disturb him. Alternatively, these patterns of behaviour may be reported by his family or friends. Neither the patient nor his family need any specialist knowledge to identify these problems. They rely upon their senses and their intuitive judgements. This means that their observations will be highly informal or unscientific. Our professional responsibility is to follow up these casual observations by introducing more formal 'tests'. These could be seen as the psychosocial equivalent of the biological and physiological tests already mentioned. These methods *should* be more reliable and objective. They should be less arbitrary and subjective. They should help us to clarify the nature and significance of the patient's problems. They should tell us 'What is wrong with this person?' and 'How serious are his problems? In a sense we are also asking, 'What does the problem *mean* for the person concerned?' I say that we should use these methods, *in principle*. It would appear that, in practice, we often continue to rely upon methods which are less than scientific; and may be heavily influenced by our own biases or prejudices.

The Assessment Process

On a technical level any assessment involves collecting data; arranging this into a suitable format; and analysing and interpreting this 'picture of the patient'. Finally, we make predictions about how the patient might function under a different set of circumstances: under treatment or 'therapeutic' conditions. My definition of assessment suggests that we need to collect fairly precise measures of the patient's functioning. We need this precise information to make some hypothesis about *why* the patient functions in this way. This represents our understanding of 'him' as an individual. Then we test out our hypothesis under treatment conditions, continuing to monitor his performance throughout. In effect, I am describing a 'scientific' model of nursing assessment. This model would, I hope, take account of the 'science of man': all that we know about the experience of being human.

The Six Honest Serving Men

In order to set up and follow through the assessment process, we

Figure 1.3: Six Honest Serving Men

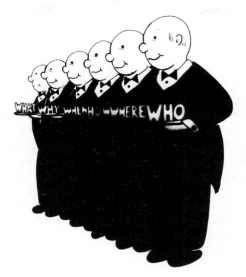

need to ask ourselves a series of simple, yet far-reaching, questions (see Figure 1.3). These are built around the 'six honest serving men' who taught Rudyard Kipling all he knew. 'Their names are What and Why and When and How and Where and Who.'[6]

(1) Why am I doing this assessment? What is the aim of the assessment? What do I want to know or find out about the patient? Am I studying him with a view to discharge? transfer to another ward? suitability for employment or resolution of specific distresses? In answering this question we give the assessment a necessary 'slant'. We are deciding what kind of assessment we are planning: one which will assess whether or not he is wrongly placed, understimulated, overworked, or otherwise in 'need' of some help.

(2) What should I assess? If you want to take a snapshot portrait of someone you must stand close enough, and must focus the camera, so that his *features* can be caught clearly on the photograph. An assessment also tries to capture the patient's important features. To do this requires some selection. You must decide what to focus upon and, by implication, what you are going to ignore or allow to merge into the background. This selection process is not always easy. The important features of the patient are those which

are related — directly *and* indirectly — to the area of 'need' established in answer to question (1)

(3) How will I get the information I need? A wide range of options is open to you when it comes to deciding how to tackle the assessment. You might interview the patient, gaining an insight on his view of the problem. You might observe the patient, building up a picture from your own viewpoint. In other cases information might be supplied by family or friends, or through the observations of other members of the care team. Within each of these general approaches lies a range of variations, from highly structured through to informal interviewing, and from fairly loose observational methods using rating scales through to 'tighter' methods using direct recording techniques. The cardinal rule is: 'Use the method which gives you the most reliable and appropriate information, for the least amount of effort.'

(4) How will I judge what this information means? The 'meaning' of the patient's functioning — or behaviour — can be looked at from a number of angles. We could ask, 'How big a problem does this represent?' This would involve evaluating the problem in terms of scale or quantity. However, before we can do this we have to find a standard, or *norm*, against which to compare the patient. Our question then becomes, 'How abnormal is the patient's behaviour?' As we shall discuss later, a single norm or standard is rarely available. Instead we use a variety of norms — determined by factors such as class or cultural affiliations, by educational background, occupation, religion or political persuasion. These different influences determine how something I might consider 'normal' might be viewed by someone else as 'deviant'.

We should also try to remember that much of our behaviour is 'expressive': through our behaviour we say something about ourselves, about our situation and our relationship with the world in general. The behaviour we show to the world often acts as a signal or symbol for what we experience on other levels of our functioning. In trying to understand what the patient's behaviour *means* we should try to judge what it might be saying about the patient and his life. What does it signify about other, more hidden, aspects of his life experience?

(5) How might the patient function under different conditions? By this stage you should have arrived at a fairly objective assessment of the patient's *present* functioning. You have described how

he functions, on as many levels as is appropriate. You have also described the conditions under which this functioning takes place. Your last task is to predict how the patient might function if any of these conditions were altered. This is the last stage of the assessment, and the first stage of the treatment plan.

These five questions will help us to decide upon the general aim of the assessment, the major objectives that will help to achieve that aim, and will help us to decide what to do in the name of care or treatment. The general aim of assessment might be to measure the patient's level of anxiety, or his level of independence, or his level of social interaction. Our objectives in carrying out the assessment again involve the use of Kipling's 'honest serving men'.

Measurement: What does the patient do? *How* often does he do it? For *how long* does he do it? All these questions will help yield quantitative measures which will help judge the scale or size of the problem.

Clarification: How does he perform these behaviours? On his own? With others? *Where* does he show these patterns of behaviour and *when*? Answers to these questions will help us understand the context — or conditions — under which these things happen.

Explanation: What is the effect of the patient's behaviour? How do others react? Can the patient explain *why* he does this, rather than that? Answers to these questions will help us to understand the possible purpose or function of the patient's behaviour.

Variation: How does his behaviour change from day to day? from week to week? or from one situation to another?

Information of this sort helps us to appreciate the scale of the patient's problems: their 'seriousness'. It also helps us to see how they may vary from time to time, or from one situation to another. This kind of overview also helps us to form hypotheses, or make up 'hunches', about why the problem exists at all. It is to this last area that we turn our attention when we start to think about using our assessment to design care or treatment. The information about the size, the nature and the variations in the problem can be used to monitor any changes which occur during care or treatment. This monitoring function helps us to decide whether treatment has been successful or unsuccessful.

Focus

Before we leave the process of assessment let us consider how closely we should study the patient. How many questions should we ask? How detailed should our enquiries be? This question of focus is of crucial relevance. We can study a flower by looking at it with the naked eye. We can also take it apart, putting each petal under the microscope. This analogy holds true for the assessment of people. We can study people in fairly general terms, making notes and observations upon what is audible or visible. We can also study the person in much closer detail, examining every aspect of his functioning, embracing the many layers of his life mentioned earlier. For example, a person who complains of 'anxiety' might be asked to rate his anxiety: to describe how he feels (an internal account). At the same time we could observe how he presents when he says he is anxious (an external account). This is the simplest kind of assessment possible. It might also, in some cases, be the best. Yet, we could also undertake a much finer-grained analysis of the problem. We might use biofeedback equipment to monitor his sweating, pulse, blood pressure and muscle tension, assessing these biological 'behaviours' across different situations. This sort of analysis would not only describe very precisely the variations in his anxiety, but would also indicate any possible 'trigger situations'. This kind of fine-grain analysis is appealing, especially to those nurses who feel the need to demonstrate the scientific status of their 'art'. However, a number of considerations need to be taken into account before we decide upon such an in-depth study. Do we have the time to devote to such a detailed assessment? Do we have access to such sophisticated equipment? Would we know how to operate it? These involve professional costs — time, resources and expertise. There are also possible costs to the patient. How will he feel if he is wired up to all this equipment? How realistic is it to expect him to move from one situation to another carrying such equipment? To what extent will the presence of all this 'hardware' influence the measures we are taking? These considerations involve balancing out the costs of the assessment, for staff and patient, against the advantages of gaining certain kinds of information. It should be apparent that the advantages of a system should always outweigh the disadvantages involved in taking the measure. However, there is an additional consideration. On occasions, we may believe that information can be obtained by relatively simple means. For example, we may believe that we can find out all we need to know by asking the patient a few simple questions. In such a case there is no need to look any further. However, such a simple form of assessment is rarely adequate. More often than not we are obliged to add additional layers of enquiry. We may need to help the medical staff take various physiological measures, such as blood or urine analysis. We may also need to collect information about aspects of biological functioning, such as thyroid function tests. We may also need to study the patient's behaviour closely: how he interacts with others and what his reactions are to everyday situations. Finally, we may need to ask much more carefully prepared questions in order to unravel the mysteries of the patient's thoughts and beliefs. These aspects of his life may be as much a mystery to him as they are to us. However, we should not assume that this kind of 'global analysis' is needed for every patient. In some cases a simple 'enquiry' may suffice, while for others something bridging a simple enquiry and this kind of global analysis is required. In general, however, if a useful picture of the patient can be achieved by simple means, why use something more complex? This is the nurse's application of the law of parsimony.[7]

Person-centred Assessment

It is almost a cliché to say that no two people are alike. Yet traditional psychiatry has often tried to deny this, searching for the similarities between patients, looking for the 'disease' which can explain their disorder, or the 'syndrome' which unites them. In our search to understand the mysteries of mental disorder we have often reduced people to the level of one stereotype or another. The world seems to be populated by a host of 'types': a plethora of neurotics and psychotics; hypochondriacs and exhibitionists; introverts and extroverts; men with mother fixations, women with father fixations; hysterical women, but rarely, if ever, hysterical men. In this male-dominated world they are usually referred to as inadequate psychopaths. I do not wish to discuss the value of such type-casting or the schools of thought that gave them birth. I wish only to remind the reader that this is the traditional face of psychiatry. A face which may mask the underlying anxiety of the field: if at first you don't understand, give it a label. Much of what follows in this book takes the line that such stereotyping may be convenient — for example in finding out how many 'schizophrenics' live in British hospitals. However, such type-casting may be less than helpful to those nurses who want to help Tom, Dick and Harry who happen to be so labelled. I say 'much of what follows' since on occasions I find myself lapsing into the vernacular and talking about 'patients' as though they were plants or some other species of life which attracts our interest. Yet, it is clear that on a few occasions it is helpful to emphasise the similarities between one patient group and another — when, for example, writing a book like this. However in most cases I suspect that assessment methods are concerned to discover the 'fact' that many problems are shared by a whole host of patient 'types'. The methods which are discussed in detail later in the book will, it is hoped, help us discover something of the uniqueness of the individual patient.

Most nurses will be sympathetic to the idea that all men and women are different. Although I have heard nurses say that a patient is a 'typical depressive', or whatever, more often I have found them scratching their heads at the apparent conflicts that exist within the patient. This conflict of diagnosis is very relevant to nursing. Over the last few years nurses have begun to realise that they are not concerned primarily with the diagnosis and treatment of illness. They are more concerned to identify the needs of individuals — who may or may not fit within a broad diagnostic category. Their first responsibility is to meet the needs of the unique person who is, temporarily, standing in a queue along with other 'patients'.

Behavioural Assessment

It should be apparent from what I have said already that I favour the description and measurement of what the patient does, rather than making wild judgements about the significance of what he is doing. I shall expand upon the use of inference and extrapolation later. For the moment let me offer some kind of rationale for emphasising the study of *behaviour*.

Recent years have seen significant developments in methods aimed at identifying and measuring discrete patterns of behaviour. These methods have largely replaced the use of projective methods, which sought to make comments upon concepts such as personality. These methods have reminded us, shoud we need such reminding, that we cannot make inferences about concepts like 'personality' without first making observations upon how the person behaves. In any situation where we observe people, we can later draw more general conclusions about the *meaning* of their behaviour in that situation, and what it says about the person overall. However, we cannot make either of these more *general* comments without first taking specific notes on how he behaves. For example, if we observed a young man who is shown a photograph of a naked woman by his friend while both of them are standing in the street, what can we say about the young man's *attitude*? Well, virtually nothing — at least until we have made some notes on his behaviour. How does he react to the situation? Does he smile, blush, laugh, look away? What did he do next? Does he take the picture to study it more closely? Does he tear it up? Does he turn and walk away? Does he say anything to his friend which can be interpreted as positive or negative comment? From these simple observations we might make some guesses — or inferences — about his attitude towards female nudity. Does his behaviour seem to suggest approval or disapproval? We might go on to make further inferences about (e.g.) his personality: does this suggest that he is shy or introverted, or gregarious and extroverted? All these sorts of 'observations' begin with an observation of what we saw the young man doing, and heard him saying. These happenings make up the basic data from which our other inferences are made. Although the kind of observations we have talked about could hardly be called scientific, they may be fairly accurate in terms of building a picture of this young man in this situation. However, we would need to see him performing under different conditions to find out if his attitude towards female nudity is a constant one, or one which is influenced by circumstances. Would he, for example, show the same 'attitude' (or behaviour) if his parents were present; or if the picture was of a member of his family, or perhaps a girlfriend?

When we are talking about the patient's *behaviour* we mean what we can see the patient doing and can hear him saying. We also mean what he can tell us about what is happening inside his body: his various thought processes and emotional reactions. Behaviour can also mean the 'hidden' aspects of human functioning which are involved in 'outward' shows of behaviour: the various functions of our autonomic or central nervous systems. Behaviour is often presumed to refer *only* to what is observable. I think that it is more appropriate, and helpful, to include the many forms of *covert* (hidden) behaviour: thinking, remembering, fantasising and imagining — among the many cognitive functions; and the action of smooth muscles and the discharge of hormones among the various functions of the autonomic system. These hidden behaviours play an important part in assisting the performance of more open or *overt* patterns of behaviour. As we shall see in subsequent chapters, our assessment of the patient often involves us in looking for evidence of the function of these hidden behaviours.

I am aware that many will disagree with my rather catholic definition of 'behaviour'. Let me simply suggest that it might be a convenient definition. In response to the question 'What do you do when you assess a patient?' we can answer that we 'begin by studying his behaviour'.

Inferences

The act of observation involves the observer using her sensory apparatus to collect information about the person under observation. The observer uses her eyes to record what she has seen; her hearing to record what the patient said; her tactile sensation to judge weight or power in a limb; and her sense of smell to note any particular odours. She might also use her sense of taste to determine (e.g.) how bitter or sweet is some food, before asking the patient to judge it in a similar manner. All the information collected here is called *data*: or rather it is usually called data when transformed into a numerical format. However, the correct definition of the term 'data' is 'the assumptions which form the basis for an inference or conclusion'. This definition is very important. It reminds us that we collect information — or data — with a view to making some more general comment, or coming to a conclusion. When we weigh a patient we arrive at some assumptions about his 'weight'. We might say that this means that he is obese: this is an inference drawn from our study of the data. We might also say that this level of obesity is pathological: here we are making a more complex inference, suggesting the possibility of an unfortunate conclusion.

You might be wondering what the relevance of all this is. I am trying to emphasise that although we often talk as if we can make immediate judgements about patients, we cannot come to any real conclusions without collecting some data. We shall use these data to make inferences about what we think is happening, and may then proceed to come to some conclusion about the situation. *Inference* is the process of reasoning by which we come to a conclusion. We cannot come to a conclusion without reasoning — without making some inferences. More importantly, we cannot make inferences without some basic data: some 'real information'.

I emphasise this point for another reason. Nurses, and indeed many other staff members, have a tendency to devote too much energy to 'making inferences', and not enough energy to collecting data. Figure 1.4. shows the levels of inference possible in making increasingly more general comments about a situation.

Figure 1.4

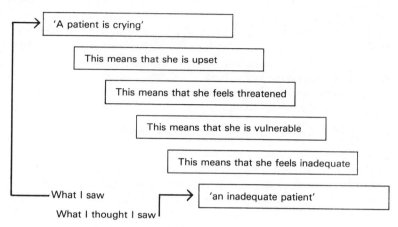

Let us take as an example the young man discussed earlier. Our 'basic data' involved notes about what he *said* and *did* in that situation. Based upon what we observed we could make a first-level inference: here we make a general comment about what we believe these observations tell us about him. Since this is only a first-level inference, the conclusion we will draw will be fairly conservative. We might infer that his behaviour showed that he was embarrassed. We do not *know* that he was embarrassed; we merely infer this from what we saw. We could take the inference game a stage further by saying that he was embarrassed *because* he is uncertain about his attitudes towards women. It is clear that we cannot really know this: again it is an inference and this time a more extravagant one. We can become increasingly extravagant in our inference game, suggesting at the next level that he is embarrassed because he has a deep-seated fear of all women, a fear which is stimulated by seeing them adopting sexually provocative poses. And so we might go on, climbing up into the clouds of 'unreason', as we move further and further away from the information which provided the starting-point. I am not suggesting that we should not make inferences about behaviour: indeed it is clear that we must, if we are to make any reasonable comment. However, I am merely alerting you to the danger of losing sight of the original data by clouding it with fanciful inferences. As I noted above, there is a tendency among many members of staff to 'jump to conclusions' about patients: they often do so because they spend insufficient time collecting basic data. A rather strict and moralistic father who observed his son looking at pictures of naked women in the street might infer that this meant that his son was immoral, or indeed had gone to the devil. We might excuse the father on the grounds that he did not study the situation closely enough, or that he had mis-interpreted the facts. We should take care that we — the profes-sionals — remember always to study situations closely, and avoid making rash interpretations.

The Normal Human: Where can we Find him?

Although we have only recently started to study the patient's behaviour in anything resembling a scientific fashion, psychiatry has always been interested in abnormal behaviour. It has been estimated that around 20 million people in the USA suffer from some disturbance of thought or overt behaviour sufficient to merit psychiatric attention. The same sorts of estimates have been made in the UK. Many of these people will refer themselves for profes-sional consultation, while many others will deny that they have any problem and may be treated forcibly by agents of the state. From even this casual observation it should be apparent that ideas about 'what is normal' can be held by the individual *or* by society. On many occasions society and the individual may be in conflict. When, for instance, a person says that he can't cope, needs help, or is otherwise distressed in some way, and we the professionals decide that he is not seriously disturbed in any psychological or psychiatric sense, then such a conflict is evident. On other occasions the roles may be reversed: we may try to impress upon a patient that he needs our care and treatment, and he may reject the service we offer him. In either example the behaviour of the patient is seen as 'abnormal': in the first case it deviates from the norm set by the patient himself; in the second from our norms — social norms.

Any pattern of behaviour — whether it involves action, thought or belief — is usually called *deviant* when it does not meet some standard, often an average for a population. We talk frequently about behaviour being within normal limits: this means the range that governs *most* of the population. People who are very tall or very short are un-average or atypical, as they fall outwith the range that covers *most* of the population. The same is true of people who are very intelligent or who are not very bright: they too fall outwith this 'normal range'. Since such people deviate, or branch off, from the 'normal standard', we could call all such people deviants. However, the term is usually restricted to characteristics that are considered to be unhealthy, unwholesome or to be discouraged in some way. Just because a pattern of behaviour is 'deviant' does not mean that it is a cause for concern. Some people dress in an unorthodox manner. In terms of the strict usage of the term they are 'dress deviants'. Commonly, we would simply call them 'eccentric', although in today's climate we would probably pay little attention to such behaviour. Other people may engage in even more unusual patterns of dressing, such as dressing up in the clothes of the opposite sex. Traditionally, such behaviour has been called a 'sexual deviation'. This simply reflects a cultural unease about such behaviour, assuming that it is in some way unhealthy, or unwholesome. As attitudes change towards sexual behaviour in general, 'cross dressing' is often seen less as a problem. From a different perspective, people who do charity work in their spare time, men who give up their seats to women on buses, or people who go to church every Sunday could also be regarded as deviants for the simple reason that such practices are not performed by anything like a majority of the population. We do not of course label such practices as deviant because, although we may not practise such behaviour ourselves, we assume that it is either noble or at least innocuous.

I have taken the view that our interest in assessment lies mainly with the study of the patient's behaviour: what he says, does, thinks, feels, etc. However, although it may be a relatively straightforward exercise to identify and measure such patterns of behaviour, it is more difficult to answer the question, 'What does it *mean*?' Once we have assessed a pattern of behaviour, how do we go about judging whether it is normal or abnormal? Arriving at such a decision is rarely easy, for the simple reason that normal behaviour can vary from one person to the next, from one culture to another, and can be influenced by different laws even within the same country. Our behaviour is, however, associated most with the culture within which we live. Most of our behaviour is learned: human beings appear to be poorly supplied with instincts, unlike our animal and insect relations. Even infants of only a few weeks old have already begun to learn how to respond to their environment: their behaviour is not pre-programmed before birth. We have no instincts or other biological endowments that help us to tie shoelaces, cook food, order a beer, comb our hair, catch a bus, or open a window for fresh air. All these mundane behaviours are acquired through learning and are all part of the culture to which we belong. If we move to a different culture — like an under-developed country or even a long-stay ward — such behaviour may not be required or may even be discouraged. The net result will be that these features of our behaviour that are normal just now may become 'abnormal', deviant or at the very least unusual.

When we come to consider the behaviour of people in the psychiatric setting there is a common assumption that their behaviour is either normal or abnormal. Although it might make our task a lot easier were this 'absolute' situation to prevail, the situation is not, however, quite so black and white. We should acknowledge this fact. As I have said, normal behaviour appears to be defined by cultures. Even within cultures, subcultures may determine different patterns of behaviour. Take, for example, the young man holding the picture of the 'pin-up girl' mentioned earlier. Within most Western cultures 'normal' male behaviour in such a situation would involve lustful, male chauvinist, expressions of sexual fantasy. Within these cultures there are, however, small subgroups of men who, for intellectual, religious or moral reasons, would refuse to display such 'characteristically normal male behaviour'. Such men might well be scorned by the majority for their soppy, effeminate un-male stance. I do not wish to discuss which of these positions is 'right'. I use this example as an illustration of the wide divergence of functioning which can exist within cultures, within subcultures, even within sexes.

There would appear to be few, if any, universal norms as far as behaviour is concerned. One might assume that murder, incest and child abuse would be viewed as unacceptable by all societies and cultures. Sociologists would argue that this is not the case. Many cultures, admittedly some of them 'uncivilised', will tolerate, even encourage, such practices under certain conditions. I take note of this simply to sharpen our focus when it comes to studying so-called abnormal behaviour within the field of psychiatry. We should not forget that even manifestly exceptional behaviour — such as the experience of hallucinations — is relatively common in some cultures. In a study in the early 1960s Lee noted that out of a random sample of Zulu women more than a third had reported visual and auditory hallucinations involving 'angels, babies and little short hairy men'.[8] In the same study he found that more than half of the women engaged in 'screaming behaviour', often yelping for hours, days, even weeks. Either of these reported behaviours would be viewed as grossly abnormal in the West. Yet few of these women showed any others signs of mental disorder. Within their own culture their hallucinations and screaming were legitimate. More recently, African psychiatrists have reported that persecutory delusions are more frequent in African, Jamaican and Caribbean subjects than in any other groups. They explain this finding by attributing the delusions to beliefs in witchcraft and voodoo, common to their cultures.[9] This has been reported by other researchers[10] who suggest that the beliefs (which we call delusions) held by West Indian psychotics are the same as those held by 'normal' West Indians, the difference between the two groups being the abnormal reaction (or behaviour) of the so-called psychotics to these beliefs. We shall return to this issue in subsequent chapters and will discuss the 'problem' of normal behaviour in the final chapter, where the ethical and moral dilemmas associated with the concept will be highlighted.

The Educated Guess

In this chapter we have looked at a range of issues in an attempt to define my objectives for writing this book. I may have patronised some readers who were already aware of many of the issues: diagnosis *versus* assessment, normal *versus* abnormal behaviour, etc. Yet it is my understanding that many of us are not sufficiently aware of the meaning of assessment. We have had little chance, as nurses, to develop experience and knowledge on the subject. If we are to develop these assets we must think about what assessment might mean in a broad sense, as well as what procedures it might contain. I have tried to emphasise the *ordinariness* of assessment. It is no different from assessing how much seed will be needed to cover the bare patches on the lawn, or how much wool will be needed to knit a sweater. Anyone might make a wild guess, and by the law of averages they could be right. But there is no substitute for the 'educated guess', made by the keen gardener or the regular knitter. The calculations here are based upon knowledge and experience. In the chapters which follow I shall try to discuss some of the facets of assessment and the experiences with patients which combine to produce an understanding of the term. It is an understanding which we appear to be constantly reaching, but which always seems to elude our grasp.

Notes

1. G. H. Jones, 'Principles of Psychological Assessment' in P. Mittler (ed.), *The Psychological Assessment of Mental and Physical Handicaps* (Tavistock in association with Methuen, London, 1974).

2. P. Ashworth, G. Castledine and J. K. McFarlane, 'The Process in Practice', *Nursing Times* (Supplement), 30 Nov. 1978.

3. In recent years in the United States there has been considerable debate over the validity and reliability of their diagnostic classification system (see Chapter 11). In 1980 the American Psychiatric Association issued a third edition of their *Diagnostic and Statistical Manual (DSM III)*.

4. F. R. Hines and R. B. Williams, 'Dimensional Diagnosis and the Medical Student's Grasp of Psychiatry', *Archives of General Psychiatry*, **32**, (1975, pp. 525-8.

5. Although we tend to talk about 'schizophrenia' and 'manic depressive psychosis', current thinking takes the view that there may be a broad range of psychotic disorders. In the *DSM III* (see note 4) as many as 15 psychotic states are discussed.

6. Rudyard Kipling, *The Just So Stories* (Macmillan, London, 1902).

7. The 'law of parsimony' is attributed to William of Occam, the fourteenth-century English philosopher. This law suggests that a more complex explanation should never be offered where a simpler one would suffice. Hence we get the idea of Occam's Razor — trimming explanations down to their bare essentials.

8. S. G. M. Lee, *Stress and Adaptation* (Leicester University Press, Leicester, 1961).

9. D. M. Ndetei and A. Vadher, 'Frequency and Clinical Significance of Delusions across cultures', *Acta Psychiatrica Scandinavica*, **70** (1984), pp. 73-6.

10. A. Kiev, 'Beliefs and Delusions of West Indian Immigrants to London', *British Journal of Psychiatry*, **109**, (1963), pp. 356-63.

2 HEAR ME, SEE ME, FEEL ME, TOUCH ME: THE ART OF THE INTERVIEW

> One of the best rules in conversation is, never to say a thing which any of the company can reasonably wish had been left unsaid. — Jonathan Swift

An old Chinese proverb suggests that to listen well is as powerful a means of influence as to talk well. More importantly, it goes on, listening is essential to all *true* conversation. This may be a good starting-point for our discussion of the art of the interview. Any interview is a kind of conversation. In this chapter I shall try to explore with you exactly what kind of conversation can *truly* be called an interview. For not all conversations are interviews, and not all interviews have the hallmarks of what the Chinese philosopher saw as 'true conversation'. In a simple sense a conversation can be seen as people talking. However, at least traditionally, conversation has been seen as something of an art form: hence the modern complaint that with the advent of television, the art of conversation has died. In *good* conversation ideas and emotions are communicated in a meaningful, creative and often entertaining manner. Where such ideas and emotions are passed from one person to another in a challenging or amusing fashion, some impact may be made upon the listener, who may be stimulated, enlightened or otherwise impressed. Verbal information, the stuff of all conversations, can assume great power when handled in a lively or creative manner. However, as the Chinese philosopher saw, the speaker is not the only influential figure. A 'good listener' has the power to draw more information from the speaker, or even to guide the content of his speech. We have all been in a situation where someone appeared not to be listening, or appeared uninterested. Our awareness of this usually results in stilted or stifled conversation. Eventually, we stop talking. Although the ability to handle words and concepts is central to the 'art of conversation', we also need to be able to flip the conversation coin, to adopt the role of a 'good listener' — someone who supports the speaker, gives his communication a good landing, and can draw deeper, more enlightening insights from the depths of his experience.

It is important that we begin our study of the art of the interview with the listening aspect. Most of our attention in this chapter will be upon talking: questioning the patient and summarising what he has said. Our efforts will, however, be wasted if we are unable to listen to him correctly, if we cannot encourage him, largely through our silence, to plumb his hidden depths. This marriage of speaker and listener has intrigued some of the great minds of all civilisations. Most of them came to the same conclusions despite being separated by time and culture. Plutarch, the Greek essayist, was a great supporter of the strong silent type. 'Know how to listen,' he said, 'and you will profit even from those who talk badly.' More recently, William Hazlitt, the early nineteenth-century writer, commented that 'silence is one great art of conversation', the other, presumably, being the complementary art of the speaker. As I have noted already, no matter how hard you try to make conversation, on occasions the listening skills of your partner will fail to satisfy you. Another such 'conversation killer' is where your partner is an impatient listener. He is so eager to put forward his point of view that he has little time to listen properly. La Rochefoucauld, the seventeenth-century French moralist, thought that 'the reason why so few people are agreeable in conversation is that each is thinking more of what he is intending to say, than of what the other is saying'. This is another facet of the poor listener syndrome. Since there is no real passing *and* receiving of meaningful information communication will be frustrated. Laurence Sterne, the Irish writer, also commented upon this traffic in conversation. In order to have meaningful conversation we must have something to 'trade': we must be able to swap or exchange ideas, emotions or experiences with our partner. If we do not reciprocate in this way we should be able, at least, to show our appreciation or understanding of what he has said. As Sterne noted, 'conversation is a traffic — if you enter into it without some stock of knowledge to balance the account perpetually betwixt you and another, the trade drops at once.' So what sort of conversational principles can we draw from these writers, which might help us in our dealings with our patients? It is apparent that we need to be able to listen. However, this is not just a passive act, sitting back and letting someone else do the talking. A good listener is a more positive force, helping the speaker to talk more; either in general, or about specific areas of his experience. We need also to beware of impatience. We need to curb our desire to give opinions or summaries before they are needed. Finally, we need to be aware that 'talking to patients' is not an activity to be taken lightly. All of us are experienced conversationalists: we can talk about the weather, our work, our families or just ourselves. Conversations with patients may need to be different from such everyday chatter. The interview is one such example: here we need to have special skills to help us interact with people who may have 'relationship' problems. We also need to have some understanding of what is taking place to use as currency in this conversational traffic. It would be wholly inappropriate to approach an interview with a disturbed or distressed patient in the same way as you would someone standing in a bus queue. Our first responsibility is to be aware of the potential importance of our interaction with the patient.

Features of the Interview

An interview is one of the simplest ways of obtaining information from the patient. It can also be one of the most complex. An interview involves asking questions from which an evaluation of the individual or his circumstances can be made. Interviewing a psychiatric patient differs little from interviewing a nurse for a post. Only the questions and perhaps the format will differ. The aim is the same: to build up a picture of the person through the medium of question and answer — through a conversation.

Interviews usually involve a face-to-face meeting between two people. Although interviews could be done over the telephone, this is hardly to be recommended. The meeting is usually arranged for formal discussion of a specific issue: in order to find out something. The important feature of the interview is the fact that it involves a pattern of interaction in which the roles of interviewer and respondent are highly specialised. We need no special qualification or training to be interviewed. People undergo interviews almost every day — when seeking employment, asking for advice from the boss, applying for unemployment benefit or a loan for a mortgage. The interviewer — by contrast — needs special training if he is to fulfil the requirements of his special position. The four main features of the interview are as follows:

(1) It usually involves a face-to-face meeting.
(2) The aims and objectives of the interview are known to the interviewer, although not always to the person being interviewed.
(3) It involves a restricted range of topics. These are controlled by the interviewer to obtain the maximum information in the

shortest possible time.
(4) Specific roles are adopted by interviewer and respondent. Often this will influence the way the two speak: tone of voice, language and terminology, as well as the degree of formality, all being subjected to some control.

In short, the interview is not just another conversation. It may look like one but for those involved it has an atmosphere of purpose, direction and business that is not found in such everyday interactions. Nurses often confuse the two, concluding that an interview involves simply 'talking to the patient about his problems'. This does not mean that a casual conversation cannot throw up useful information. However, it may not be the most cost-effective way of doing so.

The interview has three major goals or purposes. Facts or information about an individual are collected, from which a picture of the person can be developed. Nurses are not interested in John Smith 'the schizophrenic'. They are interested in John Smith 'the man', who is described as suffering from schizophrenia. I hope that my assumption is correct and that we do presume a difference between these two attitudes. The picture of the man can only be developed from a broad factual base. We need information about his physical state, his occupational skills, his family background, his leisure interests and educational attainment, his social functioning, etc. We are not just talking about his problems: we are talking *to* the whole person. The interview can also be used to diagnose the patient's disorder. In diagnosis we allocate the patient's problems to a specific category of 'suffering'. Although this is primarily a medical responsibility, nurses are often heavily involved. Many doctors rely upon nurses to provide reliable information about the patient's symptoms and how they change across time. This information is often dependent upon the medium of the interview. Finally, the interview can be used to help the patient. It can help clarify his problems and perhaps even arrive at some solutions. We can use our 'face-to-face' meetings with the patient as a major force in the helping process: we can use our meetings for 'psychotherapeutic' ends.

The Law of Parsimony

Inadequate assessment is the biggest obstacle to the presentation of successful treatment. The patient's problems must be seen in their totality: we should avoid assuming too much, and should always try to see problems against the 'backdrop' of the person involved. However, a word of caution is needed here. We can never find out 'everything' about a patient, or even about a specific problem. I should add that neither should we want to. In the past nursing assessment often tended to be overly simple or non-existent. We must take care not to fly to the other extreme. Certainly we should try to be thorough, but we must try to avoid examining areas of the patient's experience that are either irrelevant or unnecessary for our needs. Some critics of traditional 'psychiatric interviewing' have estimated that as much as three-quarters of the material covered could be left out without any appreciable loss. This view is taken on the grounds that this information plays little or no part in the plan of treatment.[1] Such 'over the top' interviewing is not only inefficient but also raises an ethical issue: what right have we to subject aspects of the patient's life to *needless* enquiry? The answer is probably 'none'. For this reason it is important that any interview is carefully planned. If we engage the patient in idle chatter we may end up asking a lot of questions about things which are of little or no relevance to his eventual course of treatment, and we may omit many of the areas which are of crucial significance. Any interview should, therefore, be a controlled exercise. The golden rule is 'Find out everything you *need* to know and *no more*.' This principle reflects the law of parsimony:[2] a law which can be useful in curbing what is often no more than our natural curiosity. Idle curiosity has no place in a professional interview.

The Structured Interview

Like a good story, a good interview should have a beginning, a middle and an end. In order to work through these stages the nurse needs a format or structure. The kind of interview which I am discussing in this chapter is one which follows a particular course of enquiry. It takes a highly specific route in order to answer the basic question, 'How can this person be helped?' The structure of the interview is a kind of skeleton. Or we might compare it to a hat-stand. The interviewer hangs questions on this framework, giving it bulk, substance or body. The design of this basic framework will influence the outcome of the interview as surely as any skeleton determines the outward shape of the person. However, this framework is flexible. It provides some guidance as to the kind of topics that might be covered. It does not dictate the kind of questions that need to be asked.

The sophisticated interviewer often looks as if he is engaging in a very casual conversation. He carries no notepad, no scribbled questions. He appears to be simply chatting to the person. The appearance may be highly misleading. The sophisicated interviewer has all his topics arranged clearly in his head. He also has a bank of questions, developed through experience, to draw upon. For the novice interviewer, who is less confident, there is no shame — and a lot of sense — in working from a framework which has been committed to paper in advance. Perhaps all of us are novices in this sense. Failure to use such a framework may result in running off at tangents, getting muddled or lost altogether. A structured interview is likely to provoke less anxiety for both nurse and patient. Structure provides security.

The Aims of the Interview

The interview can be an end in itself, but often is a preliminary for some other kind of assessment, or a preamble to the offer of some kind of help. The patient can be interviewed under a number of conditions:

The admission interview: where we try to find out who he is; where he comes from; and what are his major problems?

The preliminary interview: where we try to establish which aspects of the patient's functioning need to be followed up in more detail.

The therapeutic interview: where we try to decide upon care or treatment goals; discuss the plan of care and what is expected of the patient.

The evaluation interview: where we try to establish the process made since the last interview.

Direct versus Indirect Interviewing

Interviews, like assessments in general, can take two broad forms. We can examine the patient directly, questioning him, discussing his life, his problems and possible solutions. Or we can be more indirect, examining similar concerns through others' experience of the patient. When the nurse asks the patient's family, 'What kind of man would you say Mr Johnson is?' or when she asks, 'What do you think is troubling Janet?' she is engaging in an indirect examination of the patient. Usually this course of action is taken because the problem cannot be studied at first hand, perhaps because the patient is mute or refuses to discuss the matter. In other cases these 'second-hand' views may be sought to provide a back-up, or alternative perspective, to more direct interviewing.

The Relationship

Interviewer Characteristics

The goals of the interview can be achieved only through a carefully thought-out process. Before we go on to discuss some of the mechanics of the interview let us consider how the nurse can use her 'self' to promote these aims. If the goal of interviewing is to 'shine a light upon the patient and his problems' then clearly we want as much information as possible by the shortest possible route. How can the nurse ensure that she attains this objective? It hardly needs stating that someone who is abrupt, rude or officious is unlikely to be popular. We must assume that no nurse would dream of adopting such attitudes. Similarly, it is clear that a nurse who is cold or indifferent is unlikely to generate the trust that is essential if the patient is to talk about any delicate, or highly personal, material. Such attitudes are more likely to silence him. In many situations patients will make statements that may appear shocking to you — admissions about suicidal intent, sexual practices, past misdeeds which have inspired guilt, or bizarre delusional material. Such topics may be disturbing, especially to the novice. Any expression of surprise, astonishment, reproach or even 'stunned silence' may stifle any further admissions or self-examination. In view of the negative effect of all of these attitudes towards the patient it is generally acknowledged that *any* interviewer should strive to appear warm, friendly and accepting. These attitudes seem especially important in the psychiatric field. Your intention should be to help the patient feel that 'here is someone I can talk to'; 'here is someone who understands me; and who is not sitting in judgement over me'. It has been argued that interviewer characteristics such as empathy, warmth and genuineness can help to promote self-disclosure and self-examination.[3] However, the evidence to support this view has repeatedly been questioned. This has led some people to argue that the questions — rather than the way they are asked — are all important. This reaction seems to be unfortunate. Although such interviewer characteristics as warmth, openness, honesty, genuineness, etc. are difficult to measure in 'value' terms, this does not mean that they have no importance. I think that it may be sensible and safe to assume that the questions *and* the way they are asked are of equal importance. The nurse interviewer should set a number of targets, aiming for accuracy, objectivity and organisation — these will help her gain a recording of important information, reflecting a minimum of bias. At the same time she should try to show characteristics such as warmth, friendliness, empathy, etc., in order to encourage the patient, or his relatives, to provide this valuable information.

Reflecting on some of the points raised in the opening pages of this chapter I would suggest that the 'human characteristics' noted above are essential features of the good listener. These personal skills not only help us to achieve the aims of a single interview, but help us to build a positive relationship with the patient that can form the basis for therapy or help-giving. It is crucial that these 'conversations' with patients get off on a good footing: if we make a bad start, it is often impossible to repair the damage. With this in mind, it is apparent that we cannot take the role of our 'personal relationship skills' at all lightly.

Prejudiced before you Start?

No interview can be conducted in a vacuum. We need some kind of philosophy to guide our questioning. Traditionally, nurses have asked questions about the patient's history, trying to establish how his condition originated and progressed. This was a reflection of 'medical history-taking' — assuming that all forms of mental disorder were some kind of 'disease'. Such a theoretical stance was a kind of bias. It led nurses to ask some questions and not others. Various kinds of bias, or preconception, can influence the line that an interview takes. For instance, an ardent socialist might view the patient as a victim of circumstance. She might assume that he is depressed because of the effects of unemployment, bad housing, poor financial status, etc. This view would lead her to frame questions which would look for information to support this model of depression. Someone with more right-wing political views might assume that the patient's problems are the responsibility of the patient, and no one else. This might lead her to frame questions which would highlight the personality weaknesses of the patient: his failure to make efforts to resolve these problems; his overall 'lack of personal responsibility'. This issue of bias is another ethical problem for nurses. We all have biases and prejudices, some more strong than others. Often these biases are so much a part of us that we rarely give them a second thought. We may not even believe that they *are* biases. As I noted at the end of the last chapter, psychiatry itself has a number of biases. There is no clear model of cause or treatment for any particular condition. Instead there is a range reflecting different viewpoints or biases. Therefore, if we accept a theory which suggests that mental disorder arises out of interpersonal conflicts, we are likely to study the patient's dealings with others as the basic material of our assessment. On the other hand, if we assume that his disorder is a function of some physical cause, our enquiries will reflect this viewpoint; we will look for physical signs and symptoms. There is little I can say to resolve this dilemma. Indeed, a critique of models of mental illness is not one of the aims of this book. However, this dilemma suggests other kinds of bias and prejudice to which we can be alerted, and over which we can exert some control.

Let me assume, for the sake of illustration, that you hold strong religious views. These views may lead you to feel that certain patterns of behaviour, like suicide, homosexuality, drug abuse or even swearing are repugnant in some way. I have no way of knowing whether or not your 'attitudes' are right or wrong: like most other belief systems they represent opinions which are difficult to study in any empirical sense. However, I can predict with some confidence that unless these views are brought under some kind of control, they may prejudice your relationship with the patient. Your views may distort the 'picture of the person' which you see before you. Your beliefs, which in many aspects of your life may be wholly positive and life-enrichening, may be obstructing you in your efforts to help your patient. I use the example of religious views merely as an example. An alternative example could be someone who believes that organised religion is a disruptive social force. She believes that religion is the 'opium of the people'; that it takes away people's individual responsibility; that, in some cases, it can drive people to suicide. These are not simply examples. I have met nurses who held these very views. I highlight these extreme views simply to remind us of the need to keep our personal philosophies out of the care arena. Ideally, the nurse should act as the patient's advocate, attempting to act *for* the patient, especially where he is not in a position to act for himself. We are not supposed to act as his judge and jury, evaluating his behaviour, his life or his beliefs from the vantage point of our own personal philosophy. In this sense the profession of nursing involves sacrificing some of our personal selves. Often we need to suspend our 'personal' beliefs, at least temporarily, in order to act *for* the patient.

Accuracy

It is not enough simply to obtain information about the patient. That information should be accurate; and should be reliably recorded for future reference. How do we set about ensuring this accuracy? Some nurses have tried to resolve this problem by writing down everything which the patient says in a verbatim transcript.[4] Although most of us would not have the time to use such an approach with any more than a tiny fraction of our patients, there are some important principles inherent in this practice. First of all, research has shown that inaccuracies can creep in even when interviews are written up *as soon as they have taken place*. This means that even if we set aside time to write down what has taken place, as soon as it has taken place, we are bound to get some of this 'reporting' wrong. This may have something to do with the sheer demand of having to record so much information in what probably will be a short period of time. One way of getting round this problem is to *summarise* the interview. However, when we 'condense' the interview we may isolate and report upon certain items which are relatively unimportant; and we neglect to comment upon others which are crucial. Clearly, some kind of compromise is needed, as far as writing up the interview is concerned. Some nurses tape-record interviews with patients, using this recording as a memory aid when writing up their notes later on. However, this may be too time-consuming. Perhaps the simplest procedure is to decide in advance upon the key areas of the interview: these can function as headings, to which we can append brief notes *during* the interview. These notes can then be extended into longhand as soon as possible after the interview. We must accept that we are likely to make mistakes in reporting our conversations with patients. The reporting process that we finally adopt should attempt to reduce the risk of mistakes: it may be able to do no more.

The idea of a *verbatim* transcript is an interesting one. This means that we write down, *word for word*, what was said. We do not report what we thought the patient meant, only what he said.

In the early stages of any assessment I think that there is a great advantage in describing 'the events' of the interview, and leaving it at that. Often we are sorely tempted to *interpret* these events. Although there is a role for such interpretation, I do not think that it is in the early stages of assessment, or within the interview. Our aim in writing up a report on an interview is to have something to reflect upon, something to remind us of what took place so that we can give more thought to what was said. When we are in the heat of the interview — trying to listen attentively, making brief notes, thinking of the next question — it can be difficult to digest what the patient has said. For this reason we need a verbatim account of what he actually did say. We can then study these notes, recollecting how certain comments were made, and come to some conclusion about what it all meant. The other advantage of this verbatim account is that we can dicuss 'what the patient said' with other members of the care team. Instead of saying, 'I interviewed John Wallace today and felt that he was very depressed; almost suicidal I would say,' we can tell our colleagues that 'I interviewed John today and these were the sort of comments he was making . . .' This seems like common sense, which it is, but, as I have noted before, we often stray very quickly away from what the patient actually said, by adding layer upon layer of our 'professional' judgements. In order to maintain accurate reporting we should try to stick closely to the 'basic data': to what the patient *actually* said or did.

So far I have emphasised three key points. In order to achieve the aims of 'good interviewing' we must strive to establish a positive, therapeutic relationship with the patient. We try to gain his trust. We try to show our understanding. And most of all we try to show our willingness to listen. In preparing ourselves for the interview we try to be aware of possible biases or prejudices which might influence our perception of the patient, or might lead us to judge him by our standards — standards which may not be wholly appropriate. Finally, we need to pay some attention to how we are going to record this important event. How are we going to retain what might be a vast amount of information? I have recommended making short notes of what the patient said and did to act as a memory aid for more detailed reporting should this prove necessary. In either case these notes will remind you specifically of the responses made by the patient. I want now to consider in more detail the relationship which the interviewer has with the patient, and in turn how the patient relates to the interviewer.

The Interviewer's Attitude

In the interview you want to find out 'what kind of person is this?'
In a traditional diagnostic interview your interview would lie only
in finding out what is wrong with this person. However, I am
assuming that most nurses want, and need, to know more than this.
They want to look behind the patient label. They want to avoid
treating the patient as the mere carrier of certain signs and
symptoms. I am assuming also that patients resent being viewed
merely as a collection of symptoms, or type-cast as some classic
disorder. Maslow commented that many patients, in his experience,
dislike being pigeon-holed.[5] He suggested that they hated being
treated like some kind of specimem, declaring that 'I'm me, not
anybody else.'

It is clear that we have, traditionally, tended to make a distinction between the patient and his condition. Perhaps we have
believed that the problems that we deal with inhabit a separate
world from the person who is the patient. Cohen has commented
upon this situation within medicine by saying that '[the] doctor is
not so much interested in him [the patient] as in his malady. He
examines the patient's body as if, indeed, the patient were not
there.'[6] Sadly, this dehumanising experience is still a reality for
many people when they submit to medical treatment. Laing, the
British anti-psychiatrist, suggested that similar problems existed
within mental disorder. He suggested that we have a choice between
relating to the patient 'as a person or a thing' when he acknowledged that

> no matter how circumscribed or diffuse the initial complaint may
> be, one knows that the patient is bringing into the treatment
> situation, whether intentionally or unintentionally, his existence,
> his whole being-in-his-world . . . every aspect of his being is
> related in some way to every other aspect, although the manner
> in which these aspects are articulated may be by no means clear.[7]

The tone of Laing's argument is philosophical and perhaps may
appear a little abstruse. Yet I think that the basis of his statement is
quite simple. Patients are people before they become patients. They
do not cease to be 'people' when they enter their 'career' as
psychiatric patients. We would do well to remember this fact.

On your Guard

I have made some observations already on the building of a positive relationship with the patient. I now want to consider the sorts of actions which might prejudice that relationship, or which might not be in the patient's best interests.

Concern. In general it is important to appear *interested* and *concerned* about the patient's plight. This rule applies even where 'the problem' may appear minor or trivial. The patient may, in such cases, have a wholly different perception of his situation. In this context we should guard against suggesting that the patient's problems are 'not real' or are in some way 'imaginary'. Many psychiatric problems involve the 'experience' of some difficulty. In this sense it may appear non-existent or insignificant to others, but it is very real to the patient. Avoid embarrassing or alienating the patient further, suggesting that his problem is *not really* a problem. Instead, try always to appear interested and reasonably concerned for him.

Reaction. I have mentioned already the problem of 'shocking' or taboo material. During the course of the interview the patient may say something that might shock or surprise the nurse. Such a reaction will depend, of course, on her background and experience. However, it is important to try to avoid showing *surprise*. Following what I have already discussed above, it is also important not to show *too much concern*: this may increase the patient's natural concern. Instead, simply acknowledge what has been said, nodding, as an expression of acknowledgement and understanding, accompanying this with simple verbal encouragement — 'Yes, I see' or 'Uh huh . . . go on.' This shows that she has heard and understood. More importantly, it makes it clear that she is not judging the patient. Any judgement the nurse might make is made privately and kept private.

Sympathy. Where the patient is discussing highly distressing material — such as extreme anxiety or suicidal thoughts — the nurse should try to avoid becoming emotionally involved in this situation. However, there is a very thin line between 'overinvolvement' and 'lack of concern'. It is important to show some support for the patient in such circumstances. This should not be extended to become grave concern or unnecessary reassurance. As I noted earlier, in such instances the nurse might disapprove of the patient's actions or intentions. It is important here to *avoid appearing unsympathetic*. This does not mean that you should be 'oozing' sympathy: this may only make the patient embarrassed. Avoid what might be a temptation to *blame* the patient for his present difficulties, and fight what might be a natural inclination towards being unsympathetic.

Interpretation. There are a number of rules related to the nurse's attitude towards the material which emerges from the interview. Remember that the main aim is to *collect* information. Consequently, an *'open'* system is needed. Avoid the temptation to *interpret* what is being said. This can be done later when all the information is available. Avoid trying to 'dig' into areas of the patient, his experiences or his attitudes, that he appears to want to keep sectret — at least for the time being.

Values and Beliefs. I have emphasised the need to be non-judgemental. I have also ackowledged that the patient's philosophy of life, his values and his attitudes towards himself and others may conflict with your own. It is important to *avoid appearing narrow-minded*, especially where the patient is describing bizarre or irrational material, or even some unorthodox practice. It is also important to accept the patient's value system, even where it conflicts with your own. You are not being asked to agree or disagree, simply to acknowledge what he 'is'. In this respect it is probably a good idea to avoid discussing political or religious material. If he tries to engage you in such a debate, suggest that this is not appropriate, unless of course you have good reason to think that such a discussion is relevant. If he presses you directly for comment, admit that your opinions are not important right now. This is an 'honest' reply: you are not suggesting that you have no opinions. In this respect it is a good idea for nurses to keep their own 'selves' out of the interaction with the patient. The nurse *can* act as an important model during psychotherapeutic treatment; here she might disclose feelings or thoughts of her own, to help the patient identify with her. However, there is little room for such disclosure within the assessment stage. Discussion of the nurse's views, experiences or problems which have an affinity with those of the patient may simply be distractions. They may draw attention away from the real area of concern — the patient's experiences and problems.

Patience. Very few interviews are without difficulties. One of the main problems is the uncooperative, incommunicative or inarticulate patient. These three characteristics all combine to present one specific problem: a lengthy, and possibly frustrating, interview. Some patients are unwilling to talk about any aspect of their problem: they may have been over the same ground repeatedly, with medical staff, social workers, psychologists and now nurses. Such patients need an explanation of *why* this interview is important. But most of all they need time — time to find out about you, the interviewer, and time to change their attitude towards the interview. Other patients may find it difficult to answer your questions, as the material they wish to communicate may be too distressing, or they may find it difficult to find the 'right words'. Again, patience is essential. In other cases the patient may appear to be skirting around the subject, going off at tangents, taking a long time to answer your question, or appearing to be avoiding answering at all. These responses may be an indication of difficulty. Again the patient needs time. Avoid showing any sign of impatience: beware even of checking your watch, as you will invariably be spotted.

Conflict. No matter how hard you try, there are likely to be some patients whom you do not like. They may be the same people who exasperate you, as noted above. Or they may be people whose past actions, personalities or attitudes and values you find repugnant. I see no real problem here *providing that you do not show your intolerance.* Ideally, I would like all members of the 'caring professions' to be tolerant, accepting and non-judgemental. However, this may be too idealistic. Despite more than a century of the myth, nurses are not ministering angels: we all have feet of clay. Whilst we pursue the ideals of caring, let me make a few practical suggestions. Avoid arguing with the patient, avoid belittling him, and avoid blaming him for his failures. In general, avoid being 'punitive' or making moralistic judgements. Many patients have had more than their fair share of conflict already. What they have been, or what they are, is in conflict with what they would like to be. Avoid adding to that conflict.

Professionalism. During the course of your conversations with the patient he is likely to disclose details of conversations he has had with other staff: nurses, doctors, social workers, etc. In such situations beware of being drawn into criticism of your colleagues. Patients often say, 'This morning Sister said to me . . . what do you think of that? That can't be right, can it?' The appropriate response, as noted earlier, is 'I don't think that "what I think is important". It's what you think that is important. If you don't think that is right perhaps you had better ask Sister to discuss it again with you?' I would hasten to add that we often feel good when someone asks us for our 'professional' opinion: it reinforces our self-esteem. Such pleasures, however, may have painful consequences. Team morale and loyalty may be prejudiced by innocent, yet indiscreet remarks. The patient may also be confused by one person telling him one thing, and someone else something completely different.

In this context it is also important to emphasise the confidentiality of the interview. Somewhere at the beginning of your conversation you must reassure the patient that anything he says will be treated in the strictest confidence. There can be complications resulting from this 'confidential relationship', as I shall discuss in Chapter 11. However, you are obliged to give this assurance. Without it your interview may hardly even get started.

The Patient's Attitude

We have discussed the nurse's attitude towards the interview, and the person being interviewed. What about the patient? What kind of problems will the interview pose for him? As I have noted already, the interview is an unnatural form of conversation. This may be even more true for the patient: at least staff have a chance to become more 'natural' through practice. The unusual nature of the interview may promote a lot of anxiety. The patient may be unaware of 'why' he is being interviewed, or may simply feel uncomfortable when questioned closely about the private corners of his life. This is a natural anxiety. Most of us feel uneasy when under such 'direct fire'. The nurse would be sensitive to this, even when the anxiety is not obvious. Many people can disguise their discomfort, displaying their uneasiness more indirectly through hesitant answers, short replies, or apparent 'striving to please' — always answering 'Yes,' or agreeing with everything you say. Some of this anxiety can be reduced by the line of questioning. Always begin with non-threatening material, simple questions about who he is, where he lives, etc. These should be phrased to allow very short answers. Avoid asking for opinions or 'self-analysis' in the early stages, as it is too demanding. If the interview has progressed beyond this stage and the patient again becomes anxious, postpone the questions which appear to upset him. If the patient becomes distressed it may even be appropriate to return to more mundane topics. This will give him a chance to regain his composure. The interview can return to the 'threatening' material gradually, allowing the patient to regain his confidence through *active* participation. In some cases it may be appropriate to signal when he is 'ready' to return to such a line of questioning: 'We spoke earlier about . . . do you feel ready to return to that just now? If you don't want to discuss it just now, just say so.' Giving the patient a chance to influence the direction of the interview is of crucial importance. This way he becomes a 'partner', instead of something manipulated by the interviewer. This partnership should begin at the very beginning. The nurse's first responsibility is to tell the patient what she would *like* to do; why she wishes to do this; and what the patient's role in the whole proceeding will be. Before beginning your questions, ask the patient if he has anything he wants to ask you — about the interview — before you begin. This tactic is perhaps the best guard against anxiety, since it takes away a great deal of the threat of the 'unknown'.

There is some likelihood that the patient may not be enthusiastic about being interviewed. This is often true of newly admitted patients, who may already have seen a long line of such interviewers. The patient may be irritated at the prospect of *another* interview. The nurse should acknowledge that such irritation or annoyance is natural or appropriate. She should emphasise that she is aware of how the patient might be feeling. This acknowledgement shows that the nurse is trying to consider the patient's feelings: he is not just another name on a list. However, this interview is slightly different, as it may be helpful in ensuring that the patient gets the right kind of care during his stay in the ward. You tell him that you 'hope he will be able to help' you in this way.

In general I am talking about 'resistance' to the interview. However, instead of blaming the patient for his 'poor co-operation' I am trying to see the interview from his angle, so that we might prevent such 'resistance' developing. Some patients may be unhappy about being grilled or cross-examined. This seems to be quite a reasonable objection. Why should the interview be so unpleasant? It must be something to do with the line of questioning or the way that questions are asked. It is important that we do not assume that patients should want to answer our questions. The interview should be so designed as to encourage this 'participation'. Even where patients are not resistant they may not be overly enthusiastic. Again this may be a reflection of the interview format. Are you simply rushing through a routine checklist, ticking off answers, looking as though you have done this a hundred times before? If this is the case the patient may feel that this is not very important, and may be disinclined to 'work' at the interview. There is great value in trying to make each interview a stimulating prospect, for patient and interviewer alike. Even if this is the hundredth time this month, try to tailor the interview to suit the patient: make it something personal to him. He may appreciate it.

I have written much more about the interviewer's attitude since I am able to draw upon my own experience, my own failings. I have said very little about the patient's attitude for the simple reason that I want to make as few assumptions about patients as possible. The one assumption I have made is that all patients want to be treated as people. They want to be given a chance to be themselves — even when they feel at odds with themselves. They also resent being patronised; treated like children; or as if everyone knows what is right for them, except them. It is a sad fact of psychiatric life that, even today, few patients get reasonable explanations about what is being done to them. Few patients are given a chance to participate, even in a small way, in their care and treatment. Ironically, evidence from research suggests that such policies make life harder, rather than easier, for the care staff. In the interview context, patients become resistant, or unmotivated. In preparing to study the patient in this way we should try to ensure that we give the patient his true status as a person, as it will make the whole interview process more satisfying for him and for us.

An Overview of the Interview

So far we have talked about some of the considerations which influence the interview. Let us now discuss the mechanics of interviewing — what we need to do and how we ought to do it.

Phrasing the Question

Questions are an obvious feature of interviews, so that is where we shall begin. The first priority is to avoid confusing the patient. He may be confused or otherwise 'at a loss' already.

Specificity. The first priority in phrasing a question is to avoid ambiguity. Avoid questions which may have more than one meaning. Focus your question so that it will draw information on *one* aspect of the patient's functioning or experience. If you do not get the answer that you expected, you may not have asked the question you meant to ask.

Length. Brevity is another key issue. Avoid asking long rambling questions. Avoid making general observations about the patient or his situation, including a question somewhere within this statement.

Don't ask	*Do ask*
'You were saying earlier that you feel pretty tense all the time . . . that must be pretty awful . . . I can see that you are tense right now. You're sitting all sort of bunched up . . . is that what you mean? Like you said a moment ago I mean . . . is that how you feel . . . all tense, anxious, nervy, like you said. Is it?'	'You said a moment ago that you often feel tense. What do you mean by that?' (await reply) 'So how do you feel right now?' (await reply) 'You are sitting sort of hunched up. Is that how you usually are when you are tense?' (await reply)

The rambling question, rolled up in some observations, may be appropriate on TV chat shows. In a clinical interview it may simply lose the patient. Since the question is not direct, or specific enough, it is more difficult to answer, and may increase his anxiety. The same is true of the string of questions. Ask one question at a time, unless you have very good reasons for acting otherwise.

Time. The question should also specify the time clearly, where appropriate. 'How do you feel *now*?' or 'How have you been feeling over the past two or three days?' Where the time-scale is necessarily vague, as in 'Can you tell me what sort of things you were able to do when you were well?' or 'How did you feel when you were well?' follow up the reply by asking, 'And how long ago was that?' Be aware that many patients who are highly distressed feel that they have 'always' been like this. Help them be more objective by tightening the time focus.

Open and Closed Questions. There are two main kinds of question: those which elicit a short reply, perhaps just 'Yes' or 'No', and those which require fuller answers.

Closed question	*Open question*
'Are you still feeling down?'	'Tell me how you are feeling today.'
'Your husband left you. Do you think that made you depressed?'	'How did you react to your husband leaving you?'
'Do you hear voices a lot?'	'You say that someone is talking to you: in your head. How often do you hear voices like that?'

Closed questions may be appropriate in the initial stages of the interview, as they put fewer demands on the patient, but open questions will provide more information about what it is like to be him, about his experience.

Reflection. When the patient says something that appears interesting or significant, you may want to develop this theme, or gain more information. The simplest, and least intrusive, way to do this is to *reflect* — or bounce back — his reply. Hopefully he will pick this up, and amplify his meaning.

Example
Patient. I get so confused sometimes I just don't know whether I'm coming or going.
Nurse. You don't know whether you're coming or going?
Patient. That's right. I mean . . . I just don't seem to be able to cope with things. I feel so useless all the time.
Nurse. I see . . . you feel useless?

Emphasis should be given to certain words to show that you are phrasing a question, and not simply repeating what he has said. Reflection should also be used with discretion. If you repeatedly reflected the patient's answers he might think that he was answering the questions badly, or that you were making fun of him.

Reflection can be taken a stage further by using the patient's actual phrasing to frame another question, e.g. 'You say that you don't know whether you are coming or going. Can you tell me what you mean by that?' The key feature of reflection is that you provide the minimum of guidance. You interrupt the patient no more than is necessary. This allows cost-effective interviewing: you get the patient to give as much information as possible, for the minimum of interviewing time. More importantly, it allows the patient an opportunity to talk as much as possible, without losing the necessary structure.

Perceived Threat. Some questions will be disturbing or threatening to the patient. Avoiding such questions is not a solution. Instead questions about sensitive or distressing subjects should be carefully framed, to reduce their impact. It is not possible to list all such perceived threats. These can vary from one patient to another. However, even in today's liberated society detailed questioning about sex is often perceived as a threat. The same is true of domestic violence.

Don't ask	*Do ask*
'How often do you and your wife have sex?'	'You and your wife seem to get on fairly well. Is there any aspect of your marriage that you are not entirely happy with?'
'Do you ever beat your wife?'	'Does you wife ever lose her temper?'
	'What about you? Do you ever lose your temper? Do you ever feel that you are going to lose control?'

If the patient feels threatened by direct questioning he may simply deny the existence of any problem. By taking a more oblique line of questioning the 'glare' of the searchlight is reduced. Such 'indirect' questioning may make it easier for the patient to admit to problems of which he is ashamed.

Devising a Framework

Any interview must have a structure. This can, however, be rigid or flexible — depending on the demands of the situation. The 'structure' most commonly refers to the kind of questions which you will ask. For example, a typical interview might begin with very 'open-ended' questions, such as 'Would you like to tell me what's bothering you at present?' Grandually, more specific queries can be introduced, such as 'How often has this happened?' Eventually, the patient's perception of his 'problem' can be narrowed down to finer detail: 'How severe would you say this is at present, on a scale of 1 to 10?' These stages — beginning, middle and end — show how the interview begins with very broad concerns and gradually sharpens the focus on one or two problems. A first interview might be devoted entirely to drawing up a list of his problems. Subsequent interviews might take individual problems as 'topics', devoting the time to trying to understand each one better, through closer analysis.

In general a flexible framework, where the interviewer decides upon her line of questioning *within* the interview itself, is for the expert only. Most of us need some preparation. We need some simple framework of questions to give us some security, so that we don't get lost for words. Our aim is to have a 'conversation' with the patient. We want to talk to the patient as normally as possible. If we have a general outline of the questions we want to ask — the areas we want to explore — then these guidelines may make us feel more comfortable. We may decide to use such a framework as a guide to notekeeping during the interview, or we may simply memorise the question areas. Again, select the approach that is most appropriate to you or the patient. Some patients like to think that their problems are being dealt with seriously: a more formal interview may be appropriate for them. Others will find this uncomfortable. Finally, we must consider the needs of the nurse: what sort of format would she be comfortable with?

Interview Discipline

It is a fact of life that interviews rarely ever turn out the way we planned them. It is important that we are prepared for problems: we need strategies 'up our sleeve' to avoid getting lost, or grinding to a halt.

Failure to Respond. The patient may find it difficult to give the information you want, especially at the first interview. How far should you 'push' the patient? Should you push him at all? If the patient fails to answer 'appropriately' — i.e. to your satisfaction — it may be that the question has been badly phrased. It may be impossible to answer in its present form. Try presenting it from a different angle.

Example

Nurse. When there is conflict within the family, what kind of coping strategies do you employ under such conditions? (no answer — try again)

Nurse. Well, let me put it this way . . . when there's an 'atmosphere' at home, how do you deal with that?

Although the first example looks like a 'spoof' question, it is actually drawn from a published transcript of an interview. The second example asks the same question, but uses the language of the patient to aid communication.

Difficult to Answer. The patient may be able to answer, but may be unsatisfied with his reply. It is appropriate here to offer some words of encouragement, helping him to find the words he needs to express himself. Beware, however, of putting words into his mouth. Instead, try to shape up his answer through discreet prompting.

Example

Nurse. So how did you feel when that happened?

Patient. Oh, I don't know. Just lost . . . sort of . . . eh . . . I, oh I don't know.

Nurse. Uh huh, you felt 'lost': lost in what way?

Patient. Lost, yes. Didn't know what to do, what to say.

Nurse. Lost for words?

Patient. Yes . . . lost for words. Didn't know what to say to her. Felt powerless. No, that's not right. Can't seem to think straight.

Nurse. You were lost for words. You didn't *know* what to say to her; or you felt that you couldn't *tell* her how you felt?

Patient. Well, maybe that's true. I knew how I felt, but I just couldn't face her. I couldn't bring myself to tell her how I felt.

Refuses to Answer. Finally, the patient may not answer at all — an indication, perhaps, of his unwillingness. What should we do? Rephrase the question? Try to nudge him gently? Or simply respect his wishes, leaving this issue for another time, or another place? My sympathies lie with the last solution, although there are bound to be occasions when it might be appropriate to try the others. If I did 'postpone' a question, however, I would let the patient know why I was doing so.

Example
You don't seem to be too happy with that question. Maybe it was the way I put it. Perhaps you don't feel ready to discuss that with me just yet? Maybe we could come back to it some other time, when you think you're ready. OK? (pause) We were talking a moment ago about . . . (next question)

Tangents. You cannot expect to find answers to all your questions in a single interview. Ideally, one question leads to another and so on, and may span several interviews. In practice, however, one question usually produces a number of answers, some aspects of which are relevant, others which are less so. The nurse must decide whether or not to follow up such 'tangents', or to stick to the core questions. If she decides to deal only with some of the patient's replies she should make it clear that she is doing this. Let us take an example of a patient who is being asked how she feels about going out of hospital on a shopping trip.

Nurse. How would you feel about going into town this weekend with one of the nurses?

Sally. Oh, I don't know. I'd get terrible tense in the crowds . . . just know I would. Then there's my Cyril. I've been worrying a lot about him too. He doesn't really manage well on his own. I worry about him ever so much, and little Johnny . . . he's just eleven. How he must feel about not having his mummy with him like other children. Sometimes I just can't bear it.

Nurse. I understand what you are saying, Sally. Your family obviously mean a lot to you, and you worry about them a great deal. Maybe we should spend some time later just talking about that side of things? It is obviously very important, so we want to give it the attention it deserves. OK? (Sally nods) You seem worried about going out as well? Can you tell me what bothers you about the crowds?

The nurse had a decision to make here: either to respond to the patient's 'need' to discuss her worries about her family, or to stick to the agenda of the interview. She chose the latter, but made arrangements for dealing with the other 'worries' the patient introduced. In most situations, where time is limited, it is essential to stick to the agenda, otherwise the topics you wish to cover may be unfinished when your time runs out. But always make it clear that any 'extra material' is not being dismissed out of hand. Arrange for it to be rescheduled to another time or another place.

The Setting

We must always look upon the interview as a 'formal' conversation, since the outcome may be of crucial relevance to the patient. Interviews need not, however, be structured in a formal manner. On occasions, it may be appropriate to interview the patient in bed or at his bedside. We might also use a consulting room off the main ward, or a special 'interview room' at a clinic. These are all standard settings for conducting interviews. It may be just as practical to interview the patient in the hospital grounds, in his sitting-room at home, or whilst walking his dog in the park. The important consideration in the selection of the venue, or setting, is 'Will we have privacy, peace and quiet?' The patient is unlikely to want to discuss personal problems within earshot of other people, and may become distracted if there are repeated interruptions. In some cases 'walking in the park' may be more private and distraction-free than a ward consulting room.

The setting is also important in terms of 'putting the patient at his ease'. An anxious patient may feel more comfortable 'chatting' over a cup of coffee in the corner of the hospital cafeteria, or when walking in the fresh air. The restrictions of a small interview room may enhance his anxiety, and may make communication more difficult. However, in some cases it is appropriate to pick an awkward setting. If the patient has identified a situation which appears to 'trigger' his problem it may be appropriate to conduct the interview there. We might take someone with social anxiety out into the street. If the patient was suffering from a grief reaction, we might take him to a setting which evoked special memories of his loved one. In both examples the setting selected would serve as a trigger for certain emotions, thoughts and memories which might be less evident in a more formal interview setting.

Communicating with the Patient

Some patients do not like the idea of being interviewed. Often this stems from bad experiences in other interview situations at the hands of the over-efficient, the cold or probing interviewer. I have emphasised already the need to be warm, understanding and genuine. In addition to these classic features it is also important to talk to the patient in language he understands. He may be baffled by the language of professionals, who often use jargon, vocabulary or grammatical structures which are beyond his capabilities. In addition to easing tensions, the use of a common language — especially where the patient speaks in some dialect — may be helpful in establishing a positive relationship.

> *Nurse.* You're looking pretty down today Geoff. Would you like to tell me what's troubling you?
> *Geoff.* Oh, I'm just proper fed-up. Scunnered like. Been like this for weeks.
> *Nurse.* You feel scunnered. What, with everything?
> *Geoff.* Yeah, just sick of everything. But especially myself.

By picking up on the patient's use of the expression 'scunnered' — meaning sick, or tired of — the nurse hopes to strengthen her rapport with the patient. She hopes the patient will think, quite literally, that this person is someone I can really talk to. In the same context it is worth picking up the use of more technical terms — like 'depressed', 'anxious', 'alienated', 'paranoid', 'hostile'. These words, which have very special meanings in our professional language, have become part of the vernacular. However, we should not assume that because such expressions are in everyday use that their meaning remains the same. Where the patient uses such 'technical expressions' as part of his description of self, ask him to clarify *what he means*.

Presenting the Interview

Preparation

Whether the interview is to be formal or informal, taking place in the ward or under a tree in the grounds, the nurse should always be prepared. By preparation I mean knowing the *aim* of the interview, *how best* to conduct it, and how much *time* is available. As I noted earlier, the aims of the interview can vary enormously from one interview to another. This means that some preparation is necessary to ensure that you cover all the points you wish to cover. A general outline of what you *intend to do* is helpful for the following reasons:

(1) It acts as a guide to the line of questioning, guarding against getting side-tracked.
(2) It helps you follow a logical, sensitive line of questioning, in most cases beginning with non-threatening material, building up gradually to more sensitive material.
(3) It guards against duplication of lines of questioning followed by other members of the team: doctors, nurses, psychologists, etc. In some cases such a 'follow-on' may be recommended. Doctors and psychologists may ask nurses to pursue certain questions in an attempt to gain more information.
(4) It guards against taxing the concentration of the patient, e.g. by being unduly long, and guards against time-wasting, e.g. by spending too much time on general issues, before reaching the key questions.

It is also a good idea to prepare to conclude the interview at least ten minutes before you need to. This allows the patient time to regain his composure or to ask any further general questions.

The Plan

We have already discussed various ways of phrasing the questions. It is also helpful to break questions down into higher- or lower-order groups.[8]

Lower-order Questions. There are four main kinds of 'lower-order' questions: in general, these are simpler forms of question. The first involves the *recall* of information. Here the patient might be asked, 'Have you ever felt this bad before?' — to which he can answer 'Yes' or 'No.' Alternatively, he might be asked to recall more information: 'When did you last feel this bad?' The second kind involves *rephrasing* or 'rewording' certain concepts or ideas: 'Can you tell me in your own words what you mean by helpless?' In the third class the patient is asked to *compare* or *contrast* situations or experiences: 'Which situations do you normally feel worst in? Can you tell me, then, where you would feel OK?' The last class of lower-order questions invites the patient to present *alternatives* to what they have done in the past: 'How could you handle that differently? Given what we have just discussed, how would you tackle that situation in the future?'

Higher-order Questions. This class of questions involves more complex answering. First of all the patient may be asked to *analyse* a situation: he is required to give some indication of *why* something happened. These motives or causes cannot, of course, be drawn simply from memory; the answer needs to be more 'creative', and is therefore more difficult. 'Why do you think your wife stopped talking to you?' or 'How do you think you came to be depressed?' This class also contains questions which require the patient to make *predictions* or to discuss *complex ideas*: 'What would happen if you did that?' or 'What would be so bad about that?'

Ideally, the plan of the interview should begin with lower-order questions, which require the patient to 'dip into' his memory or require simple problem-solving answers. As the interview progresses, or as the patient becomes more comfortable, the more complex questions, relying on complex reasoning, may be introduced.

Seating

The classic interview usually seats the interviewer behind a desk, with the interviewee facing him, at the other side of it. Research suggests that this 'job interview' arrangement is wholly inappropriate in psychiatry. Where two people face each other it may appear 'confrontational'. Where a desk is used it may appear to represent a shield or barrier, placing the interviewee at a disadvantage. The height and design of chairs are also important. If one person sits on a higher chair, this may appear to give him an advantage. If the patient is given a stiff, high-backed chair, while the nurse sits in an easy chair, again there may appear to be an advantage, the person in the easy chair appearing more relaxed and comfortable. In general, both nurse and patient should sit on the same kind of chairs, at roughly 60 degrees to one another. This allows easy eye contact and orientation, such as is found in most normal social interaction.[9] The seats should be close together, registering the privacy and intimacy of the conversation. If they are far apart, this may be interpreted as a 'gulf' between nurse and patient. However, as with other aspects of the interview, check with the patient that such an arrangement suits him before beginning.

Opening

The nurse should begin the interview by preparing the patient for what is to follow. She should tell him first what she is *going* to ask him. She will then proceed to conduct the interview, finishing by trying to summarise some of his answers. In her opening remarks the nurse should explain her 'aims', asking the patient if he has any queries or objections.

Example

Hello Mr Smith, I'm Jennifer Masters, the Staff Nurse on this ward. (pause) I know that you have just come in and probably you are a bit tired of people asking you questions and fussing over you. However, I would be grateful if we could spend just a few minutes getting some more details about yourself. Just a few minutes, that's all we'll need. OK? (pause) I'd like to ask you a few questions about where you live, your family, and a little bit about what led up to you coming into hospital. (pause) If you have any questions for me — or if you don't understand what I'm asking you — just stop me. Is that OK with you?

Here the nurse is making it clear *who* she is and *what* she wants to do. She also tries to acknowledge that the patient may feel inconvenienced, and tries to encourage him to question her if he wishes. She also tries to make the whole affair as non-threatening as possible, by giving him 'permission' to interrupt. She pauses briefly throughout her introduction, giving the patient time to speak, or to allow her words to register. This kind of honest opening may reduce the patient's natural anxiety. The emphasis upon a kind of 'collaboration' may also raise the patient's self-esteem.

The Core

After this simple introduction the interview proper can begin. Here also it is important to emphasise the structure, marking clearly the beginning and end of each section; and summarising where appropriate.

Example

(A) To begin with, I'd like you to tell me a bit about yourself.
   (This general question is followed immediately by a series of

specific queries: 'Do you live on your own? Who does your shopping for you? Where did you work before you retired?')

(B) Good. That seems to cover everything there. Maybe we could talk for a moment about how you came into hospital? Now you said that you lived alone . . . (By recapping on some of the points covered in (A) above the nurse might move on to more open-ended questions: 'When did you first feel that you needed help? Who did you discuss these problems with? How did you feel about being on your own?')

(C) That's fine. I have found that very helpful. Perhaps we might discuss some of the problems you have mentioned in more detail? Are you ready for that just now? (If the patient agrees, further questions of a 'who, where, when, what, how and why' variety might be asked: 'Where did that first happen? Were you on your own at the the time? What would be so bad about that? Why do you think that *that* is a problem?')

(D) From what you have said a number of things appear to be a problem to you just now. First of all there are these worries about your son? . . . (The information collected can now be summarised briefly. At the same time the nurse can check that her interpretation of the 'facts' is correct.

Helping the Patient

As we noted earlier, the nurse must present a certain 'image' in order to encourage the kind of positive relationship essential to the success of any interview. So far we have discussed only the 'verbal' aspect of the relationship with the patient. I should like now to pass comment on some aspects of the 'non-verbal' interaction between nurse and patient.

Many of the characteristics of the 'good' interviewer will be expressed through her non-verbal behaviour. Or rather, the patient is likely to perceive the nurse positively or negatively, on the basis of observation of these subtle characteristics. When we find people 'likeable' or 'unpleasant', rarely is this because of what they have said. More often it is the outcome of the way they said it, or some even less specific factor — 'It's something I can't put my finger on.' We should be aware that the 'impression' which the patient forms will be based largely upon how we stand, sit, use our hands, look at the patient, etc. It is not possible to cover all aspects of non-verbal behaviour here: I shall simply review some aspects of 'body language' which are helpful to the interviewer.

Spatial Behaviour. I have already mentioned the need to sit close to the patient, on an equal footing. This signifies the removal of status. If you wish to 'control' the other person, you try to look down at him, or sit behind a desk. The side-by-side orientation recommended earlier will probably communicate your 'liking' for the patient and may give reassurance.

Posture. The nurse should always try to appear relaxed and comfortable during the interview. This should communicate 'confidence'. It may be appropriate to change posture during the conversation, leaning forward if the patient is discussing confidential material or is distressed, or settling back in the chair if he appears able to talk at length. These posture changes may communicate a willingness to be confidential, or a willingness to listen. In general it is appropriate to sit turned slightly towards the patient, leaning slightly in his direction.

Facial Expression. Our faces provide a regular commentary on our speech, as we 'flash' our eyebrows, smile, frown, grimace, etc. The nurse should attempt to follow the patient's conversation by showing appropriate facial expression. However, this should always be controlled, otherwise it may look theatrical and insincere. For instance, if the patient is discussing a harrowing incident it may be appropriate to acknowledge this by furrowing the brows *slightly*. Interest or mild surprise can be communicated by a slight raising of the eyebrows. If the patient says something amusing, or laughs — even nervously — it is appropriate to smile, acknowledging his communication of humour. In these examples I am suggesting that the nurse *partner* the patient, by showing that she appreciates the meaning or significance of what is being said.

When meeting the patient for the first time, even the first time each day, it is important to smile slightly. This should be enough to signal confidence or a positive attitude only. A beaming smile, of the 'have a nice day' variety, is not recommended. The patient may interpret this as patronising, or dismissive of the severity of his problems.

Eye Contact. Usually, we look at other people in order to pick up the non-verbal cues just mentioned. However, gaze has another function: it adds emphasis to our speech and can be used to 'reply' to the other person. Although the amount of eye contact varies from one situation to another, rarely do we ever gaze constantly at the other person, except when we are madly in love, or enraged with anger. 'Normal' gaze patterns involve looking and quickly looking away, resulting in about 75 per cent of the time spent in eye contact. If we give more than this amount of eye contact we may appear 'confrontational' or aggressive; less, and we may look embarrassed or ashamed. Many nurses think that they should 'study' the patient all the time. If they try reversing roles for a few minutes, they will soon find out how uncomfortable this can be.

Gestures. We use our hands, like our eyes, to add expression to our speech. Gestures can play an important part in any interview, for example when we 'wave' to the patient *inviting* further comment, or signal for him to stop for a moment. These gestures are direct signals, from the nurse to the patient. We can also 'signal' our attitude: for example, drumming our fingers on the chair or twiddling a pencil may signal impatience; resting our chin on our hands may signal 'thoughtfulness'. (I have a habit of stroking my moustache or pulling the end of my beard. This has been interpreted variously as 'a thoughtful look' to 'complete boredom'. I mention such 'autistic gestures' simply to remind you that you may be giving signals which you would rather omit.)

We also gesture by nodding or shaking our heads. The head-nod is a valuable gesture, indicating agreement, acknowledgement, and also serving as an encouragement for the patient to continue talking.

Physical Contact. Contact between nurses and patients — especially male nurses and female patients — is often seen as taboo. However, when carried out appropriately it can be a helpful adjunct to speech. It is important to recognise that the West is a 'non-contact' culture: we only touch people anonymously — bumping into people in a crowd — or in highly ritualised situations such as the handshake. This convention extends to the psychiatric field and is broken only under certain conditions. If the patient is very distressed reassurance can be conveyed effectively by gripping him lighly on the forearm or resting your hand on his shoulder. I hesitate to suggest further in the case of adults, although in the case of some children much more contact may be considered appropriate. However, in the case of some children this may be highly undesirable, for example 'autistic' children.

Abuse of the Interview

I have suggested in this chapter that the interview can be used to elicit all kinds of information from the patient, from identifying who he is to asking him to comment on his role in life, if not his thoughts on an afterlife. Interviews are not restricted to the assessment phase, and may figure in the treatment phase itself, or even in the follow-up, for example when a community nurse visits a patient at home after discharge. At each end of the care spectrum questions are asked to elicit information about the patient's history, his expectations of treatment, his attitude to treatment received, his relationships with family, friends or other patients, his anxieties about the future or his plans for life after discharge. The uses to which the interview may be put are probably endless. However, in all these situations the interview is designed to achieve the following:

(1) To provide a situation where nurse and patient can get to know one another — or can re-establish relationships of a positive nature. This is the rapport-building level.
(2) To gain basic information to help orient the care staff towards the patient, placing him in identity, time, place, etc. This is the history-taking phase.
(3) To collect detailed information of a qualitative or quantitative nature which will help us plan the kind of care he needs.
(4) To help the patient assess or evaluate himself and his life situation by helping him to look at facets of his own functioning and relationship with his world.
(5) To help the patient feel that he is part of his care and treatment. To make him feel that we are interested in him as a person, not as a rag-bag of disparate psychiatric symptoms.

I summarise these aims to remind myself that many interviews fail to achieve these fundamental goals. These aims are not in any way idealistic, and I am sure that many more refinements and additions could be suggested. The main aim of this kind of interview is to provide a supportive, reassuring, non-judgemental environment in which the skills of the nurse and the assets of the patient can combine to shine some light on the mystery of the patient.

It is quite easy to turn the interview, from this positive, creative exercise, into a third degree inquisition. Although in some cases it may be necessary to look at aspects of the patient's life he might rather leave alone, we should avoid making him feel worse. Providing that awkward or threatening material is handled sensibly and sensitively, the patient may even feel that he has achieved something by confronting his problem. There is, however, a danger in taking such a 'confrontational' approach to extremes. Indeed, nurses often hold extreme views on the issue of upsetting patients. Some, who have had experience of certain brands of psychotherapy, believe that all patients should be confronted with their problems. I am not sure that such a generalised attitude is ever sensible. Other nurses might take the opposite view, believing that they should never upset any patient, in any way. Again, this extreme view seems illogical. By way of practical advice, I would suggest that we should only stimulate strong emotion in patients *if* we have reason to believe that we can handle this, and that the patient can emerge from the trauma with some definable 'gain' from the experience.

In many interviews it is likely that the information you desire may not be forthcoming. It is important here to avoid becoming frustrated, exasperated or downright angry. It is not necessary to remain forever tolerant and smiling. However, allowing your emotions to surface 'under their own steam' is to be discouraged. Instead, give the patient some 'feedback': let him know that you do not seem to be getting the information you want. Does he not wish to answer these questions? If necessary, tell him that you are getting lost, finding it difficult to conduct the interview — even that you are becoming frustrated, or annoyed. Better to tell the patient intellectually than to let him experience this emotionally.

In some situations the information the patient offers you could be interesting for reasons other than professional curiosity. Where the patient describes some behaviour, belief or emotion *which is strange to you*, resist the temptation to question him further simply to satisfy your own curiosity. This problem seems particularly prevalent where sexual behaviour and marital relationships are under discussion. In the same vein it is important not to stray to the other extreme. Some nurses are afraid to ask any sensitive questions about sex or relationships. The rule is, only ask about what appears to be relevant to the problem in hand. We might avoid such abuse of the interview if we were more knowledgeable about our own motivations before we began to study those of the patient.

In order to achieve the basic aims of the interview, we must guard against these three examples of abuse. We must beware of using the interview as a means of dismantling or devaluing the patient, as we should be concerned only with his development. We must beware of becoming emotionally entangled in the interview process, especially where it begins to fail us. Instead of using our status as 'interviewer' as an excuse to ventilate our feelings, we should try to construct solutions through more reasoned 'contracting' with the patient. Finally, we must beware of idle curiosity. We must acknowledge the responsibility vested in us to probe and pry no more than is absolutely necessary.

Summary

In this chapter I have discussed the use of conversation to gain insights into the unique world of the patient. I have emphasised the need to focus the interview on the person behind the patient label, studying his experience; what Laing would call his 'being-in-his-world'. The basic interview format needs to be adapted to suit the patient. Factors such as age, sex, cultural background, values, beliefs and presentation will influence how we prepare or conduct the interview. These adaptions influence the structure of the interview, what we do and say, how long it lasts, where it takes place and how we record the outcome. The interview has no single purpose apart from eliciting information. It may be used for a multiplicity of purposes, from finding out who the patient *is* to evaluating how he thinks he has changed. Throughout this range of conversations some basic principles remain constant. The interview should be seen as a two-way process and the patient should be given every encouragement to collaborate. He should also be kept informed of the progress of the interview, and in some cases informed in advance of 'what is coming next'. I illustrated how the patient should be encouraged to participate in the control of the interview: in certain cases he might be asked to decide when he is ready to discuss certain aspects of his situation. Of supreme importance is the need for the interviewer to be unbiased, isolating any preconceptions or prejudices hidden in her view of the patient. Instead, the patient's value system should be accepted, although this need not mean that it is given active approval. The patient's perception of his world and himself is used as the vantage point for the assessment. The interviewer tried to see the world through his eyes, at least for the time being. Later, in the treatment phase, it may be decided that his view of the world *is* his problem.

I have paid some attention to the mechanics of interviewing. Various ways of eliciting the patient's thoughts, feelings and beliefs were desribed briefly. These responses are used to supplement the nurse's observation of the patient's presentation. Emphasis was also given to the need to be as unobtrusive as possible. The patient should be given every opportunity to speak. This rule is amended only where he is uncommunicative, where there is an expressed need for a talkative interviewer.

The interview can be a highly sophisticated interaction. In many ways it can also be therapeutic. If handled properly the patient may discover aspects of his functioning of which he was unaware. Sometimes these revelations can be traumatic, the 'gains' often being seen as 'facing up to the problem'. In general, I have defined a 'good interview' as one that will ultimately benefit the patient. Even a difficult or distressing interview yields an abundance of such fruits. I warned, however, against possible abuses. The status of the nurse should never be used to manipulate the patient. Destructive interviews should be avoided at all costs. Finally, we must take care not to allow our natural inquisitiveness to dominate our clinical judgement.

Notes

1. D. R. Peterson, *The Clinical Study of Social Behaviour* (Appleton-Century-Crofts, New York, 1968).

2. This principle was noted briefly in Chapter 1. The principle as stated by William of Occam is known correctly as 'Entia non multiplicanda praeter necessitatem': 'Entities ought not to be multiplied beyond necessity.' As an example of this principle Robert Bierstedt mentions the experience of two seventeenth-century chemists, Stahl and Becher, who proposed a theory of combustion according to which something called *phlogiston* is present in the fire to make it burn. When Priestley discovered oxygen the phlogiston theory was no longer needed and was dropped as an explanation of combustion. Bierstedt notes that Occam's Razor is used, one might say, to shave the metaphysical stubble off the physiognomy of science. See R. Bierstedt, *The Social Order* (McGraw-Hill, New York, 1963), p. 21.

3. For a detailed discussion see C. B. Truax and R. R. Carkhuff, *Towards Effective Counselling and Psychotherapy: Training and Practice* (Aldine, Chicago, 1967).

4. Altschul has described the 'practice on which much of American psychiatric nursing is based; that of one-to-one establishment of relationships, usually of a psychotherapeutic nature . . . Some half-hour of a one-to-one session between patient and nurse requires verbatim record keeping, termed a "process recording". Each half-hour session requires about two hours work subsequently from the nurse and a further 1–2 hours from her supervisor.' She goes on to say, 'I believe that

this practice is good for nurses, but I don't know if I still believe it is good for patients.' A. Altschul, 'Does Good Practice Need Good Principles: II', *Nursing Times*, 18 July 1984.

5. A. Maslow, *Toward a Psychology of Being* (Van Nostrand, London, 1962).

6. J. Cohen, 'The Relationship of Psychology to Medicine', *Imprensa Medica*, **23** (1959), pp. 113–15.

7. R. D. Laing, *The Divided Self* (Penguin Books, Harmondsworth, 1965), p. 25.

8. This format is adapted from F. S. Hewit, 'Communication Skills: Questions and Listening', *Nursing Times*, 25 June 1981, pp. 21–4.

9. For a detailed review see M. Argyle, *Bodily Communication* (Methuen, London, 1975).

3 THE WEB OF LIFE: TAKING THE HISTORY

History is neither more nor less than biography on a large scale. — Alphonse de Lamartine

In this chapter I want to discuss the construction of some kind of history of the patient's present and past life. As I shall discuss later, I have some reservations about the role of the 'history' in care planning in psychiatry. I am also undecided, as yet, about how it should be done, if at all. However, given the traditional role of history-taking in all spheres of health care, I would be foolish to neglect what is, at least administratively, an important subject. I am also aware that other members of the health care team take 'histories' of patients. The 'psychiatric interview', conducted by the doctor, is an extensive history. Social workers, psychologists and the various paramedical groups all complete histories usually as a reference point for more detailed examination at some later date. Nurses have also conducted truncated histories as part of traditional practice. With the advent of the 'nursing process' we have all been urged, especially by our American colleagues, to be more holistic, which usually starts with extensive life-histories. It would be foolish of nurses to conduct their own life-history survey if it simply reproduced information already available either in medical or some other 'file'. However, in some settings nurses may be able to gain more information than other professionals on the patient's life-style. As a result, they may be the best person to conduct the 'history', but I see no sign that such a history will ever replace the psychiatric interview. Even if nurses do not complete histories as a matter of routine, it is important that they should be aware of its contents. The information contained in the history will be of crucial relevance to nursing care planning. It is irrelevant *who* took the history in the first place. In many settings nurses may be asked to follow up certain facets of the patient's life-history, perhaps where multidisciplinary teams operate, each member of the team contributing some information to the final history.

The Biography

Although I have admitted my reservations about the history, it is clear that we cannot assess the patient further without knowing something of who he is. The history of the patient is a badly written biography, drawing together important milestones in the patient's life, identifying his interests, his obsessions, his work, his family. Since the field of psychiatry is concerned primarily with human weakness, the history may pay scant regard to the patient's assets. The history is an important starting-point for subsequent assessment since it is here that we begin to understand the relationship between the patient and his life. As Goethe, the great German poet observed, 'Life is a quarry, out of which we are to mould and chisel a character.' Our intention in trying to unravel something of the patient's past is to try to understand how he became what he is now. This experience may be of value in the future. 'I know the past,' wrote Shelley, 'and thence will essay to glean a warning for the future, so that man may profit by his errors, and derive experience from his follies.' The history should never be a 'routine administrative chore': it should aim to search out something of the *real person*. As Bulwer-Lytton, the nineteenth-century novelist, observed, 'There are two lives to each of us, the life of our actions and the life of our minds and hearts. History reveals men's deeds and their outward characters but not themselves. There is a secret self that has its own life, unpenetrated and unguessed.' He wasn't talking about the kind of history we have in mind here, but the words are wise none the less.

I shall divide this chapter into three sections. First I shall discuss the broad content of the history, then I shall suggest where it might lead us, in terms of further assessment. Finally I shall discuss the concept of the nursing process, since the taking of a history, or the execution of any subsequent assessment, must be seen as part of some 'process of nursing'.

The Organisation of the History

The Admission Profile

In this section I shall review those aspects of the history which should be taken on admission. Of necessity, this discussion relates only to 'new' patients. The admission profile represents the *basic history*: details of the patient's identity, and status necessary for administrative purposes. Since there are regional and national variations on the recording of such information, I shall not describe this in any detail.

Whom to Interview? Patients may be admitted to hospital by a variety of means, accompanied by relatives, professionals or alone. They may present variously as lucid, mildy anxious, or floridly psychotic. Common sense dictates how the admission profile should be completed. The patient will be interviewed if willing or able, or failing this, a member of his family or whoever accompanied him — friend, neighbour or some professional. In some cases community nurses 'admit' patients who are on their list. In such cases this nurse can provide important information, and would be a key liaison agent during the patient's stay in hospital.

Where to Conduct the Interview? Ideally, the information should be taken as soon after admission as possible. The interview should be taken in private, except where a chaperone is thought advisable. The patient should be encouraged to see, from the outset, that he will be handled with dignity and confidence in an atmosphere of privacy and confidentiality. Background details may be available either from the admitting agent or from earlier records if he has previously been in the hospital. Where such records are available, these should be checked to rule out any change of circumstances, or omissions.

Content. The patient's *identity* should be carefully recorded: all Christian names, including a check on spelling and pronunciation. If the patient has an unusual name it may help to establish rapport if you ask him how he prefers that it is pronounced. It may also be appropriate at this stage to ask him how he would prefer to be addressed: e.g. full Christian name, abbreviation, some nickname, or a full title such as Mr Smith.

Age, Sex, Marital State. The patient's date of birth should be carefully recorded along with a note on gender identity: this is important for record purposes where the patient's name may not indicate sex, e.g. Frances, Vivian. Enter also whether married, divorced, separated, widowed or single. In this context it may be appropriate to ask women how they prefer to be addressed in writing, e.g. Miss, Mrs or Ms. Some married women may have retained their single identity.

Family. Details on the patient's family should be briefly recorded. Does he have any children? Do they live with him? Details of age and sex. Does he live with parents? Does he have any brothers or sisters? Is he a member of an active 'extended family'? Whom does this include?

Domestic. Where does he live? Is this his own house, rented, a sub-let, etc.?

Occupation. Is he employed at present? Where does he work and what is the nature of his job? What occupation did he last follow?

Socialisation. Does he have any close friends? Does he have other acquaintances or relationships? Is he a member of any clubs? Does he attend church regularly?

Financial Status. Does he have any money with him? Other funds? Does he have any outstanding bills at present? Make a careful record of any money handed over for sake keeping.

Personal Belongings. A record should be made of significant items of clothing, jewellery and other possessions carried by the patient, especially if these are handed over to staff.

Medical Cover. Name and address of the patient's physician (and social worker if appropriate). Is he currently taking any medication? Has he been receiving any other form of medical or psychological treatment?

The purpose of this initial interview is largely to establish the identity of the patient. Although this information can be obtained in a few minutes, in some cases even this will not be possible, and the nurse may have to await the arrival of relatives to furnish these details. Most of the details fulfil administrative requirements. Other details, such as occupation and home background, give a broad indication of class background. Identification of marital status, family situation and relationships are important for identifying people who may visit him shortly. If the nurse can quickly become acquainted with the patient's family and cultural background this may enhance her status in the eyes of the patient. Advance knowledge of this nature also helps avoid making *faux pas*, e.g. asking 'Will your wife be coming to see you today?' where the couple are separated. This information helps build a simple sketch of the patient, from what he likes to be called to whom may need to be contacted regarding his care.

In taking these notes it is important to emphasise that all such information will be kept strictly confidential. Many patients are rightly suspicious of such documentation. Similarly, patients or their relatives should always be *invited* to offer information — especially about relationships and finance. At no time should they feel that they are under any obligation to supply such details, however inconvenient this may be to staff. The nurse should also make it clear why *she* wants this information, not just for records, but so that she can get to know the patient better, so that she knows who to contact if he becomes ill or needs someone, and so that she can learn to help him during his time in her care.

The Presenting Problem

The initial interview of the admission profile involved simple questions of a factual nature. The second part of the history involves looking at the patient's problems, necessarily a more complex affair. This interview may follow from the admission profile, or some time may be allowed to elapse to let the patient settle down before further questioning. The aim in this next stage is to identify the patient's problems, and to find out how they relate to various aspects of his life.

The Problem. Some idea of why the patient is in hospital, or why he feels that he requires care or treatment, is needed. This can best be answered by asking him, 'Can you tell me what has brought you into hospital?' This direct question is perhaps appropriate only for the patient who is not overtly distressed. The nurse must judge in advance whether or not the patient can handle such an open-ended question. If he appears to need some help or reassurance the following, more indirect, approach might be tried.

OK thanks for giving me all this background information: that was very helpful. Now I'd like to ask you a few questions about how you are feeling just now. Is that OK? (patient nods) Well, how are you feeling right now? (following reply) . . . All right, now I know that you have been having some problems at home, before you came in. Do you think that you could tell me a bit about them? (following reply) So, from what you have said, you seemed to be having difficulty with . . . . . . and . . . . . . Are they the cause of you coming into hospital? Or do you think that something else is to blame?

The aim at this stage is merely to get the patient to specify, in fairly broad terms, the nature of his problem, e.g. 'Couldn't cope any longer' or 'Couldn't stand the voices' or simply 'I just don't know what is happening to me'. The nurse should try to guide the patient to reveal more details of his problem, using the following factors as anchors.

Functioning. Has he noticed any change in his bodily function — the use of his limbs, speech, memory, eyesight, etc.? If so, what is the nature of these changes? How does the patient contrast what he is like *now*, with what he used to be like?

Behaviour. Have any noticeable changes in his behaviour occurred? Is he concerned about things he *used to do*, or even things which he has *never* been able to do? (E.g. he used to be a 'good mixer', but since he moved to a new job he doesn't seem 'to fit in'.) Is he doing things now which are upsetting to himself, or other people?

Affect. Does he experience any specific feelings associated with these problems: anger, sadness, fear, tension, threat, confusion, excitement, etc.? Can he describe *how* he feels these sensations: do they involve his body or his mind, or both?

Cognition. Does the patient have any specific thoughts about these problems? Does he spend time ruminating? If so, what does he think about? Does he have any recurring thoughts, which just 'pop into his head'? How do these thoughts present themselves: as words, images, memories or day dreams?

Beliefs. What does he think these problems mean? What does he believe is happening to him: e.g. does this mean he is going mad? being punished? or being rejected?

Physical. Has he experienced any physical problems associated with these difficulties: pain, loss of appetite, loss of sleep, listlessness, decline in weight and loss of interest in sex?

Relationships. Have his relationships with family and friends changed recently? Does he attribute this in any way to his 'problems'?

General Orientation. Have any changes occurred in the patient's relationship with himself? Is he concerned about losing touch with reality? losing sight of his former goals? changes in his personality? losing contact with friends, neighbours, etc.?

Expectations. What does he think is going to happen to him in hospital? Is he going to be cured? have his problems taken away? learn to come to terms with himself? with his fears? Or does he want to change the way he lives? Does he expect to be involved in his own care and treatment? Do his family and friends have any expectations of him, or the hospital?

The first review of the patient's situation is unashamedly 'problem-oriented'. Later it will be necessary to build a more balanced view of the person. However, for now, it might be inappropriate to study his assets. The patient might even think that the nurse was afraid to grapple with his problems. Although I have discussed this interview in terms of a hospitalised patient, the same format would apply to a 'new case' on a community nurse's caselist, or a patient seen at a day hospital or psychiatric clinic.

Developing the History

The information detailed above might be collected in the early days following admission, or as part of the initial assessment in the patient's home or at a clinic. The next phase of the assessment involves the development of this thumbnail sketch. The nurse now tries to expand the material, beginning with a look at his past history, his present circumstances and the way his 'problem' interferes with these aspects of his life. Depending on the setting and the resources, this interview might take place within the first week of admission or at the second appointment — at home or the clinic. This interview will try to develop a more balanced view of the person, emphasising his positive features as well as his difficulties. Again, I shall discuss the interview under topic headings. There is no need, however, to follow these in strict sequence. The sophisticated interviewer may well 'hop' back and forth across topics.

Education. A brief description of his schooling at basic and advanced level, especially his attitude towards his education: was it an enjoyable experience? Does he still enjoy learning? Did school put him off the idea of education? Since some aspect of the patient's 'therapy' may involve learning, in one form or another, these questions are of vital importance. Knowledge about educational background is also important in terms of judging his capabilities, e.g. for filling in questionnaires, handling abstract concepts, etc.

Occupation. Further details about his present job or his previous employment. In some cases 'work aspirations' may be a more appropriate topic. Did he select his present occupation? past occupations? Was he forced into it by family or financial circumstances? How does he feel about his present job? Is there something else he would rather do? Is he proud of his position or indifferent? Does his present problem interfere in any way with his capacity to work?

Social Network. Is the patient a 'social animal'? Does he enjoy going out: cinema, clubs, dining out, the local pub? Can he describe his friends and acquaintances in terms of a network, extending from very close ties through to casual acquaintances? What kind of social life would he prefer, if any? Part of this line of questioning should refer to the patient's sex life. What are his attitudes towards monogamous versus casual sex, for example? Is he happy with his sex life? (Note: we should not assume that, because the patient has no sex life, he is unhappy.) What improvements would he like to see in this area? Is there any way that his 'problem' interferes with any of his relationships with people?

Recreation. How does he use his free time? Does he have any hobbies or preferred activities — from passive ones (watching TV, listening to records) to more active ones (working for a political party, visiting old people)? Is he happy with his recreation? In what way would he like to see it change or develop? Does his present 'problem' interfere with this in any way?

General Health. How has the patient's health been during his life? How is it at present. How does he view his health: does he 'run to the doctor' with every complaint? or does he tend to 'put up with things'? Does he try to maintain his health: through diet, exercise, moderate drinking, etc.? Does he see his health as his responsibility, or merely the 'luck of the draw'?

Drugs. Does the patient take any drugs? Are they prescribed, self-selected or illicit? How does he feel about taking drugs? How would he describe his use: regular, habitual or a last resort? What other 'drugs' does he use: cigarettes, alcohol, coffee? Has he ever tried to stop taking these drugs? Has he ever experimented with drugs? What was his reaction? Does his present 'problem' cause him to use any of these drugs more often?

Past Treatment. Apart from drugs, has the patient had any other form of treatment for his 'problem'? What effect did this have? Did he think that this treatment was appropriate? What did he think that he needed at that time? Is there any form of treatment that he wishes he had received?

Coping. The patient meets with 'problems' on an everyday basis. How does he cope with these upsets? Can he provide details of how he stops himself doing things, or how he prevents problems preying on his mind? How does he think that he is coping with his present 'problem'? How could he handle it better?

Outstanding Problems? Are there any aspects of his 'problem' which he feels are beyond solution? Has he ever felt that he couldn't stand things any longer? How did he feel like reacting — showing his anger, killing someone, committing suicide?

Patient's Role. Who is in the patient's family at present (recap on first interview)? Are there members of his family whom he rarely sees? If they are important to him — such as daughter in Australia — how does he feel about them? How does he get on with his family: how would he describe their relationships? Do they have arguments? Does he think that this is a good thing? Do they spend much time together? What are his thoughts on this? In what way has his problem prejudiced relationships with his family?

What about his original family: what was it like to grow up in that family? Was his family similar or different to his 'own' family? Does he model himself on anyone from his original family? What was important about this person that he wishes to copy?

How would he describe his role in relation to either or both of these families? Is he an important, or an unimportant, figure? Why does he think that? What do other members of the family think of him? How does he relate to in-laws where appropriate? Does he make rules and regulations for the family? Does he keep these himself?

The admission profile and initial 'problem analysis' are akin to a skeleton. In the development interview we attempt to put some flesh on these bones. By trying to establish some details of how the patient functions and what his attitudes to himself and his world are we grow to 'know' him a little better. This biographical interview is in no way peculiar to psychiatry: some journalists, even television chat-show interviewers, do this very well. In the space of a few minutes — providing the patient is willing — we have located him in time, place, context, culture and role. We should not delude ourselves that this is anything other than a further character 'sketch': we have done little more than scratch the surface of his life. However, a good interview, like a 'good' portrait sketch, often catches something of the sitter which disperses some of the mist which enshrouds him. Such carefully rendered features provide something of an insight into his character. So far, we have asked a few questions and made some notes about the answers. A well-designed computer could have kept up this pace. We can take the history a stage further by making some observations on what takes place within the interview.

The Nurse's Observations

In addition to the information supplied, the manner in which it is offered may also be important. The nurse needs to make detailed 'mental notes' during the conversation of how the patient appears, judging how he behaves, feels and thinks.

Appearance. The nurse should make a note of the *general* presentation of the patient: any specific deformities or disabilities? Does he appear healthy, wasted, undernourished, overweight? What is his approximate height and weight? (These may be checked later at a physical examination.) How is he dressed: not so much in terms of fashion, but in terms of appropriateness to the situation? Finally, some notes on his interaction during the interview need to be made. How did he look at the nurse: avoiding eye contact? staring? appearing distracted? What about his general posture? Did he appear tense, relaxed, edgy? Was he willing to converse? If he appeared resistant, in what way did this show?

Behaviour. Notes on his behaviour during the session should also be made. Did he use many gestures? Were they appropriate or manneristic? In terms of his overall activity level did he appear restless or relaxed? How did he walk — hurried, limping, with any peculiar gait pattern? What about his speech? Did he speak audibly, too loud or too soft? Did he speak too fast or too slow? Did he display any interruptions: stuttering, stammering, long pauses?

Affect. More detailed judgement of the patient's affect should be made during the interview. Here we are interested in the patient's emotional state. Please note that I am discussing only the patient's mood or feelings *during* the interview: this might differ markedly from his mood at other times. How appropriate is his mood to the situation? This must be related to the topics under review. Does he appear serious when discussing serious material; relaxed when discussing lighter material — perhaps even showing humour? Or is his mood incongruous: not in keeping with what he is saying? There is a wide range of mood states that we might judge under the affect heading. The nurse should avoid looking only for stereotyped emotions such as depression, anxiety, etc. Below I have noted just a few of the possible emotions which might be expressed by patients:

'Sometimes I just feel like crying. Like right now' (sadness)
'I guess that I enjoy life.' (smile) (happiness)
'I feel trembly all over. See, look at my hands.' (anxiety)
'I'm worried about what is going to happen tomorrow.' (apprehension)
'What do you mean? I just told you, *twice.*' (anger)
'I'm scared right now.' (fear)
'I just feel lost. Out of touch.' (alienation)
'I just can't be bothered.' (apathy)

Although I have noted verbal associates of these emotions, it is possible to detect emotional state by non-verbal means. Excitement is often shown by speed of speech and movement, rather than content; pain, by ways of holding parts of the body; hostility, by subtle looks or sidelong glances. Finally, in addition to noting how appropriate, or *congruent*, is the patient's emotional state, the nurse should note the main affective theme. What is the main emotion shown? What is the main emotion that is voiced?

Cognition. It is a truism to say that most of the interview is a reflection of *how* the patient thinks or indeed *what* he thinks. We are not dealing with factual material. Instead we are inviting the patient to give a report on certain aspects of his life. Some kind of judgement must be made as to the relative accuracy of this information. Is it true or false? Might it be distorted by his interpretation of the facts? The patient's thinking — or cognition — can be considered in two ways: the *way* he appears to think, and *what* he appears to think about. Form and content.

Form. The form of the patient's thinking can be looked at from a number of angles. I do not wish to encourage nurses to repeat the psychiatric interview. The psychiatrist's interview is designed to ascertain the form and content of the patient's thinking. However, the nurse's interview should also include some observation on the patient's thought processes. This may reinforce or help to modify the other opinion, or provide information to help the nurse's evaluation of progress at a later date.

Among the general characteristics that might be judged are the following:

How *fast* does the patient appear to think? Does it appear excessively fast or slow? Is he easily *distracted*? Does he flit from one idea to another as he talks?

To what extent does there appear to be *continuity* of thought? Is he able to link the various themes in his conversation?

Does he appear *alert*: sensitive to the line of questioning? Or does he appear dulled in some way?

Does he volunteer answers in a *spontaneous* manner? Or does he continually wrestle with himself, looking for the 'right word or expression'?

Is his speech *coherent*? Or does it appear fragmented? Or with parts of words fused together?

Does he show any *perseveration*? Repeating statements or words over and over?

Does he appear to get 'stuck' on a single theme, mulling it over 'in his head'?

Does he suddenly *break off* in mid-sentence, showing 'blocking' in his thinking?

Does he seem unable to draw out ideas or be specific? (commonly called 'overinclusiveness')

Is his speech disrupted by *disruptions* to the normal association of ideas? (commonly called 'knight's-move thinking')

Is he unable to think — or discuss ideas — in *abstract terms*?

(commonly called 'concrete thinking')
Does he *coin new or unusual words*? (neologisms)
Does he 'invent' material as a false recall for *failed memory*?
Does he constantly introduce highly *personlised themes* which appear to reject reality? (commonly called dereistic or autistic thinking)
Does he find it difficult to *concentrate* upon the interview, or to *recall* information?

I need hardly remind the reader that, important though these 'observations' are, they can be wildly inaccurate. Some of the disorders of thinking that have been noted briefly are very subtle. It often takes a highly trained interviewer to spot them. However, I do not think that this is very important. One would expect that someone else, in another interview, would pick up these subtleties if they are present. What is more of a problem is the danger of 'finding' something through the simple act of looking for it. If we applied these notes to an analysis of a conversation over coffee, or in a pub, I am sure that someone, somewhere, could be called 'thought-disordered'. For this reason I urge caution, and conservatism, in interpreting the patient's thinking.

Content. The major consideration regarding content involves the patient's major themes. What does he spend most time thinking about, or talking about? Are these both the same? How does he think about himself? Does he evaluate himself positively or negatively? To what extent does he believe that he has a problem? This is especially important in the case of the patient who has been admitted against his wishes, or is being treated compulsorily. I am unhappy about the use of the term 'insight'. Often we accuse the patient of lacking insight because his assessment of the 'facts' does not match ours. However, providing that we use it in its proper sense — meaning the extent to which the patient is aware of what is happening to him, and can think about these events — then it is permissible. On a similar level we should consider the patient's ability to *judge* the significance of what is happening to him, has happened in the past or might occur in the future. What thoughts does he have about these aspects of his life?

What are the patient's major *worries*? These may not be the same as his presenting 'problems'. Does he worry about things that have happened in the past, are happening to him or might happen? Are these worries real or imaginary fears? Is he afraid of going mad? The patient may also describe material of a 'delusional' character. It is important to be scrupulously objective here. Many people have beliefs or ideas which are 'strange' to me. Does that mean they are delusions? Obviously not. We are concerned here with beliefs which have no discernible basis in reality. It is easy to spot such delusions when they are extreme, but less easy to judge subtler variations on the delusional theme. For instance, if the patient believes that he 'can't cope with life', and the facts suggest that he manages tolerably well, is he deluded? Perhaps again, 'obviously not'. The patient may also refer to 'hallucinatory material', hearing voices or sounds, seeing sights, of which other people are unaware. Again, I hestitate to say that these are *not* real. In the case of delusions and hallucinations I think the solution is simply to report what the patient says. Rather than 'labelling' the material, let it speak for itself.

The patient may also have various vague fears that preoccupy him: fear of dying, of impending doom, or of nothing in particular — just 'everything in general'. He may be preoccupied with performing certain mental rituals in order to prevent disasters occurring. His thinking may also project ideas about himself which appear extreme, either overinflated, grandiose or unnecessarily worthless. In this context it is important to identify any sign of suicidal thinking, which may be explicit or veiled. Is he preoccupied with morbid thoughts? Does he think a lot about death or dying? Does he ruminate about the trappings of death — funerals, death notices, graveyards? Or is he preoccupied with extreme religiosity? It is worth asking the patient directly whether he has ever considered killing himself. Although many professionals still believe the myth that questioning a person about suicidal ideas may 'put the idea into his head' or make it more acceptable, if he is already thinking about it, the reverse is the case. Encouraging a patient to discuss such ideas often offers some degree of relief. In addition to asking whether he has ever considered harming himself, has he ever thought about harming anyone else? What is his reasoning for this?

Finally, the nurse should try to judge the patient's contact with reality. Typically, this can be tested by reference to the year, day, date, etc. This will be discussed in Chapter 5. It may be more appropriate to try judging his orientation to events that have occurred in the distant and more recent past, such as dates of weddings, starting a new job, period of last illness. This may be less obtrusive than a formal 'reality orientation' test.

The Concept of Personal Norms

The information drawn from this development interview should help the nurse to summarise the patient's problems, using the life-history of the person as a backdrop. We have found out a little of the stages in his life, the framework of his life, and what it means to him to operate under the name of John Smith, or whatever. We may also have discovered how his perception of 'John Smith' has changed during the course of his life. We have found out something of his problems: how they relate to various facets of his life; whether they are new or repeats; how they developed. We may have some idea of the kind of person he was before these problems emerged, and how they have grown, diminished or remained static over time.

The use of the personal history is, in one sense, less useful than it is in general medicine, and in another it is a crucial part of the assessment process. In general medicine, if a professional footballer breaks his leg, it is clear that rehabilitation of this injury must aim at restoration of his former athletic ability. Most medical treatment involves this *restoration* process: find out what he could do before he became ill, and we will restore him 'to health'. In psychiatry, the problem may not be so simple. In many cases it is not advisable for patients to 'go back'. It may be that their life-style before their illness was a contributory factor. Perhaps the solution is to help the patient to 'move forward', rather than backward. However, the personal history is most helpful in helping us to understand the patient's 'personal norms'. The 'disorder' which the patient presents with today may be an exaggeration of his normal behaviour. However, his normal functioning might be viewed as 'pathological' if it was shown by someone else. For instance, a patient who has always been independent, free and easy, with a joking manner, suddenly becomes indecisive. He starts to have problems at work, feels obliged to plan everything very carefully, and becomes very sober in his manner. He 'looks' just the same as his colleague, with whom he shares an office: indeed both behave in exactly the same way. But even he is saying, along with the rest of the work-force, 'What's the matter with you, are you nuts or something?' Many of the problems we meet in the psychiatric field are not pathological, in the sense that oedema or diplopia are pathological. These problems represent signs of an underlying disorder which would constitute problems for most people. Changes in a person's psychosocial functioning may constitute a problem for him because this is a sign of a disruption of his 'personal norms'. Such problems may be unremarkable when found in someone else.

I said at the outset that I had reservations about the 'history'. As I have noted above, I consider the history an invaluable *part* of the assessment process. My reservation is that some nurses — indeed some doctors too for that matter — seem to think that they can base care or treatment on this single assessment strategy. I have even more reservations about some of the narrower 'life-histories' which abound in clinical practice. Although it is far from exhaustive, the history model I have outlined tries to be comprehensive. It avoids looking at the patient as though he were a 'one-dimensional man'. All the questions I would like to ask have some bearing on the 'problem': they either reflect ways in which the 'problem' intrudes on the patient's life, or they highlight assets which might be conscripted to help solve the 'problem'. Of supreme importance is the recognition that the patient is defined largely by the social order around him: how he relates to this social world and the demands it makes, and the restrictions it imposes upon him. Unless this reciprocal relationship — the 'patient-in-his-world' — is described in some detail, the history will be largely useless. The patient does not inhabit a vacuum. The history must illustrate something of the richness of his past and present experience.

The history can tell us a lot about the patient and his world. What it does not tell us may be more significant. The main weaknesses of the history are that it 'quantifies' so little, and that what it does quantify could be so much fantasy. The problem we face in using the history as the sole assessment vehicle is that we have little of a measurable nature. How do we judge the size or scale of the patient's problems? How can we use what amounts to an extended 'conversation' as a means of evaluating progress? The second problem involves the medium of the interview. The patient may present an image of himself here which is in stark contrast to his other 'self'. Either he may heighten the intensity of his problems, or he may underplay them. Although nurses often make great play of being 'non-judgemental', this stance can be taken only so far. We do not pass judgement when the data are being offered to us.

But once the information is in our possession it is our responsibility, often an awesome one, to judge its validity. If we fail to honour this responsibility the patient, or some significant other, may unwittingly prejudice the course of care and treatment.

Opening Doors

The nursing history can be seen as a way of gaining an overview of the patient's problems, against the broader canvas of his life, his world. This picture can hardly be anything but impressionistic, given the crude nature of the interview method. This is not to say that it is not important. We need this character sketch to help us judge what we euphemistically call his 'mental state'. Without this judgement we could hardly proceed. We need to proceed further with our 'picture' of the patient. So far we have a sketchy outline of his problems, seen against the perspective of the world he inhabits, and interacts with. From this overview we can decide where we should focus our attention. Which part of his life needs to be drawn into tighter focus? We cannot, indeed should not, study closely every facet of his being. We shall use the history as a springboard for further, more detailed, enquiries. The history will help us to plan the rest of the assessment. Using some of the functional problems discussed in the later part of the book I shall now discuss briefly how the history can open doors into the patient's life.

The Person who is Dependent. A key feature of severe mental disorder is the loss of independent functioning. This is most evident in the chronic patient, who has become heavily dependent on family, support services or the hospital routine. Such people may suffer more from these secondary handicaps than from their original disorder. The history may reveal dependence as one problem area of significance for the patient. His reliance on others, to help perform tasks or to make decisions, may emerge from this introductory profile. This should lead us to consider assessment of independent functioning as a key target. We need to know: to what extent can he perform everyday routines? To what extent is he capable of, or motivated to, make decisions affecting his life? Although people who are handicapped in this way are likely to have many other problems, loss of independence may be a key area for closer study. This topic is discussed in Chapter 5.

The Person who is Anxious. The experience of anxiety is natural to all animals. Without it we could not survive. We only stop to consider it when it gets out of hand, when it becomes unnatural. Anxiety can be a problem for a wide range of patients. It is not restricted to those with so-called 'anxiety neuroses'. The history may reveal situations in which the patient is unable to cope with work, relationships, stress or the myriad other 'threat' factors found in our environment. This may suggest that we need to look more closely at this experience of 'threat': what are the situations in which he feels anxious? how does it manifest itself for this patient? and how severe is this problem? We also want to know: what is the effect of anxiety upon the person? his dealings with others? his life in general? This topic is discussed in Chapter 6.

The Person who is Depressed. The person who experiences a disturbance of the elevation of his mood — occasionally feeling low in spirits, or swinging to the other extreme of euphoria and excitability — is the partner to anxiety, as one of the commonest *emotional* problems. Depression of mood is the commonest problem and can also be seen in a range of patients, including those not diagnosed specifically as 'depressives'. The history may reveal situations where the patient becomes depressed in the event of some noticeable 'loss': bereavement, financial crisis, failed opportunities. Often no obvious cause is evident. The interview with the patient may reveal evidence of depression, shown perhaps more by his presentation and lack of motivation than by any verbal signals. This may suggest a need to study this area of his emotional functioning more closely. How can we gauge the changes in his affective state? What relationship do such changes have to his observable behaviour? In what way is this 'depressed' state a function of events in his life? To what extent does it interfere with the everyday living of his life? These topics are discussed in Chapter 7.

The Person with Relationship Problems. Any of the people mentioned above might also have problems involving their interaction with other people: other patients on the ward, family, spouse, friends, neighbours, individuals or groups. Since much of the history focuses upon the reciprocal relationship between the patient and his 'significant others', any problem met in this area should emerge quite quickly. This might lead us to study at closer range the exact nature of such problems. Does he feel anxious in company? Does he feel 'unprepared' to deal with certain social situations? Does he have difficulty making friends or sustaining conversation? The relationship problems may be specific 'disorders' of psychosocial functioning. They might also be part of a larger problem: depression, anxiety, schizophrenia. Either way, there is some advantage to be gained from defining and measuring more specifically the nature and function of such problems. This topic is discussed in Chapter 8.

The Person who is Out of Touch with Reality. This is a rather poor alternative to the title 'someone who is psychotic'. I use this euphemism in order to include others who may appear to have major perceptual disturbance, but who might not be diagnosed as psychotic. People who see things, or hear voices which do not appear to be there, or who discuss ideas which seem bizarre in the light of our experience, might be included in this category. As my overview of the history suggested, such characteristics may be evident from our conversation with the patient. Alternatively he may tell us about his experience of such 'unreal' phenomena at other times in his life. As with the other problems mentioned, it may be desirable to collect more specific data on this problem. What exactly does he see, hear or think? Are other people aware of his bizarre status? How can we begin to measure what appears to be a facet of our higher consciousness? This topic is discussed in Chapter 9.

I have by no means exhausted the possibilities of 'doors' which might be opened. The corridors of psychological distress are long indeed. There are people who engage in sexual deviations, and those who cannot engage in sex at all. There are those who prejudice their health by eating too much and those who starve themselves to death. There are patients who attack and maim others, and those who enjoy the experience of being brutalised. The list appears endless. The illustrations of 'problems' which I have selected for the second part of this book are significant in two ways. First, they can be viewed as 'problems of living' as opposed to specific disorders: I have suggested this already by pointing out the way such problems may occur across a range of patient populations. Second, these problems appear to establish links, one with another, in many patients.

The Case of Harry. Harry was a young man of 25 when he was made redundant from his job in a tyre factory. He had a wife and two young children to support, and little money to do it. Two years later he had run up a pile of debts through trying to own what he couldn't afford, and was finally evicted from his flat for non-payment of rent. His wife returned to her parents, taking the children. Harry moved into a friend's house, leaving after a few months to lodge at a men's hostel. The hostel was for sleeping only, so Harry tramped the streets by day, avoiding any old friends or acquaintances, manifestly depressed by his downfall. Gradually, he stopped visiting his children on Sundays. Visiting his in-laws only induced great anxiety beforehand; leaving his children afterwards induced a raging despair. As his relationships dwindled he began to lose confidence. Even 'signing on' at the labour exchange became an ordeal. He thought that the clerks were laughing at his shabby appearance, talking about him behind his back. When he was called before a DHSS panel, he felt he was being victimised. It was an elaborate plot to bring him finally to his knees. He began to drink heavily to relieve the depression. He drank alone. He drank to forget. When the anger inside him couldn't be stifled any longer he slashed himself repeatedly with a broken bottle, to ease the tension. The punishment was almost at an end.

The problems that we pick up in the history may be circumscribed. More often than not they will be diffuse, or linked tenuously with other disorders. In Harry's case his 'career' was almost predictable. The loss of something prized leads to the loss of self-esteem. The loss of self-esteem leads to the loss of motivation. Loss of motivation leads to loss of action. When we fail to act, events overtake us. When the world starts to run over our heads, we are under threat. When we are under threat we need to do something to resolve the distress which threat brings. Hiding, avoiding, abusing drugs and eventually opting out of life are fairly common strategies for coping with such distress. Why mention Harry here? Well, he was one person whom I would have liked to do a complete history on: but sooner.

The History in the Process

Some years ago Annie Altschul commented that the nursing process was 'the current vogue in nursing circles'.[1] Seven or eight years on she remains sceptical about its validity as a mechanism for organising nursing care.[2] Whether care is to be 'well organsied "good care"' or 'well organised "bad care"' seems to depend more on the skills at the nurse's disposal than upon any 'process' she uses.

The development of the nursing process is an American tale with some Canadian inflections.[3, 4] The development emphasises the planning of more individualised care and a move away from task-oriented nursing. In the United States at least, this has had led to the formation of the concept of holistic care.[5] Nurses have always used a planning and execution model, even for the execution of tasks. The history of nursing would suggest that little attention was paid to the orientation of this model to individual people, with individual problems. The concept of the nursing process is heavily imbued with mystique. It is heavily laden with 'scientific' jargon and 'humanistic' concern. At its root, however, the concept is simplicity itself. It may be the walking personification of 'good old-fashioned common sense'. As Altschul has pointed out, we must use a 'process' when planning an evening's entertainment for friends. We need to decide what they should eat and drink, and which music to play. We try to present a 'programme' which will meet general needs — promoting conviviality and satisfaction — and will also meet individual needs, such as dietary prejudices or the execution of deviant behaviours, such as smoking. The hostess who devises the evening's entertainment makes judgements about which 'needs' to satisfy, and which she will ignore. She may make a no smoking rule, or may try to introduce an ardent carnivore to the pleasures of a vegetarian dish. Here the hostess is not blindly accepting that all her guests' needs should be met. She makes her own 'value judgements'. These may turn out well, or may be a disaster. The smoker may feel insulted, or may be happy that some-one is trying to help him kick the habit. The carnivore may enjoy the nut cutlets, or may find his appetite unsatisfied. Where 'needs' are not met directly, such an unpredictable outcome is likely. At the end of the evening the hostess will evaluate the outcome of the party. What evidence was there that people were happy? What steps could be taken to ensure that the next soirée will be better?

The planning of nursing care, '*à la* process', seems little different from the plan of this evening's entertainment. We assess the patient, in order to identify his 'needs': these form the basis of the care plan. We then decide whether or not we should try to meet these needs. In some cases, one patient's needs may infringe another's, as in the case of the smoker. In other cases there may be an ethical objection to meeting a particular need. Finally, there may be the consideration that the needs of the majority will prevail over those of the individual. Once we have decided which needs to meet, we plan how to do this and, having done it, we evaluate its success. Have the patient's needs been met? Is he satisfied? Have we achieved our nursing goal?

A Popular Nursing Process Format

This book is not about the nursing process. However, assessment is part of 'the process', thus making a brief discussion relevant. One of the more popular, and practical, formats is the SOAPE model described by Desmond Cormack.[6] Based on an original model described in the United States,[7] this model cites five stages. First, information is collected about the patient's complaints. Subjective information, supplied by the patient (S), is paired with objective information, supplied by the nurse (O). From these two categories of information an assessment is made (A). Cormack calls this the 'nursing diagnosis'. Then a plan is prepared — what the nurse will do to meet the patient's need (P). Finally, the plan is evaluated, by hypothesising what *should* happen as a result of the intervention (E).

SOAPE is rational, systematic and straightforward. Consequently it should be easy to use, at least with simpler, specific problems. Where the problems are more diffuse — or like Harry's mentioned earlier, 'interconnected' — difficulties might occur. I have serious doubts about deciding on an action to meet such individual problems. separately. Take, for example, a patient who is depressed. He may show a wide range of problems:

'affective': he complains of being unhappy
'behavioural': he speaks very slowly, gives poor eye contact
'motivation': says, 'I can't be bothered trying any more.'
'cognitive': thinks, 'I'm all washed up.'
'physical': eats little, sleeps even less

Most of these problems are interconnected. Instead of individual solutions perhaps we need a 'build-up plan', one which begins with motivating the patient to become more active, which may have a spin-off to his affective level, and may help improve his physical problems. Becoming more active may also reduce his low self-esteem. The next stage might involve tackling his negative affect, improvements in this area improving his behaviour, and raising his self-esteem. Then we might move on to look specifically at the cognitive problems, which might lie at the core of his difficulties. I should emphasise that my suggested care plan here is not of a different order to SOAPE, but simply an alternative formulation. I simply have an anxiety about drawing up lists of problems where they occur in a complex form, and proceeding to 'pick them off' like plaster ducks in a shooting gallery.

Altschul, as we know, has reservations about 'the process'. She is particularly concerned that the care delivered by nurses should continue to 'express' the inputs of other professions. She emphasises that the care offered by nurses cannot be divorced from the inputs of other staff. Altschul is concerned, too, about tabulating long lists of problems which nurses 'pick off' without due consultation with other members of the care team. As I suggested with my 'depression' example, some problems will resolve themselves, at least partially, as a function of gains in some other area. Where the patient presents with highly complex problems, the basic nursing process model requires major revisions. Perhaps , however, the major problem lies in the nurse's working relationships with other professionals. Can she promote a 'nursing' process which is *not* wholly congruent with the 'medical, psychological, social work, physiotherapy, etc.' process?

Baker, Baker, Bake Me a Cake

In closing this brief discussion I should like to make my own contribution to the 'nursing process' models. This is an idea which might help to understand the design of nursing care, and which takes into account the roles of professions allied to nursing. It is also a little 'lighter' in tone than some of the more 'scientific' pronouncements about the 'process'.

In Figure 3.1 I am drawing an analogy between meeting patient needs and baking a cake. As I have discussed, meeting such needs can be a complex business, but it is apparent that we must begin by deciding what kind of cake we want. I am a strict vegetarian. So if you were baking the cake for me you would need to make sure that no animal products were included, to meet my philosophical as well as dietary needs. Therefore, deciding what kind of cake is needed represents the *assessment* phase. We then have to decide how we

Figure 3.1: 'Baker, baker, bake me a cake'

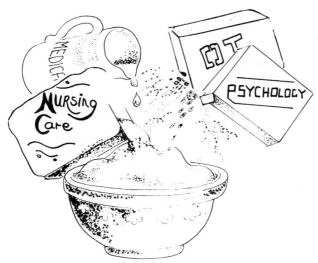

meet my nutritional needs. My illustration shows how this *plan* is concocted. A number of different personnel are represented by different ingredients: mixed peel, drops of water, grains of salt, pounds of flour, etc. Not that the contributions vary enormously in weight. This is like the care situation. A doctor, who may only see the patient fleetingly may, none the less, make a very important contribution. He adds that small dash which gives the cake its special flavour. The social worker is a regular contact: he provides a large helping of sultanas. The psychologist offers help with things of which others have only limited knowledge: he offers some spices from the orient. The domestic staff offer irregular but honest support and reassurance: the salt of the earth and the milk of human kindness. So far we have a pretty indigestible mess. We need something to bind my cake (care) together. We need some dough. Metaphorically speaking, this is the nursing contribution of time and effort, which also acts as a catalyst in the oven: our symbolic 'melting pot' of psychiatic care and treatment. The evaluation, of course, takes place after the first slice has been tasted.

The Concept of Need

Most nursing theorists base their models of practice on the concept of fulfilling needs. One of the goals in the history, which figures centrally in the 'process', is the identification of the patient's needs. Where I have talked about 'the problem' we could easily substitute the term 'need'. Before we close this chapter perhaps we should consider the concept of need.

It is apparent that people have basic physiological needs for food, drink and warmth. Without these the biological self suffers and may die. We also have basic needs for comfort, shelter from the elements and security from danger. These are also concerned with preservation, and maintain the basic quality of life. Much of 'basic nursing care' is concerned with meeting these needs. We assume that a patient 'needs' a drink when he says he is thirsty or appears dehydrated. Usually we plan to meet these needs in advance, preventing desperate needs arising. Similarly, we arrange certain kinds of seating, or help non-ambulant people to move around, to avoid pressure sores, thus meeting the twin needs for comfort and physical exercise to stimulate circulation. In any 'basic care' situation we meet basic needs for food, drink, warmth, ventilation, comfort, avoidance of pain, injury, etc. However, the concept of need can at times be a different concept. To begin with, it is largely hypothetical once we go beyond the stage of basic needs. What other kinds of needs do people have? A need for sex; need for success; need for recognition; need for friendship; need for control over situations; need for happiness; need for freedom from worry; a need for freedom itself. These needs are much more vague and subjective. I could give you a list of 'my needs': what I think I must have satisfied to lead a full, satisfying life. Does this mean that all my needs *must* be satisfied, simply because I have said so?

Consider for a moment a patient who experiences severe anxiety whenever he goes out. This anxiety makes him avoid leaving his house. He says that he feels insecure whenever he is far from home. He stays at home because it makes him feel secure: it satisfies his 'security need'. If a community nurse asked him how she could help, he might say, 'Arrange for my shopping to be done, and for my friends to call round, so that I needn't go out.' If we did this we would meet his 'need for security'. It is clear that we would not have helped him. A similar problem might occur with the patient in hospital who is depressed. Each time he thinks about a distressing situation he feels the 'need to cry'. When asked how we might help him he says, 'Just leave me alone, I need to be on my own. I need to cry.' Again question-marks hang over whether or not we should meet these needs for privacy and emotional expression. Our great need in such situations is to be aware of the possible outcomes of providing the 'help' the patient asks for. Such awareness will help us to judge which needs to satisfy and which to ignore.

When we start identifying the patient's 'problems' in the history we start to make judgements about what he *needs*. Someone needs to learn how to pay a compliment without feeling embarrassed. Someone else needs to learn how to cope with anxiety; to control anger; to ease the distress felt when thinking about unhappy events. In each case we are talking about the necessity for some change in the patient's functioning. This is our judgement. The patient may not see these needs at all. We might say that our housebound patient needs to be able to go out without experiencing crippling anxiety. He sees his need for staying indoors, his need for security. The depressed patient we see as someone who needs to be able to look at his life problems in a more objective manner. The patient sees only the need for privacy and emotional expression. I raise these points as a way of rounding off our discussion of the history. In the history we identify the patient's problems. We see these problems against the backdrop of his life. I am suggesting that it may be incorrect to assume that the problems we identify represent needs in the patient's eyes. In many cases what we see as 'needing' to be done may be the reverse of the patient's need-goals. When our assessment is translated into the 'process of nursing', the needs that we identify *in* the patient exist solely in our professional, clinical judgement. Our view should be influenced by the available body of knowledge about the identification and resolution of psychiatric distress. The needs of the patient, and the needs we attribute to the patient, may well be in conflict. There is no obvious solution to this conflict. This is just one nettle of the assessment process that we must grasp without too much trepidation.

Summary

In this chapter I have discussed the role of the life-history in assessment. Some attention has been given to the general structure of history-taking, suggesting that three stages are evident: the administrative 'admission profile'; the problem-oriented interview: and the development interview, where more comprehensive coverage is attempted. I have compared the development of this history to the construction of a skeleton, followed by a gradual shaping of the human figure, who is the patient. This kind of assessment is based entirely on the conversational elements discussed in the last chapter. Information is supplied in response to questions, the nurse making objective judgements all along the route. From this combination of 'subjective' and 'objective' data emerges the picture of the patient: necessarily crude, but a representation none the less. This picture can help us to open doors which, I hope, will lead to closer examination of important facets of the patient's problems. Finally, the profile, and all subsequent assessment data, need to be compiled in some kind of format which will allow them to be manipulated as a care planning and care evaluation method. Some consideration was given to the role of the 'nursing process' concept in this respect.

Notes

1. A. Altschul, 'Use of the Nursing Process in Psychiatric Care', *Nursing Times*, 8 Sept. 1977, pp. 1412–13.

2. A. Altschul, 'Does Good Practice Need Good Principles?', *Nursing Times*, 18 July 1984, pp. 49–51.

3. V. Henderson, *Basic Principles of Nursing* (ICN, Geneva, 1960).

4. D. G. Little and D. H. Carnevali, *Patient Care Planning* (J. B. Lippincott, Philadelphia, 1976).

5. C. M. Beck, R. P. Rawlins and S. R. Willams, *Mental Health Nursing: A Holistic Life-cycle Approach* (C. V. Mosby, St Louis, Mo., 1983).

6. D. F. S. Cormack, 'The Nursing Process: An Application of the SOAPE Model', *Nursing Times*, Occasional Papers, 30 Apr. 1980, pp. 37–40.

7. L. Weed, *Preparing and Maintaining the Problem Oriented Record: The PROMIS Method* (The Press of Case Western Reserve University, Cleveland, Ohio, 1971).

4 THE STUDIED GAZE: SOME METHODS OF ASSESSMENT

Method will teach you to win time. — Goethe

It has often been said that 'method' is like placing things in a box: a 'good' packer will get in half as much again as a 'bad' one. In this chapter I want to discuss some methods of assessment and ways of gaining information about the patient for the minimum of effort. I want to consider some ways of obtaining a 'good' assessment, but I do not intend to discuss any of these methods in any great detail. Some of the important methods will be discussed again in subsequent chapters. Neither do I intend to cover all the possible mechanisms of assessment. Instead, I want to discuss some of the differences between various methods in common use, emphasising their advantages and disadvantages.

In the last chapter I discussed ways of describing the patient and his life from the perspective of his personal history. This relies upon the collection of information through interviewing: the patient, or his family, is asked to report what he believes to be 'the truth'. This picture may be broadened by including observations made by the nurse: what she perceives to be the truth. I need hardly comment upon the weakness inherent in relying upon the history as the *sole* method of assessment. Not only may the final picture of the patient be of doubtful accuracy, but it may also lack the fine detail necessary for planning care or evaluating progress. In this chapter I want to move forward to consider some of the methods which can add detail of a more precise and accurate nature.

The need for some kind of 'system' for studying a situation is taken for granted in scientific or technological circles. In the past, many nurses have been unhappy with the concept of 'scientific method'. Often it has been seen as in conflict with the 'art of nursing', an activity that operated outwith the narrow confines of science. Nursing was often thought to be too flexible and pragmatic — not to say creative — to be defined in any systematic or scientific way. However, without science our view of the world would be uninformed or idiosyncratic. We take for granted our use of scientific principles and knowledge in our everyday life. My labelling and interpretation of certain atmosphere events at the beginning of

Chapter 1 may be simple, but are scientific none the less. The influence of science on our perception of the world is noted by Bronowski and Mazlish.[1] Commenting upon the way in which our view of the world changes in the light of scientific discovery, they argue that science influences our 'concept' of the world.

> A medieval traveller was not unobservant when he described what is obviously an elephant as an animal with five feet, one of which the animal uses like a hand. To us the traveller's tale is ridiculous, because to us the elephant fits into the order of mammals and the unfolding of evolution . . . but to medieval men, the world had a different set of inner connexions; it was organised differently.

So our conception of the world, how we think about it, is influenced by what we know from the world of science. In considering how we conceive that part of our world, inhabited by our patients, we must ask, 'What can science offer by way of a positive influence?' In many instances, our view of our patients is often 'medieval' in character, so removed is it from the influences of contemporary scientific thought.

However, the need for some system, or systematic way of working, is not peculiar to the scientist. Even writers like Samuel Taylor Coleridge commented that 'the first idea of method is a progressive transition from one step to another on any course'. Joseph Addison, the seventeenth-century essayist, remarked wisely that

> irregularity and want of method are only supportable in men of great learning or genius, who are often too full to be exact, and therefore choose to throw down their pearls in heaps before the reader, rather than be at the pains of stringing them together.

It is clear from the advice of these two eminent minds that *method* is an essential part of writing. It should also be clear that it must also be an essential part of the assessment of psychiatric patients. As I noted earlier, we must give assessment the status it deserves. It is also clear from Addison's comments that the vast majority of us simply cannot afford *not* to be methodical. Assessment involves collecting information so that we can construct some image of the patient. That image is then communicated to others. We must be at pains to describe exactly what is there, within the parameters of a rational, scientific, view of the world, so that others may appreciate what we have witnessed.

The General Approach

Information can be collected in two ways. We can ask the patient to *report* on his situation, which might involve simply answering questions, or filling in a record we have devised. In either case we need to be confident that the patient is willing and able to provide such subjective reports. We also need to be assured that he has no reason to wish to mislead us. If we do not possess such confidence or have this assurance, then the report method may be worthless. The alternative is to invite other people to make observations on the patient. It may be appropriate to ask members of his family to use their 'proximity' to the patient to study him at close quarters. However, in practice we use nursing staff and other members of the care team — doctors, psychologists, physiotherapists — to provide such 'objective reports'.

Selecting the Channel. Any of the methods dicussed in this chapter could be used as subjective or objective reports. Wherever possible, information should be obtained direct from the patient, either by direct 'subjective reports' or direct observation — by studying him closely. The 'second-hand' observations often obtained from family and friends come a very poor second in this respect. We should be aware, however, that the patient may mislead us — intentionally or unwittingly. In some cases the patient may be unwilling or unable to provide the information you need, requiring you to fall back on the reports of others. The comments and observations of other people can serve an important function, providing information which may be known only to them, or as corroboration or contradiction of the story offered by the patient. For instance, junior nurses on a ward may have much more contact with the patient than the senior staff. Consequently they can offer insights into his behaviour, known perhaps only to them. Where the patient describes a specific problem it is often helpful to ask 'significant others' to comment upon this, such as family, or friends who know him well. Their report may reinforce his description, or may cast doubt upon his story. Even where the patient's report is not substantiated this may also be significant: it *may* suggest that this is the way the patient perceives the situation.

Collecting information from the patient or his 'significant

others' usually involves some 'informal' method of assessment. Information taken from staff is more likely to be 'formal', involving the use of some standardised method of observation or recording. The aim of the assessment will determine which information channel is selected.

— If you want to know how the patient thinks or feels, or if you wish to identify his values or beliefs, ask the patient.
— If you want to know what other people think or feel or believe about the patient, ask those other people.
— If you want to know how the patient behaves under certain conditions, *either* ask him to study his own behaviour *or* ask someone else who is available to study him in these settings. It should be apparent that these two options may provide completely different reports.

The Methods

1 Interviewing

Although interviewing was covered in Chapter 2, let us refresh our memory about its nature and function before we contrast it with other methods. In an interview the nurse questions the patient about his feelings, his thoughts, his behaviour or his beliefs. These questions may relate to his life in general, or may be specific to things like his current course of treatment. Figure 4.1. illustrates how, at one extreme, an interview can simply mean 'sitting down and chatting to the patient'. At the other, the patient is simply asked to answer 'Yes' or 'No' to a series of questions on a checklist. These represent highly unstructured and highly structured formats. Somewhere between the two lies the semi-structured interview. Here the patient is asked a range of exploratory questions on various topics. His answers may generate some additional questions which need to be answered before moving on to the next topic. The unstructured 'chat' may be too rambling to lead anywhere conclusive. It may also make the patient uneasy, since he may feel that the conversation isn't going anywhere. By contrast, the highly structured 'quizzing' of the patient may appear impersonal and officious. The patient may feel that he is being processed: he has no part to play in this other than to supply these highly specific replies. The semi-structured format is my own preference

Figure 4.1

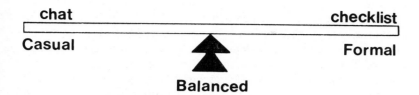

for virtually all situations. The conversation is orderly, without being regimented. There is room to break off at a tangent where appropriate, without losing one's place. This allows the conversation to 'flow', giving both nurse and patient some security.

Advantages of the Interview. The popularity of the interview can be attributed largely to its simplicity. Many nurses can 'converse' with patients with little or no training. Suffice it to say that they might converse a lot better if they were properly trained. The interview may be most appropriate where the patient is unable to use any kind of self-assessment. This is especially the case where patients are illiterate, or can speak the common language but may have difficulty in interpreting it in writing, such as immigrant populations. The interview also allows us to check the patient's understanding of a particular question. If he appears hesitant or puzzled we can rephrase it or amplify it in some way, to help him answer. This is not possible where the patient is left to fill in a questionnaire or rating scale. The interview also allows the patient to give as much detail as he thinks is necessary. The semi-structured format described above allows the patient to develop a theme that may not be possible by any other means. Of course such a development is only possible if the nurse has the ability to recognise 'something significant', and can encourage the patient to amplify his response. Finally, the interview usually allows the nurse to design the rest of the assessment. Interviews are often the first 'port of call' in the assessment process. We may have no idea of what we should be studying until we have conducted a preliminary interview. This may give us the clues we need to introduce either other interviews, or other methods.

Disadvantages. Interviewing can be very time-consuming. In a difficult, or badly handled, interview, a lot of time may be spent for little reward. A successful interview may be equally costly: a lot of time is spent preparing the ground, asking general questions, probing the details, and recording the patient's replies. This does not take account of time lost following up 'red herrings'. Secondly, the interview can be very demanding in terms of expertise. I noted above that many nurses are obliged to assess patients in this way with minimal training. Where the patient is very confused or otherwise distressed we must challenge the wisdom of this policy, not to mention the ethics. Where the patient is not distressed, but is anxious to resolve his problems, this may also tax the expertise of the nurse. Intelligent and articulate patients can be as demanding as those who are less gifted. In either case the nurse may need considerable skill to cope with difficulties or high expectations. One way to resolve this problem is to allow junior staff to develop their interviewing skills gradually, beginning with the highly structured 'quiz' which usually greets the patient on admission, working gradually towards a more semi-structured format. A third problem is that the nurse may have a 'negative' effect upon the patient. Some patients become anxious during interviews, especially when they are uncertain about the aims of the interview, or find it difficult to supply the answers. They may also be anxious about how their replies may be interpreted. It is clear that similar anxieties may be present when a patient is asked to fill in a form. However, interview anxiety seems to stem from being looked at, when the patient may feel that he is being 'scrutinised'. Although I suggested ways of offsetting this anxiety in Chapter 2, it is clear that the interpersonal nature of the interview may cause problems for some patients.

2 Logs, Diaries and Records

A more formal way of collecting information from the patient involves asking him to record details of his behaviour, feelings or thoughts *as they occur*, during the course of everyday activity. A log or a diary will provide details of the patient's actions and experience more or less as they occur. The diary may be completed once a day, such as the evening. Or the patient may fill it in at 'rest points' in the day: lunchtime, at the end of the afternoon, before retiring to bed. In Figure 4.2 I have illustrated a typical diary sheet kept by a hospitalised patient beside a similar format kept by a

Figure 4.2

Daily Diary   NAME...Terry Molloy..................... Wk. Beg. 2/Feb.

MAKE A NOTE OF WHAT YOU ARE DOING
AND HOW YOU FEEL EACH DAY

	MORNING	AFTERNOON	EVENING
MON	SAW DOCTOR WENT TO O.T. FEEL TENSE.	WENT FOR WALK WITH SALLY. STILL TENSE	READ. CAN'T CONCENTRATE. WENT TO BED @ 8 DEPRESSED.
TUE	WENT TO O.T. (CAN'T CONCENTRATE) CAME BACK TO WARD	LAY DOWN ON BED WOKE @ 4 FEEL DEPRESSED.	
WED	TALKED TO NURSE T. WENT BACK TO O.T.	PLAYED SCRABBLE MADE TEA DEREK	DEREK GONE TO BERWICK. (TENSE) TOOK TABS. @ 8 OO.
THU	WOKE EARLY - ANX. SCRUBBED KITCHEN WASHED CLOTHES HAD A SHOWER SCRUBBED BATHROOM.	HAD SHOWER - ANX. POLISHED BED. FLOOR WASHED CURTAINS EDGY FEELINGS.	HAD SNACK WASHED DISHES POLISHED SINK CHANGED BEDCLOTHES
FRI	WOKE EARLY - EDGY. HAD SHOWER. CLEANED FRIDGE TENSE FEELING ~ 11	FEEL TENSE - TOOK MORE TABLETS WENT TO BED	(BAD DREAMS) WOKE @ 9.00 JITTERY WATCH TV
SAT	TOOK MABEL TO DOCTOR (SCARED ON BUS) SHOPPING	SHOPPING in CAFE "NICE" BUS	HOME @ 6.00 PHONED DEREK. (CRIED ON PHONE)
SUN	8.30 - RANG DEREK (CRIED) HAD TO GET OUT	WALKING WORRYING MET ARCHIE IN PARK (NICE)	HOME AT 7.30 DEREK IN. CAN'T TALK. FEEL AWFUL.

Figure 4.3

ACTION	EMOTION	THOUGHT
(MON - 12 MN) MARY DIDN'T COME HOME TILL LATE	FELT ANGRY + ? JEALOUS	MAYBE SHE'S SEEING SOMEONE
(TUES - EVENING) MARY NOT SPEAKING BECAUSE I SWORE AT HER	ANGRY / NERVOUS	I CAN'T STAND MUCH MORE OF THIS
(TUES - LATE) COULDN'T SLEEP GOT UP MADE TEA.	TENSE / DEPRESSED	I DON'T KNOW WHAT'S HAPPENING TO ME

patient who was being visited at home by the community nurse. In both examples the patients were asked to record what they did during the day, and any significant emotions or thoughts that accompanied these actions. In a sense these diaries are no different from the traditional diary format. This 'self-study' format can be formalised by breaking the diary down into sections, allocating space for action, emotion and thought, for example (see Figure 4.3). This format might make it easier for the patient to know 'what to record'. For example, if a patient described a feeling of anxiety that came and went throughout the day, it might be helpful to monitor this. If the anxiety appeared to prevent him from doing things, the nurse might ask him to record any activity which was

Figure 4.4

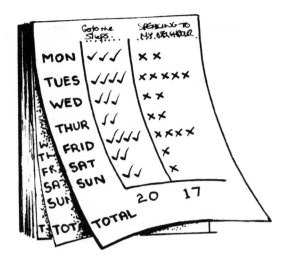

disrupted, when the anxiety began and ended, and how severe he felt it was. Such information not only provides more details about the presenting problem, but can be used to evaluate progress at a later date.

Even simpler log formats can be used to record specific problems. In Figure 4.4 I have illustrated a small notebook that a patient used to record certain 'obsessional' thoughts, and the number of times he avoided doing things. The patient had tried unsuccessfully to use the diary format described above, but the A4 size sheet was too large to carry around with him. This small notebook, measuring 70 × 100 mm, was substituted. The patient carried it in his shirt pocket, using it to record each time he 'had the thought' or 'avoided an activity' by simply entering a tick in the appropriate column. Although this recording method did not provide details of where, when or how these incidents occurred, it allowed the patient to participate in his own assessment. This was significant, given his earlier failure with the diary format. Since the problems tended to occur in a variety of places, at all times of the day, this method — which emphasised the size of the problem — may be the most appropriate.

Figure 4.5

DAY	Where was I ?	What was I doing ? What was happening?	How did I feel ?	What was I thinking ?
Monday	At work	Girls in canteen made fun of me.	Quaking Awful	Wish I could run away
	In the bus queue.	Asked a woman for change.	Embarrassed. (Giggly)	She thinks I'm stupid.
	On bus	Just sitting	tense frightened I would do something silly!	Everyone is looking at me.

Advantages. The main advantage of these diary formats is their simplicity. They can also be seen as 'cost-effective' since they can reveal a wealth of information for minimal staff time. This information can be 'qualitative', as the diary examples show, or 'quantitative', as in the case of the simple record book. Where the patient is already a diary keeper, these notes may be seen as a simple extension of routine 'self-study'. Where the patient is less confident about committing his experiences to paper, it may be necessary to tailor the format to suit him. An example is given in Figure 4.5. In some cases the patient may make suggestions of his own as to how he might study his life experience. A young patient who had been studying for an engineering degree used his home computer to design an elaborate daily diary, which included schedules for completing various activities, ratings of performance and satisfactions, as well as a section for 'failures'. This format was interesting since it was a more 'positive' record: it laid out what he *wanted* to do — as a result there was less emphasis given to the things he failed to do.

Disadvantages. Although these diary formats require little investment of nursing time to complete, they can be costly in terms of analysis. This is the case where the patient commits a lot of information to paper, some of which may be of little relevance. If the nurse asks the patient to study only one area of his life experience, this advice may influence the patient's observations. This is commonly called 'observer effect'. For example, if the patient is advised to make a note in his record each time he feels anxious, he may record more instances of anxiety than he was previously aware of. The simple act of 'looking for' anxiety increases the patient's awareness of his feelings, thereby increasing the severity of the problem. Alternatively, if the patient is asked to record the number of times he avoided a situation or lost his temper, he may record less of these than we might expect. Since he is aware that these actions are 'undesirable', this awareness reduces his performance of such behaviour. On a more positive note it should be apparent that, if used correctly, these self-study methods may reduce problems *before* treatment even begins. A further disadvantage with these methods is that, because they are so simple, even commonplace, the patient may forget to complete them. If this is the only information that is being collected then the assessment of the patient can be delayed considerably. In this context it

Figure 4.6

```
Please answer YES or NO to the following questions.

If any of the situations have never happened to you try to suggest how
you would react in such circumstances.
```

Yes/No

YES   1. If you found out that a friend had be**trayed a confidence** would
you challenge him/her about this?

No   2. If someone took your place in a queue would you point this
out to him/her?

NO   3. Do you enjoy meeting new people?

YES   4. Are you able to compliment people on their work or appearance?

No   5. If a neighbour borrowed something and forgot to hand it back
would you remind him/her about this?

No   6. Are you able to introduce new material to a conversation?

YES   7. Do you prefer being on your own, to being in company?

No   8. If you were lost in a strange town would you ask a passer-by
for directions?

may be helpful to design diary systems to suit individual patients. If
the format is seen as 'their special diary', like my engineering
student, this may encourage them to be more fastidious.

3 Questionnaires and Rating Scales

This class also involves written formats. However, these differ
from the simple methods described above in the way they have
developed. Questionnaires and rating scales are designed to gain
specific measures of a *problem area*. (As we shall see later, this
general rule can be broken.) These methods are usually developed

Figure 4.7

Name .... Date........

	Correct	Incorrect
A What is your name?		
How old are you?		
What is the name of this place?		
How long have you been here?		
What is the name of the town near here?		
B What day is it today?		
What month is this?		
What year is this?		
What time is it just now?		
C What is your next meal?		
When will you be having it?		
What was your last meal?		
When did you have that?		
Where do you have your meals?		
D What time did you go to bed last night?		
What time do you get up in the morning?		
Where do you sleep?		
Where is the toilet/bathroom?		
E Do you know who that is? (point to nurse)		
What does she do?		
Do you know who that is? (point to patient)		
How long has he been here?		
Score		

from research projects. Various 'drafts' of the measuring devices are tried out on a sample population, revisions or modification being made depending on its success. When the research is complete, the questionnaire or rating scale should provide a reliable measure of a specific problem for the minimum of effort. A vast assortment of such methods has been developed to assess 'depression, dependency, disorientation, or social competence'. I put these 'problems' in inverted commas since each one is an idea rather than a reality. Each problem may be composed of a number of behavioural, emotional or cognitive 'problems'. The questionnaire or rating scale gives only a global, or general, estimate of its severity.

Questionnaires. If the nurse wants to collect information on one aspect of the patient's functioning, a questionnaire might help her do this for little effort. In Figure 4.6 I have illustrated a 'socialisation' questionnaire. The patient is required only to answer 'Yes' or 'No' to the questions. This will provide a 'total score' for socialisation, a score which can be compared with those of other patients, or 'normal' subjects. The questionnaire can be completed by the patient alone, or as the basis for a structured interview. In Figure 4.7 I have illustrated a questionnaire which is used by the nurse to assess the patient's orientation to reality.[2] The nurse asks the patient to answer each of the questions, indicating whether his replies are 'true' or 'false'.

Rating Scales. The rating scale also tends to specify a problem area. However, instead of answering 'Yes' or 'No' the patient is asked to rate the *severity* of a problem; or to rate his *performance*; or to indicate the extent to which he *agrees or disagrees* with certain statements. In Figure 4.8 I have illustrated a rating scale which uses a set scale to assess how the patient would perform under certain conditions. This scale asks a range of questions about social functioning: the patient is required to indicate whether they would 'always do it' or 'never do it', using the scale provided. In Figure 4.9 I show a scale which tries to measure certain beliefs about the patient's illness. Again a scale is provided, against which the patient is asked to note her agreement or disagreement with the various statements. Although there can be some variation from the standard procedure described, all scales result in a numerical score. This will reflect the level of 'anxiety, depression' or 'the presence or absence' of a skill.

Figure 4.8

Listed below are a range of everyday situations. Please indicate how you would react to these situations, using the following scale.

1 = Never
2 = rarely
3 = sometimes
4 = often
5 = always

If any situation has never happened to you, indicate how you think you would deal with it.

Rating

__2__ 1. If you found out that a friend had betrayed a confidence would you challenge him/her about this?

__1__ 2. If someone took your place in a queue would you point this out to him/her?

__3__ 3. Do you enjoy meeting new people?

__3__ 4. Are you able to compliment people on their work or appearance?

Advantages. The major advantage in using one or other of these *standardised* formats is that a fairly exact picture of a problem area will be reached for the minimum investment of time. We could spend 20 minutes interviewing a patient about 'what it feels like to be depressed'. Perhaps even more information can be obtained through use of a rating scale, and requires only a few minutes' explanation, and a further few minutes' scoring. Since the same facets of the problem are assessed in each patient, some comparison can be made between one patient and another. Most published questionnaires and rating scales include 'norms', reflecting the range of scores obtained from the study of different populations — e.g. hospitalised patients, 'normal subjects', etc. It is possible, therefore, to compare the score one patient gains on the measure

Figure 4.9

	I agree strongly	I agree a lot	I tend to agree	I tend to disagree	I disagree a lot	I disagree strongly
When I become ill it is because I have not taken enough care of myself.				X		
People who never become mentally ill like me are just plain lucky.	X					
I am the only one who can be responsible for my mental health.				X		
If I want to get better I can only do what the doctor and nurses tell me.	X					
With mental illness you just never your going to be affect						

with the available norms. It is possible, then, to say that 'this patient is very dependent, depressed or anxious'. This judgement is not your opinion; it is made in the light of available knowledge regarding how other people function. A third advantage is that these standardised methods often break a 'problem' into various facets. A scale measuring 'depression' might cover aspects of the patient's motivation, mood, interest in sex, appetite, etc. An anxiety scale might measure the patient's experience of a range of anxiety-related factors: feeling tense, panic attacks, sweating, urge to pass urine, etc. These analyses of various classic problems are not simply whimsical exercises, as the various items on the scale or questionnaire have been arrived at through careful study and experimentation. As I noted in the opening chapter, these methods are the psychological equivalent of the measuring tape, the thermometer and the sphygmomanometer.

Disadvantages. The main disadvantage is that both of these methods are rigid, not allowing the flexibility found in direct interviewing. The patient may gain the impression, once again, that he is being 'processed'. We are interested only in certain facets of his problem, and we spare no time in establishing these facets. A further disadvantage is that many people find it difficult to express themselves using a structured format. They may want to enter 'sometimes' or 'just in the morning'. The scale, however, may make no concession to these varieties of experience. Finally, it is apparent that some patients are unhappy with the written format. The demands of the exercise may throw them completely, adding to their distress. For this reason it may be necessary to select patients carefully, where questionnaires or rating scales are involved.

4 Direct Observation

This last category involves the most rigorous and methodical of the methods described here. Direct observation can be carried out by the patient himself, where it may be called 'self-monitoring', by members of the staff team, or, less frequently, by members of the patient's family. Although the principles behind the two approaches are the same, I shall discuss them separately to aid clarity.

Self-monitoring. This approach is an extension of the diary/log format. However, here the self-assessment is made more formal.

The patient is helped to identify specific 'targets', which are defined clearly and unambiguously, so that some kind of measure can be taken across time. The patient can self-monitor any aspect of his experience, but in practice specific motor behaviours, discrete thoughts and clearly defined feelings may be appropriate targets. Following the intitial assessment the nurse discusses the patient's problems with him, selecting the targets for self-monitoring. A decision must be made regarding the kind of measure to be taken. This usually involves an estimate of *frequency* or *time*. In the frequency count the patient records each occurrence of the target. I noted earlier how a patient recorded each time he experienced an 'obsessional thought' and each time he avoided doing something. These recordings can be tallied up each day to give a daily score for each target. The patient might be asked to record each time he had a panic attack, drank alcohol, felt angry, spoke to a stranger or finished a task. The only requirement for this technique is that each incident should be similar in size or severity to the others. Before beginning the exercise it may be appropriate to ensure that the patient can distinguish 'anger' from 'jealousy' or even 'annoyance'. The easiest way to ensure this is to define what the person *might* do or say when he is angry, jealous, annoyed, etc. It might be appropriate to distinguish (e.g.) between *feeling* angry and 'losing his temper'. In some examples the definition can be quite specific: 'drinking alcohol' can be defined in terms of units of alcohol consumed, rather than glasses of beer or gin and tonic. 'Speaking to a stranger' might be defined in terms of the sort of interactions which could be included, which might be many and varied, and might need to be listed to exclude any inappropriate behaviours, such as 'saying "Hello" to a neighbour'. In other cases this list might be necessary to ensure that all necessary behaviours were recorded: 'This is only a half-pint of cider, it doesn't count.' The best targets for a frequency count are those actions which have a clear beginning and end. The patient might be asked to record every time he:

> drinks one unit of alcohol
> introduces himself to a stranger
> swears at his wife
> slaps his son on the arms or legs
> smokes a cigarette
> thinks to himself 'I'm a failure'

eats a sweet biscuit
refuses to do someone a favour
thinks he heard the voice of his dead mother

All these 'actions' have fairly clear-cut beginnings and endings. Some are perhaps more independent than others. However, it will be possible for the patient to distinguish each occurrence of these actions, thereby ending up with a frequency count of at least one facet of his 'drinking', 'bad temper', 'greed' or 'unassertiveness'.

In the case of other behaviour patterns it may be more helpful to measure how long the patient spends engaged in the action. This is indicated where on some occasions the action may be short-lived (shouting for a few seconds), but on others it may last much longer (e.g. a violent argument lasting 20 minutes). Instead of counting the number of times the patient loses his temper, washes his hands, checks the doors and windows, or has a conversation with a work-mate, he is asked to note roughly how long he spent engaged in the activity. These are usually called *duration* measures.

In a few cases a slightly different kind of time measure may be appropriate. Where the patient is particularly slow at doing something, such as 'summoning up the courage to say "Hello" to someone', or making decisions, it may be appropriate to measure *how long he takes* to complete these actions, from the time he started the action. This is often called a *latency* measure. In any situation where the patient appears to take a long time to do something, this kind of measure is appropriate. He might be asked to record how long he takes to:

get up in the morning
get dressed
answer a question
select a particular brand of peaches
sit down to dinner
answer the telephone

These examples were all problems for one patient. He described the problems variously as 'I can't be bothered getting up,' 'I don't know what to wear,' 'I can't think of anything to say,' 'I can't make up my mind,' 'I'm too busy, I'll be with you in a minute,' and 'I'm frightened who might be on the line.' Although these problems could be described variously as apathy, indecisiveness, insecurity, obsessional routines and anxiety, they all boil down to the same common denominator: the patient takes a long time to do any of these actions.

Self-monitoring is rarely an easy exercise. The patient is required to 'keep an eye' on himself virtually all day long. If he has too many things to monitor, the activity may simply overwhelm him. If the exercise requires him to make detailed notes of his behaviour, it may interfere with his work or his social life, and he may abandon it. In both cases selection of appropriate assessment targets, and a simple observational method, are of crucial importance. The patient may be given a tally counter to carry in his pocket. He can clock up every 'worrying thought' or each time he 'thought people were laughing at me', without anyone noticing. Other ideas for frequency measures might be placing ticks on the inside back page of a diary; at the top of a newspaper; on the back of his hand with a felt-tipped pen; or on the corner of a desk blotter. These 'ticks' can be tallied up at the end of the day or week, whichever is appropriate. I once worked with a patient who carried a plastic container of tiny cachous. Each time he felt 'gripped by panic' he would suck one of the cachous. He counted the number of sweets in the box each morning and night, and with a little subtraction was able to record his frequency of panic attacks. Time measures are more complex on a practical level. However, with the advent of the micro-chip almost everyone is now sporting a stop watch within their wristwatch. Providing that he remembers to set and stop it, highly accurate timings are possible. These can then be transferred to the top of the newspaper, back of the hand, etc. Such self-monitoring is unlikely to be noticed since most people fiddle continuously with 'chronographs' anyway. However, just because a simple measurement system is selected, this offers no guarantee that the patient will continue with the self-monitoring. Unless he already is an avid 'self-watcher', such as a diarist, he is likely to tire of the chore. Consequently it is necessary to provide regular boosts of encouragement or offers of alternative ways of collecting the information. Otherwise the exercise may simply become another problem, on top of many.

Staff Monitoring. The three simple methods described above can also be used by staff where self-monitoring is impossible or inappropriate. Take for example the case of Jeffrey, a patient in a long-stay ward.

It is 9.00 am. Jeffrey leaves the breakfast table and walks across to the toilet area. Here he remains for the next few hours, pacing back and forth on the tiled floor. Every so often he stops and rushes over to the window which he opens and closes repeatedly for several minutes. His pacing is accompanied by rhythmic waving of his arms, which he raises aloft. He talks aloud to himself, occasionally making a strange 'barking' sound over and over again. At less frequent intervals he stops, puts his hands over his ears, and sways backwards and forwards on the same spot.

What can we make of this behaviour? Is this some kind of psychotic manifestation? Is he engaged in some strange obsessional ritual? As I noted in Chapter 1, our task in assessment is, first of all, to collect some information about what is happening. Only when we are in possession of such detailed information should we begin playing the 'inference game' — drawing conclusions about what the information means. Earlier in this chapter I suggested that we might help the patient to study how problems come and go during the day, by noting when they began and ended and what was happening at those times. This simple analysis would be our first 'port of call' in the assessment of Jeffrey. We would be interested to know what he does, and the things that are happening around him, as he performs these various actions. In Figure 4.10 I have illustrated how a nurse spent 10 minutes observing Jeffrey in the toilet area: these observations were repeated at random intervals over a period of a week. The aim of the observations was to find out whether his behaviour varied from one day to the next; to draw up a list of behaviours that might be studied in detail later; and to try to establish whether any events preceded or followed any particular pattern of behaviour. As the figure shows, the nurse recorded what Jeffrey was doing in the B category — his behaviour. She also noted what was happening around him in the A category — the antecedents of his behaviour. Finally, when he stopped doing something she noted any events which followed — possible consequences of his behaviour. This A B C analysis tries to make sense of Jeffrey's behaviour by trying to detect any 'cues' within the environment which might play a part in signalling the beginning of a behaviour, and any events which might lead to the termination, or maintenance, of the action — possible 'reinforcers'.

Figure 4.10

A	B	C
3.20 JEFF. ALONE IN	PACING — SLAPPING FACE. OCCAS. SHOUTING	JOHN T. TOOK HIM AWAY FOR TEA.
4.15 SEVERAL PATIENTS WASHING AT SINKS	J. SWAYING IN MID. FLOOR — HANDS OVER EARS	GERRY G. SWORE AT HIM. TELLING HIM TO BEHAVE HIMSELF
5.00 J. ALONE	PACING — WAVING ARMS IN AIR.	
5.30 GERRY G. SHOWING	J. OPENING/CLOSING WINDOW	G.G. PUSHED J AWAY FROM WINDOW

So what do these notes tell us about Jeffrey's behaviour? We might assume that he goes to the toilet area for 'a bit of peace and quiet'. Certainly, every time someone comes in he either begins swaying and covering his ears or heads for the window. However, I do not wish to discuss possible inferences or interpretations here. I wish only to note that through such structured observations a picture of Jeffrey's behaviour can be built up. This might prove helpful in trying to establish 'why' he does this or that. However, even where such an explanation proves elusive, these few observations will help us decide which aspects of his behaviour we might study more closely, perhaps through some frequency or duration measures.

The simple frequency, duration and latency measures could be used to quantify Jeffrey's behaviour. However, this would require a nurse to 'shadow' him constantly, clocking up each time he

Figure 4.11

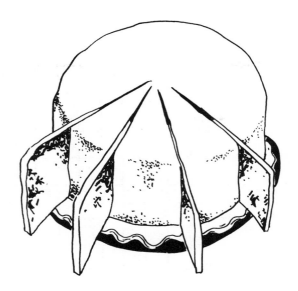

opened the window, or how long he spent pacing the floor. In most situations such a detailed picture, although desirable, is an impossibility. One alternative is to take 'samples' of the patient's behaviour. This is analogous to taking very thin slices out of a fruit cake, at regular intervals. These slices give us an indication of what the whole cake is like, although only a tiny proportion of the whole cake is sampled. Such a sample is reasonably accurate (see Figure 4.11). However, it would be acknowledged that, depending upon where the slice was taken, a juicy currant or glacé cherry might be missed. The same is true of the *time sample*. This involves taking very quick observations of the patient at regular intervals. The nurse acts like a camera, taking a mental snapshop of what the patient is doing at the very instant that she looked at him. These observations give us a flavour of the patient's overall behaviour. If, however, the observations are too widely spaced, important pieces of behaviour — like the cake's glacé cherries — may be missed.

In the checklist in Figure 4.12 I have shown how the time sample method might help us to collect some detailed information on how Jeffrey behaves each morning in the toilet area. The checklist is so arranged that a picture of the main classes of behaviour, noted

Figure 4.12

Date: 25/8/85

Time: From – 10·00   to – 11·40

	1	2	3	4	5	6	7	8	9	10	%
Standing at window			X								10
Pacing the floor	X	X							X	X	40
Lying down				X							10
Sitting on radiator					X	X	X	X			50
Waving arms		X					X		X	X	40
Opening/closing window			X								10
Slapping face	X			X							20
Combing hair					X			X			20
Speaking to self		X	X				X			X	40
Speaking to others					X	X					20
Making barking noise	X			X					X		30

in the narrative notes made earlier, can be measured. In each of these classes of behaviour the individual actions exclude one another. Jeffrey cannot be standing at the window at the same time as he is pacing the floor. He cannot be shaving himself when he is waving his arms in this rhythmic fashion. The behaviours are, therefore, said to be mutually exclusive. In these observations the nurse would visit the toilet area at regular intervals: let us assume every 10 minutes. She looks at Jeffrey and immediately notes which *general* motor behaviour he is showing; which specific motor behaviour he is showing; and whether or not he is showing any verbal behaviour. She ticks the appropriate boxes, leaves the area, returning at the next time period — in 10 minutes — to repeat the procedure. If we were to study Jeffrey in this way a picture of his behaviour, in a specific setting, could be obtained for little effort. If we observed him every 10 minutes between 8.30 (leaving breakfast) and 11.50 (preparing for lunch), 20 observations could be taken. By use of simple arithmetic we could calculate the *proportion of the observation time* Jeffrey spent in each of the behaviours listed. As the illustration shows, we can work out that some behaviours occur more often than others. This information may be important when we come to evaluate the effect of different kinds of treatment or management. Although these measures do not represent real time or frequency, providing that the observations are done in the same way, each day, comparisons can be made between one day and the next, and one week and the next. Since each observation takes literally only a few seconds, the picture of the patient is gained for very little effort.

So what are the disadvantages with this method? Like the slices of the fruit cake, it measures only the behaviour shown where the sample is taken. Important behaviours may occur between the samples. Ideally, time sampling should only be used to study behaviour which lasts for at least a few minutes at a time. If the interval between samples is geared to the shortest behaviour under review it may be possible to 'catch' all behaviours. Another disadvantage involves the need for designing new formats to suit each patient. The time sample method used for a range of patients will be the same. However, the list of behaviours to be studied and the time between samples must be worked out for each individual. This often deters a lot of nurses, who would like a standard format for all patients. Since each patient is likely to show different patterns of behaviour, at different intervals, this is not possible. It is clear, however, that with a little effort a simple observational format can be worked out which will collect a lot of information for little cost in terms of nursing time.

The frequency and duration measures mentioned earlier are best used for single behaviours: counting the number of times a patient loses his temper, refuses to go to work, answers a question in an interview; or timing the length of conversations, hours spent working, or how long he can stand beside some feared object. In certain cases it may also be interesting to time how long a patient takes to answer a question, get dressed, remember his name, etc. These measures appear so simple that nurses are often blasé about their use. Although they require little effort in their application, some planning and preparation are necessary to ensure that each nurse observes the patient in the same way, and records the information reliably. Many nursing reports describe the patient as 'very disturbed this morning, hallucinated and agressive'. These observations may be accurate, but because they do not quantify his behaviour in any way they serve little purpose in evaluating change in the patient. Indeed they are *not* observations. They are interpretations of something the nurse observed, but has not written down. By using frequency, duration and latency measures the nursing team may be able to discuss exactly what the patient did this morning. The report might then read: 'the patient was observed to shout and scream three times this morning. He also paced back and forth, gesticulating and muttering to himself for half an hour before sitting down.' Alternatively, the report might simply record: 'shouting/screaming' — 3; 'psychotic behaviour' — 30 minutes. This would be appropriate providing that all the staff agreed what 'shouting and screaming' and 'psychotic behaviour' comprised.

Valid and Reliable?

I have described a few methods which illustrate the major differences between the main classes of assessment. I began with the most open-ended kind of observation, the interview, and ended with some fairly tight measures of discrete behaviours. Before looking at the use of these methods I have two questions that are worth considering. They may prevent you from wasting time using a method which is not suited to the problem in hand or which does not give you reliable results.

Will the Method I have Selected Measure or Assess what I Want to Measure?

It is always good policy to play your own devil's advocate. By being sceptical about what you are doing, you may see weaknesses that you might otherwise miss. Try looking at what you are about to do through the eyes of someone who is less committed to the idea than you are. Let us assume that you have decided to interview the patient, to find out how he feels. You have selected this approach because the patient is fairly talkative, is intelligent, appears 'insightful', and appears to like being questioned about his problems. But will this approach tell you what you want to know? How the patient feels when he is under pressure at work or alone at night? The patient may be able to recall how he felt at these times. But is his memory of the event the same as his experience? In the same vein, it is clear that what people *say* they have done, or are about to do, may not match their behaviour in real life. Helpful though the interview may be, it may only assess 'interview behaviour'. Let's take another example. Let us assume that we want to assess a patient's social skills. We decide to observe his interactions with other patients in the day area of the ward. We rate the content of his speech, his non-verbal skills, and we count the number of times he initiates conversation. This is a complex piece of observation. But are we measuring his social skills? Or are we simply noting how he functions under very special circumstances? Will this information tell us anything about how he interacts with family, friends, neighbours, workmates, authority figures, etc. Scepticism on this level is useful. It helps us judge the true merits of the assessment method. Both approaches illustrated have points in their favour. But both could benefit from some extension, either the addition of another technique, or broadening the format to cover more situations.

The question raised concerns *validity*. How valid is the information we are collecting? What does it really tell us about his feelings, social skills, etc.? One of the big problems in psychiatric assessment is the use of what the American, Robert Mager, called 'fuzzies'.[3] These are the vague concepts which professionals and laypeople alike bandy about with gay abandon. They are called 'fuzzies' because they are ill-defined, unquantified and unobservable. Mager popularised the use of the 'Hey Dad' test. Children tend to ask their parents to explain things to them, from their background of experience and greater knowledge. In the 'Hey Dad' test Mager illustrated how a 'fuzzy' could be distinguished from a 'performance', the performance being a description of something which is discrete, observable and quantifiable. Below I have listed a number of 'fuzzies' which are in common use in psychiatric nursing. Beside each 'fuzzy' I have tried to restate the concept in performance terms. The novice nurse might, looking up respectfully to her patriarchal male tutor, say, 'Hey Dad, show me how I can . . .'

Fuzzies	*Performances*
assess this patient's personality	observe what he says and does under a range of set circumstances

study staff morale	observe attendance at work and requests for transfers
establish meaningful relationships	listen to the patient without interrupting or looking bored
help this patient get better	set goals for him which can be monitored and evaluated
help him understand his illness	identify his thoughts, emotions and behaviour, and how they relate to various factors in his environment
help promote my own personal growth	graph the number of times I use a performance description instead of a fuzzy and see if the trend is upward.

We use fuzzies all the time, mainly because they are convenient shorthand. If we are pressed, most of us could tighten up a vague concept. We could translate it into performance terms. Sometimes, however, we do not take the time to do this and *invalid* observations or assessments can result. At a case review the nurse-in-charge discusses a patient with her staff.

Beryl has become more dependent over the last few weeks. (murmurs of agreement) She is also acting out quite a bit. On other occasions she doesn't say anything but she is very hostile. (nods of agreement) I think that we should do a careful assessment of her, and report back to Doctor Black on Monday. Any questions? Good. Pamela, Jackie and Eric. Could you three take responsibility for this? OK.

Similar conversations can be overheard in the medical, occupational therapy and psychology meetings. In each of them, although there is agreement that a problem exists, one is uncertain as to exactly *what* it is; or if everyone is murmuring or nodding their agreement in response to the same mental picture. Unless this meeting ends with a clear statement of the goals of the assessment — in clear performance terms — the reports of the three nurses on Monday could differ enormously. They may all have ended up looking at completely different patterns of behaviour. It does not matter *how* you intend to conduct the assessment — by interview, rating scale, questionnaire, direct observation or all four. The first step must be to define, unambiguously, what the target for the assessment is.

Will the Method Give me the Same Information Each Time I Use it?

This question is about reliability. By reliable I mean *consistent*. When you use a measuring or assessment technique does it give the same results each time you use it? If it does, then it is reliable. It is like a good friend: it can be trusted. If it doesn't, it is unreliable. Let us take a simple idea to explore this example. A clock is a measuring device. It measures time. To be a valid timepiece it must always show the correct time — day or night. Therefore, in order to be valid, it must always be reliable. If it sometimes goes slow and sometimes goes fast, it is unreliable. You can't trust it to tell the right time. Therefore it is not a valid timepiece, because it is unreliable. However, it is possible for a measuring device to be reliable — and yet still be invalid. The clock which *always* runs three minutes slow is reliable. You can trust it to be three minutes out — every time you look at it. However it is not a valid timepiece, because it does not measure the correct time.

Let us consider some examples of patient assessment. If we give a patient a questionnaire to fill in, we can judge its reliability by giving it to him again, the next day, and checking whether the answers are the same. If the patient repeatedly gives the same answers we can assume that the questionnaire is reliable. This is *not* the same as saying that it is valid. The patient may be trying to please or annoy us by his answers, which may not represent 'the truth'. To return to the case of Beryl, the nurses might decide to use the time sampling technique described in the case of Jeffrey. They might record specific behaviours that they associate with dependence, hostility and agression. Because they are short-staffed they decide to take these time samples every two hours. Initially, two nurses conduct the observations together, each independently observing and noting the patient's behaviour. The records are compared and analysed and it is found that each nurse has recorded much the same behaviour. There is a high degree of reliability between observers. Does this mean that the observations reflect a *valid* picture of Beryl's behaviour? Possibly not. Because of the wide gaps between observations, which are few in number anyway, the information is too selective to make any firm conclusions about the patient.

The issue of reliability in nursing assessment gained prominence a few years ago when a study found that thermometers in daily use gave a wide range of readings. In effect they did not measure temperature correctly. Some of the thermometers were highly consistent: they always recorded temperatures which were too high, or too low. They were not unreliable. They were simply invalid. It is of little comfort to know that a measuring device is consistent. We also need to know if it is accurate: does it measure what it says it will measure? Many of the standard methods that I shall describe in the second part of the book have been published along with reports of the validity and reliability of the technique. Although careful scrutiny of such research reports is not yet a popular pastime in psychiatric nursing, clearly it should be. Before we decide to use an assessment method we should try to find out whether it will do the job we want in a consistent, reliable manner.

Assessment Goals

Assessment can be a many-headed monster, or it can be a bag of tools which can serve us well in unravelling the mysteries of the patient. Assessment does not involve only one function. We can assess people to find out who they are — as in the life profile. We can also assess them to find out their problems — the problem oriented interview; or their assets — the global assessment. We can also try to assess the scale of these problems or assets; here assessment becomes an evaluative tool, judging whether problems (or assets) appear to be diminishing, increasing or remaining at the same level. Common to all these areas is the hope that through assessment we might grow to understand the *meaning* of the patient's problems. Historically, in many areas of psychiatry there has been an assumption that the patient's behaviour is merely a signal or outpost of some greater distress. I do not wish to debate this issue here. I believe that it is possible to follow this line of thinking only if we assume that the patient's problems are encompassed by an *idea*. This idea may be held by the patient, by us or by society at large. However, it is not a reality of itself. The fact that many people believe in the idea of 'latent hostility' or 'repressed anger' does not make this idea any more *real*, only popular. Many of the problems which we are required to deal with in psychiatry involve ideas: 'manic-depressive psychosis; inadequate personality; agoraphobia; psychopathic disorder'. These ideas exist fundamentally in our thinking and reasoning. In a sense they have a vicarious existence: they exist only through the behaviour of people whom we call 'manic depressives', etc. It is for this reason that I have emphasised the assessment of behaviour. Since the behaviour of the patient is the stimulus for the generation of ideas about 'illness, disorder', etc., the behaviour of the patient, and the real world that it inhabits, should be our primary target in the assessment process.

Stages of Assessment

We have discussed a number of ways of describing the person called 'patient'. Through interviewing we build a picture of how he functions on various levels of experience, and how he and others perceive that functioning. This is the least specific form of assessment, and by implication the most general. An unstructured interview will elicit a vast range of information about the patient, his interactions with others, his past and hopes for the future. Most of this information will be non-specific: it will be a catalogue of 'fuzzies'. A structured interview will begin the process of defining the patient and his situation more clearly. Our interest in the patient's stream-of-consciousness begins to wane as we start to narrow our focus — looking for more specific kinds of replies. We are beginning to structure the situation so that his replies become more pointed, more specific and perhaps even more considered. Naturally, the patient's 'freedom' to talk begins to be curtailed.

By the end of the structured interview we should have identified the areas of the patient, and his life, which interest us. We may now wish to describe these significant aspects in more quantifiable terms, perhaps beginning by asking the patient to summarise aspects of his life, his behaviour or his beliefs (his thoughts) through rating scales or questionnaires. These may produce a quantifiable measure of a certain idea, e.g. anxiety, social interaction, independence, depression, etc. These will reflect either how the patient sees himself, or how he is perceived by others. These are only indirect measures. They are based upon the patient's perception of himself. At a stage slightly beyond this lies the perception of the patient held by others, e.g. staff, family or friends.

At the next stage in the assessment we can tighten the focus further by assessing the discrete patterns of behaviour that have been highlighted by the indirect methods. By studying what he does, where, when and with whom, we can begin to quantify in greater detail the 'personality' before us. Staff or members of the patient's family might record how often, or for how long, he engages in certain patterns of behaviour, under different circumstances. This would bring us closer to the target: the patient's experience of these events. This is finally achieved when the patient learns how to study himself closely under a range of conditions. Using logs, diaries, self-ratings and any one of a number of simple self-monitoring techniques, he can begin to describe himself in terms of his functioning in different settings. Crude though these methods may be, they represent a form of 'personal science' where the patient studies himself in much the same way as a naturalist might study him. Of course he has an advantage over the naturalist, as he can assess his thoughts and feelings as well as his behaviour.

Conclusion

In this chapter I have given an indication of the kinds of methods which may be used to look at different aspects of the patient's life. Through these methods the process of assessment can range from the broadest description of many aspects of the patient's functioning, obtained through interviewing, to a close-up study of one specific problem by the patient himself. In selecting these methods an effort is made to pick the approach that will do most justice to the problem in hand. Examples of the use of these methods with a range of problem areas will be given in the later part of the book.

When nurses talk about *assessment* I often get the impression that they assume that it is just one thing: a singular noun. Ideally, assessment should be seen as a plural noun meaning 'a range of methods used to describe and measure the problems and assets of the patient'. Many nurses appear to be involved in some kind of search for their Holy Grail: *the* single method, preferably encompassed by no more than two pages of paper, which will tell them everything they want to know about the patient. I exaggerate, of course. Yet, like most exaggerations, there is an element of truth. Largely because of the lack of any serious assessment tradition in nursing, nurses tend to be unhappy about completing one assessment method, never mind two or even three. Yet that is what assessment should mean: a range of methods, each with a different purpose and each producing a slightly different picture of the patient. I doubt whether nurses will ever find the Holy Grail of assessment. For the patient's sake I hope that they don't. His best interests will be served by exposure to a variety of assessment methods, presented by a variety of people, from the interview taken by the student nurse as the patient has a bath, to the psychologist's highly orchestrated cognitive function test. These are obviously quite different, one from the other. Yet each has something very important to offer in the description of the patient. When we talk about assessment, we should try to think of a battery of methods, each highlighting different facets of the person. The assessment battery should become our Holy Grail.

Notes

1. J. Bronowski and B. Mazlish, *The Western Intellectual Tradition* (Penguin Books, Harmondsworth, 1963), p. 134.

2. This reality orientation questionnaire was developed by my former colleague, Jim McGlynn, as part of an unpublished research project involving psychogeriatric patients (1977).

3. R. F. Mager, *Goal Analysis* (Fearon, Belmont, Calif., 1972).

5 EVERYDAY LIVING SKILLS

> Happy the man to whom heaven has given a morsel of
> bread without laying him under the obligation of thanking
> any other for it than heaven itself. — Cervantes

One area which nurses have traditionally seen as their preserve has been helping patients with the activities of daily living. First suggested by the American Virginia Henderson in the early 1960s,[1] the nurse's role in the promotion of these activities has become a byword for nursing care across a range of nursing situations with various patient populations. Commonly, this relates to the assessment of the patient's physiological and psychosocial functioning: gauging the extent to which he is independent in areas such as mobility, nutrition, safety, personal hygiene.[2] But what does the concept 'activities of daily living' mean within psychiatric nursing? And what do we mean by the terms 'dependence' and 'independence'?

The State of Independence

Most of us take our independence for granted. Perhaps we equate independence with the state of being adult: a complete, personally effective, all-round worth-while individual. In adopting such a philosophy we are following in the tradition of people like Jeremy Bentham who believed that 'the word independence is united to the ideas of dignity and virtue; the word dependence, to the ideas of inferiority and corruption'. Although he was not talking about independence in the way we are here, as we shall see later, some of his comments have considerable relevance. Popularly, the term 'independence' is often reserved for political purposes. We talk about nations being independent, making their own laws, being self-governing. In this context another English philosopher, James Martineau, argued that 'the moral progression of a people can scarcely begin until they are independent'. The same principle seems to hold true for individuals. Can we really begin to understand ourselves, be ourselves, until we are in a position to exercise control over the everyday routine of our lives?

However, the search for — or belief in — *absolute* independence is often illusory. Can any of us say that we are truly independent?

126

Dependent on no one, at no time, for anything? The reality for most of us is that independence is a very relative state. We are more or less independent than we were. Or, we are more or less independent than others. We are never absolutely independent. Acknowledging this, the English writer William Cobbett wrote, 'It is not the greatness of a man's means that makes him independent, so much as the smallness of his wants'. Indeed, we assess our independence in terms of how much we rely upon others. This situation is highlighted when we fall sick, and someone has to pay our bills, do our shopping, fix our meals. Then, we often feel hopelessly dependent. However, the balance of dependence and independence operates within us like yin and yang, our strengths and weaknesses, our happy side and our sad side. As Wordsworth noted, 'these two things, contradictory as they may seem, must go together, manly dependence and manly independence, manly reliance and manly self-reliance'. Were he here today he might feel obliged to embrace women more specifically within this philosophy.

The Skills of Everyday Living

In this chapter I am taking the view that all of us need a certain level of proficiency in certain skills of everyday living in order to be independent. I favour the use of the word 'skill' — rather than 'activities' — since, as I shall describe later, the patients we are interested in may need help to learn or re-establish these everyday behaviours. It is not simply a case of performing them or not. They need to become more skilled in their execution, so that these skills can strengthen the fabric of their lives. However, it is clear that many people appear heavily dependent on others — such as the physically handicapped. However, such people can achieve high levels of independence in other areas of their lives (such as decision-making) which more than compensate for their physical dependence. In a sense I am saying that we should assess a person's independence in terms of what is possible for that person, in terms of his own potential. This seems a more practical proposition than trying to locate people on some absolute scale.

Speaking of 'absolute scales', I have illustrated in Figure 5.1 the independence-dependence continuum. This is the imaginary path we follow as we grow as individuals. In this chapter I am concentrating upon fairly basic skills. I shall emphasise the need to be able to attend to our physical requirements in order to stay alive, or otherwise in good biological working order. I shall discuss the kind

Figure 5.1

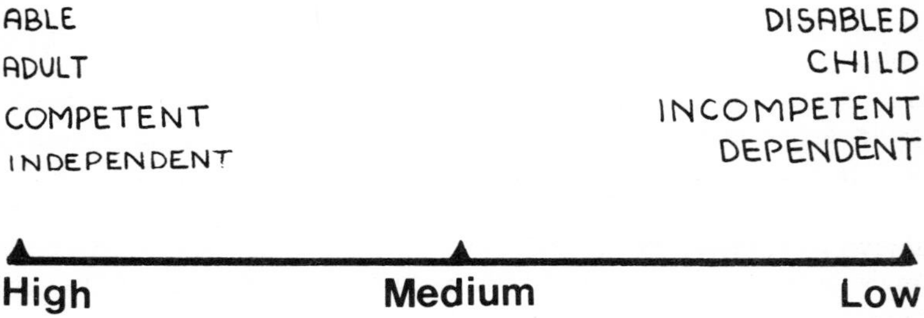

ABLE	DISABLED
ADULT	CHILD
COMPETENT	INCOMPETENT
INDEPENDENT	DEPENDENT

High   **Medium**   **Low**

DEPENDENCY LABELS

of social skills necessary for establishing various kinds of relation-ships with people. These skills help us to adapt to our social environment, the complex world which is often dictated more by the activities of other people than by the forces of nature. All the skills which can be located on this continuum are fairly concrete, observable activities. We should be able to study their presence, or absence, in our patients. I am not saying that these skills represent, in any way, the whole of our life experience: far from it. I am discussing only those aspects of our life which have a bearing upon the concept of independence.

In nursing, the term 'dependency' is used to describe the extent to which we need to care for patients, and the extent to which they can look after themselves. As a result, we often talk about 'high', 'medium' and 'low' dependency patients. Although these rather broad dependency ratings do not refer specifically to the absence of the kind of skills under discussion here, the principle holds true. The more skills a person has — or the more proficient he is in the performance of one or more of these skills — the less dependent he is upon the assistance of others. The importance of such skills cannot be overemphasised. As Bentham remarked, the person who is lacking in such skills may be regarded by others — or even himself — as *inferior*. If he can improve upon these skills he is likely to be afforded more respect and treated with more dignity.

He is likely to experience a boost to his self-esteem as a result.

We are interested in the range of skills required to lead an independent life. But what are these skills? And how many do we need to be reasonably independent? Sadly, I have no short answer to these questions. I can only offer some suggestions. I am taking the view that we can identify certain *crucial* skills which, if they are lacking, will weaken the person's 'independence quotient'. Many of the other skills I shall discuss are very relative: if they are missing or underdeveloped the person may still be able to lead a normal or acceptable life. However, if they are present, the quality of his life may be significantly improved.

The Builder's Craft

Before we go on to discuss the assessment of everyday living skills, it may be helpful to look at the concept from another perspective. I have said that we need to study the patient's independent functioning in order to assess the kind of care he needs. Do we give him more help? Or do we release him from our care? The skills we are considering are wide-ranging. They cover everything from being able to move limbs to being able to 'self-medicate'. Within each of these skills lies a range of performance. There are basic and advanced versions of each skill. For example, some eating skills are fundamental, such as eating with a spoon. Others are more sophisticated, such as using a full range of cutlery in a restaurant. However, they are both the same skill, eating, separated only by the concept of sophistication.

I have tried to illustrate how we acquire, or develop, these skills by drawing an analogy with the building of a house. The builder begins with a very basic structure, an outer structure called 'the house', within which are various sub-structures. These are designed to meet certain needs: a bathroom to wash in; a dining-room to eat in; a staircase to allow access from one part of the house to the other. The *basic* structure of the house comprises the four walls, the rooms within it and the basic amenities: plumbing, lighting, heating. These are analogous to the basic skill areas of communication, self-care, mobility, recreation, orientation, etc. A child growing up in this house will not become sophisticated in any one area at once. Instead, he will develop his skills gradually: learning the rudiments of communication in the living-room; learning to eat in the dining-room; learning how to dress in the bedroom and to play in the playroom. He also learns to climb the stairs, giving him

Figure 5.2

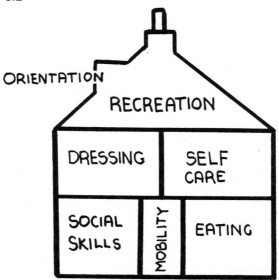

the power of mobility to transfer his activity from one area to another. As he grows, he will develop these basic skills to a more sophisticated level. He will also learn new skills. For instance, he will start to orientate himself more fully to his world within the house — knowing where everything is and what it does; and out-with the house — gaining insights into the working of the outside world through the window (see Figure 5.2).

When we develop as individuals it is usually across several areas at once. This is similar to the craft of the builder. He starts with the basic amenities — the walls, roof and room units. Then he begins to develop within these basic amenities, adding light fittings, fitted wardrobes, blinds, etc. The house does not become a 'home', however, until the family that lives within it gives it their stamp of individuality, influencing the décor, furnishings, pictures, ornaments, etc. The same holds true for our analogous child. As he grows, he develops skills that are very similar to those of other children. By the time he has matured he will present those skills in his own inimitable fashion: walking and talking, lifting and laying, acting and reacting, within the confines of his own personal 'style' — a style that bears the stamp of his own identity.

Key Skills. The building analogy is helpful also when we come to consider 'key skills'. These are skills which play a big part in the survival or promotion of other skills. These are like the foundations of the house, upon which the whole building rests, or the lintel that supports the brickwork above the window. If these foundations or supports are weak, then the rest of the assembly will be prejudiced. So what kinds of skills are key elements in the concept of independence? Communication and comprehension are two key skill areas. If we cannot understand information being relayed to us, or cannot communicate our wishes, then many of the other skills will be significantly weakened. This does not mean that we have to be able to speak fluently: perhaps a sign-language system would be adequate. The ability to move around, from place to place, and the ability to manipulate our environment, with our limbs, are two other key skills. Again, we do not need to be fully ambulant, as a wheelchair, walking stick or some prosthetic support may help us get where or what we want. All the other skills, which are dependent upon certain motor movements, or information-processing, are dependent upon these skill areas. These are our foundations. It is encouraging to note that nurses spend a lot of time promoting these skills. Almost by intuition, they are aware of their key role. It is worth noting that some other skills can play similar key roles. A colleague of mine discovered some years ago that the ability to care for personal hygiene and to dress appropriately were key factors in deciding whether or not discharged psychiatric patients survived in the community. He followed up a sample of patients who had been discharged from a rural hospital and was surprised to find that psychiatric symptoms were viewed as less important determinants of a return to hospital. Everyday skills like bathing and dressing appropriately seemed to make the patient more acceptable in his 'new' community. Other skills, like handling his own money and cooking his own meals, made him relatively independent. There may be an important moral here. If the patient is not sufficiently skilled in the art of personal hygiene, all the social graces in the world may not save him from rejection, and relegation to a status of inferiority.

The Assessment of Skills

Every day each of us is required to undertake a wide range of activities that are necessary either to keep us in the best of health, such as attending to our diet or personal hygiene, or are part of the price we pay for living in an allegedly civilised society, which requires us to dress in a particular way, or to handle our cutlery according to some convention. Everyday living skills are a combination of the *routines* necessary to keep body and soul together, and the *rituals* of civilised society. Admittedly, not all of us peform all of them, all of the time. Often we take a holiday from them, especially from those of a ritualistic nature. As we go about these activities few of us even spare them a second thought. Although these are the activities upon which our life is founded, they hardly constitute 'our life' as such. We prefer to believe that that is an altogether more intangible experience.

The Skill-deficient. Not everyone can afford to be so casual about everyday living. A wide range of people meet with considerable difficulties in the accomplishment of such skills. Although such problems are not peculiar to psychiatric patients, this group figures prominently. So who is lacking in such skills? An important group is the elderly. Many people begin to lose control over the performance of even basic skills as they age, finding difficulty in eating, dressing or going to the toilet. These problems may result from the ageing process itself, or they may be accelerated by the over-caring attitudes of hospital staff. Either way we have a person who has started to lose, or has significantly lost, the degree of independence he once possessed. If this loss is from a key skill area, the loss may be even more significant and far-reaching.

The long-stay population is another group which often presents with skill deficiencies. In some cases the patient may never have acquired certain skills. This is true of many who were hospitalised in their youth, before they matured as individuals. Others have lost their skills *en route*. In many cases this deterioration is a function of the restrictive regime of the total institution. Patients who are shaved by staff, day in and day out, eventually lose the 'art of shaving'. Patients who began their 'careers' with interpersonal anxiety related, perhaps, to the process of schizophrenia, may end up years later devoid of any of the skills which contribute to the concept of social competence. There appears to be ample evidence to support the view that these *secondary handicaps* were developed, albeit unwittingly, by the process of institutionalisation.

In addition to these two key groups there are myriad other

populations who experience difficulty in living their lives from one day to the next. People with learning disability — the so-called mentally handicapped — figure prominently in this group. Since such people may be resident in various 'psychiatric' settings, or may also be psychiatrically disordered, they are worthy of mention in this respect. We should not forget the physically handicapped, who can be a subgroup of their own, or a facet of any of the three populations mentioned above. People with mental or physical handicaps may have problems with independent living that may play a part, no matter how small, in the creation of a psychological disorder, or in the aggravation of a more serious psychiatric disorder.

Psychological Effects. Since we take our everyday living skills so much for granted, we should be keenly aware of what their absence might mean to others. But how can such skill deficiencies help to produce psychological disorder? Try considering for one moment how you would feel if, for whatever reason, you become incontinent, couldn't fasten the buttons on your clothes, or were unable to make a sandwich when you felt hungry. Would you continue to be your usual bright and cheerful self? Or would you become frustrated, angry, even depressed? There is no doubt that some people cope with the loss of independence remarkably well. That does not mean that such 'loss' does not hurt. What is more important is that many are visibly hurt. To return to a point I made earlier, it is not enough simply to look at people according to some standard scale of independence. There is little value in saying 'Well, this patient is no more dependent than others (in this psychogeriatric ward).' We should be trying to evaluate what independence means for the person concerned. If he is frustrated or upset by his loss of independence, it is because he is thinking, 'This is me this is happening to — not anyone else!'

An Assessment System. The Everyday Living Skills Inventory (ELSI) was designed to help in the assessment of independence across a wide range of skill areas (see Figure 5.3). ELSI was designed by nurses with various nursing settings and problems in mind. It was also prepared to help nurses who were all too aware of the weaknesses of available systems.[3] Many of the skills contained in ELSI could be called 'key skills'. They either maintain our survival or promote out social acceptability. However, exactly how much ability, and in which areas of competence, has not been established. So far, research suggests that factors such as the patient's diagnosis, where he resides, and the cultural group to which he belongs influence strongly the view of his dependence/independence.[4] However, the general nature of the scale suggests that it can be used with almost any population, in any setting. Over the past six years I have studied its use with mentally handicapped children and adults in hospital, hostels and at home; long-term psychiatric patients in special treatment settings, 'back wards' and hostels; and the confused elderly, primarily in psychiatric hospitals. I would emphasise that the scale is of *most* use when an individual evaluation is undertaken, trying to judge the significance of the assessment for the particular patient concerned.

A key feature of the assessment is its positive emphasis. Most nursing assessments or diagnoses, as we noted in Chapter 1, tend to concentrate on the negative features of the patient. They are interested only in what is wrong with him. In terms of judging how many staff are required to care for a certain number of patients, we categorise the patients according to 'dependency' criteria. These criteria emphasise the patient's deficits. They may also be vague and ridden with value judgements. More importantly, they are not concerned with the ideal of 'patient-centred care'. ELSI was developed to try to restore the balance. Certainly, the scale can be used to identify the patient's weaknesses — his skill deficits. It can also be used to draw up a list of his strengths — his assets.

The Care Planning Assessment

The overall aim of ELSI is different from many of the other forms of assessment covered in this book. It is true that this format allows us to gain an overall picture of the patient's functioning. It is also possible to compare one patient with another, using this format. However, the main aim of the assessment is to identify the patient's strengths and weaknesses, in terms of everyday living. This knowledge is used to construct some form of 'care plan' in order to encourage progress and improvement, or simply to slow down deterioration. ELSI is different in the sense that it is not concerned with assessing psychiatric disease, disorder or illness. The package focuses upon areas of personal, interpersonal or more general social functioning. These areas of behaviour may be related to specific psychiatric disorders. They may be the 'secondary handicaps' mentioned earlier, or they may be aspects of adaptive functioning which, if missing, may contribute to the onset or repetition of some psychiatric breakdown.

ELSI measures skills: the extent to which the patient can perform independently various everyday behaviours. From another angle, the assessment tries to judge how much help the person *needs* in order to complete these routines or rituals. The inventory includes patterns of behaviour which are fundamental to survival, such as eating, drinking, eliminating. It also covers those which contribute to that ephemeral concept, the 'quality of life'. This area might include care of personal appearance, interpersonal skills, leisure activities. The level of independent functioning across these general areas shows the extent to which the patient relies upon others to organise the framework of his day, or to complete the 'menu' of skills which makes up his daily plan.

The Assessment Targets

The concept of 'activities of daily living' within nursing has tended to concentrate upon basic skills: eating, breathing, eliminating, etc. ELSI broadens this concept to include the kinds of behaviour in which people engage on a regular daily basis. Ten major areas of behaviour are specified in the inventory, each of which includes a number of specific activities.

(1) Communication: aspects of communicating, either verbally or non-verbally.
(2) Comprehension: those behaviours that are related to the patient's ability to understand and respond to information stemming from his environment.
(3) Physical development: the patient's sight, hearing and mobility.
(4) Personal hygiene: basic self-care skills.
(5) Toilet usage: elimination and accompanying hygiene.
(6) Dressing: formal dressing, fastenings and clothing selection.
(7) Eating: use of utensils, eating in public and diet selection.
(8) Domestic skills: a range of skills involving looking after personal belongings and the 'home' environment.
(9) Community living: orientation to the outside world; self-catering and awareness of public information.
(10) Social and recreational skills: varieties of social interaction, individual and group recreation.

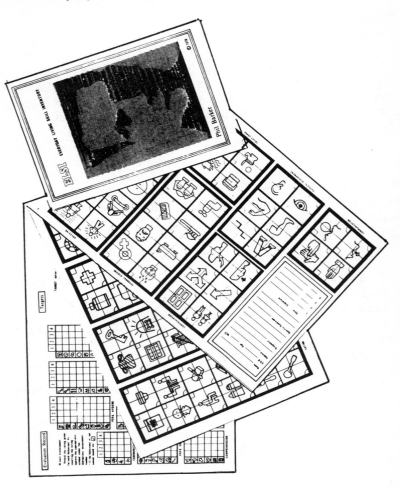

Figure 5.3

Figure 5.4

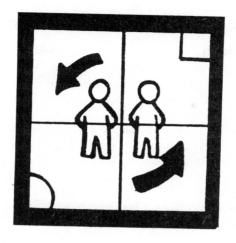

Although high-level performance is not essential across all these areas to guarantee everyday survival, or even a satisfactory quality of life, it is clear that the greater the range of proficiency, the greater the degree of freedom, range of choice, and overall independence of the person.

Using the Inventory

The ELSI package is made up of a scoring manual, two profile sheets and an evaluation record, which is also used for writing targets — the short-, medium- and long-term goals. These are all contained within an envelope folder, which fits into the patient's case file. On the first of the two profile sheets simple biographical data are recorded: name, date of birth, sex, address, diagnosis and accompanying handicaps (e.g. blindness, deafness, hemiplegia). In this section, which occupies the top corner of the profile sheet, a record is also made of the dates of each assessment. The name of the nurse conducting the assessment is also recorded. Our research suggests that where the patient is involved in direct skills training, the assessment should be repeated every four to six months. In other cases an annual assessment may be more appropriate.

The assessment package looks at 86 areas of behaviour. Each of these is assessed in the same way, using a seven-point rating scale

(0–6). In some behaviours the patient may be fully independent, requiring no help from others to complete the action. In these areas he would score the maximum rating of 6. In others he may need some kind of assistance in terms of instruction, degrees of physical assistance or supervision. Here he is obviously less independent, and scores lower on the scale. In some of the areas the patient may require no 'social assistance', but may need the use of aids or appliances, or may operate at a slower pace or to a limited degree. In these situations the patient would score less than the maximum.

The Skill Symbols. Each of the skill areas is composed of a number of specific behaviours, or sub-divisions, of the main concept. For example, under 'communication' there are four such subdivisions:

(1) The ability to use *simple gestures* to communicate needs, wishes or general information, e.g. pointing to mouth, meaning 'drink'.
(2) The ability to use *complex gestures*, communicating through the use of some standard sign language.
(3) The ability to use the *speech mechanism*, communicating audibly and clearly through the spoken word.
(4) The ability to use *speech content*, communicating at various levels through the use of language.

Each of these individual areas is represented on the profile sheet by a symbol (see Figure 5.4). This symbol is located within a grid format: this format is used for the translation of the numerical ratings into the 'visual profile'.

The Scoring Method. Each of the 86 areas of behaviour is defined in the manual, beside descriptions of various 'levels' of functioning (see Figure 5.5). As the figure shows, the ratings 0–6 are accompanied by descriptions of how the patient *might* perform the action. The nurse's task is to select the description that most closely fits the present level of functioning of her patient. Once this 'matching' has been done, the rating can be entered on the recording sheet. It is not necessary to complete each one of the 86 areas of behaviour. In some settings for the elderly, where the patients never leave the ward, it would be a waste of time giving scores for community living. Only those areas of functioning in which the patient presently engages, and which are of relevance to his overall

Figure 5.5

26. <u>SHAVING</u> : Shaves using an
    electric or soap and water
    razor as necessary.

<u>Rating</u>   Shaves self ....

6   ..... independently.

5   ..... independently – under <u>supervision</u>
              e.g. for safety.

4   ..... only when <u>told in advance</u> what to do.

3   ..... only when <u>instructed and supervised</u>
              throughout.

2   ..... only when instructed and <u>shown</u> what to do.

1   ..... only when given <u>physical assistance</u>.

0   ..... does not shave self even when given
              physical assistance.

N   ..... Does not have the opportunity to shave OR
              wears beard.

assessment, are completed. Having said that, for the majority of
psychiatric patients completion of the whole assessment is most
desirable.

The Visual Profile. Although ELSI provides numerical information, or data, in the form of the ratings described above, the visual
profile is the distinguishing feature of the assessment. This format
was developed in response to requests by nurses for a simpler way
of recording performance and monitoring progress. Nurses who
were unsophisticated in the use of standardised rating scales often

found it difficult to interpret the results of such scales. At the time many found the scoring of the scales difficult simply because such measures seemed unrelated to their experience of the patient. The visual profile was developed in an effort to make the patient's level of functioning visible, *at a glance*. Nurses who wished to interpret the meaning of the various ratings could refer to the visual profile for a graphic representation of different degrees of competence.

The visual profile format was developed for the following reasons. First, I was aware that most assessment systems relied upon either written information or numerical codings. The written systems that many nurses use gave a picture of the patient, but did not allow comparison with others, or even serious evaluation of progress made. Systems using numerical codings were more reliable, but appealed to only a small proportion of staff. To others, such methods looked 'too statistical'. As a very poor mathematician myself, I understood what they meant. ELSI was developed to provide an assessment format that would meet the needs of the very wide range of people who routinely work with the psychiatric population. By simplifying the system of assessment and interpretation of results, ELSI tried to cater for those staff who had no real training in assessment methodology. My second reason for adopting the visual profile format was an economic one. I had observed many of my colleagues using standardised rating scales and found that almost all of them found this a time-consuming activity. Not only did they need to spend a lot of time doing the assessment, but they often needed as much time again to analyse what it meant. As I noted above, for many staff this meant that they could fulfil no real function in the assessment of their patients. I also observed some of the difficulties involved in using standardised assessments at case review meetings. Often the scores would be passed round the group. Each person would nod knowledgeably, but I often doubted the level of understanding. ELSI manoeuvred this communication problem by presenting an alternative to numerical data. The ratings were duly recorded on the evaluation sheet for close examination. However, for the purpose of general discussion, such as takes place in a case review, the visual profiles provided an overview of the patient's functioning, one that could be taken in at a glance.

Translating the Scores. Each of the scores on the seven-point rating scale can be translated on to the symbol of the profile sheets.

Figure 5.6

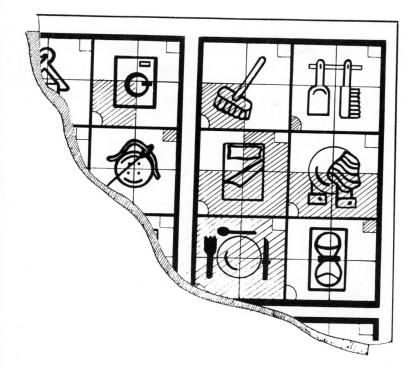

Most of the ratings are translated by shading in a part of the symbol. Where the patient scores 0 the symbol is left blank — indicating the lowest level of performance. Where the patient is given a score of 6, the complete symbol is shaded in. The scores 1 to 5 are translated by shading in progressively more and more of the symbol. Figure 5.6 shows a section of a profile sheet. It should be apparent that the pictures with the *least* shading represent areas where the patient is deficient in the skill, whereas pictures that are shaded more fully represent areas where he is partially or fully competent, When the assessment is interpreted overall, the more shading there is the higher the level of independence; the less shading, the greater the degree of dependence.

No Opportunity. The scale also includes a 'no opportunity' category. This is used where the patient is restrained from practising a skill. He may be restricted by lack of facilities — many patients do not display certain patterns of table etiquette because napkins and side plates may not be available. He may also be restricted by rules and regulations, as many patients are not permitted to bathe alone, shave themselves, or travel unaccompanied on a bus. It would be incorrect to say that they cannot perform these skills, but since they have no opportunity, the nurse has no way of gauging their ability. In either case it is appropriate to record their lack of opportunity. The only alternative is to set up a test situation, to evaluate the patient's skills in these 'new' areas.

The Evaluation Record. The profile sheets provide an assessment of how the patient functions at present. Although it is possible to judge regression on the visual profile, this is not the main function of the profile sheets.[5] Instead, progress or regression is evaluated from the evaluation record. This details the actual ratings given for each skill area across each assessment. Scores for each of the major categories — dressing, community skills, etc. — are also available, as totals of the individual scores. The nurse can check here whether the overall level of performance has improved or declined, and where such progress or regression has been made. This sheet is also used to summarise the training targets for the patient. By studying the assessment the nurse can draw out areas of behaviour in which the patient is either deficient or could benefit from an increase in skill. These are arranged in order of priority, representing short-, medium- and long-term targets. As I noted at the beginning of this chapter, there is a need to select targets which are important for individual patients, in the light of their present position or future prospects. Space is also provided for a short summary of 'how' the training targets will be achieved.

The Procedure. At the first assessment the nurse completes the biographical details. At this, and every subsequent, assessment she will sign and date the assessment. She then turns to the scoring manual, reads the definition of each skill area, and then reads through the performance description for each level on the 0–6 scale. She then selects the level which most closely approximates the current functioning of the patient under review. The manual recommends using the *average* performance over the week leading up to the assessment as a guide. Once she has selected the appropriate rating, the nurse enters this in the appropriate box on the Evaluation Record: noting either N (for no opportunity) or one of the 0–6 ratings. She then translates the score on to the appropriate symbol of the visual profile, either shading in the symbol or leaving it blank as descibed above. She then proceeds to the next behaviour in the manual, repeating this process until the assessment is complete.

It should be apparent that it is possible to complete the ELSI only if you know the patient. New staff on a unit will need time to collect the store of information necessary for the completion of the assessment. However, even staff who have worked with the patient for some time may find it difficult to rate certain items. Either they may be unsure — 'Should it be a 4 or a 5?' — or they may simply not know whether he performs this behaviour at all. In either case some direct tests are recommended: observe the patient in an appropriate situation on at least three occasions before arriving at the rating. Knowledge about the patient raises the issue of junior staff once again. It is almost a cliché to say that staff in training, or untrained nurses, often know the patient better than the nurse in charge of the ward. The reason is simple. Senior staff spend a lot of time on administration, consultation and various other office tasks, which keep them away from the patient. Junior staff have no such restrictions. Their regular and close contact with the patient often makes them the ideal assessors. As I noted earlier, such staff are usually debarred from the assessment process, because the method is too obscure. Our research has shown that untrained nurses and nurses in training can use the ELSI with *no tuition*, save for a couple of readings of the introduction to the manual. Perhaps of greater importance was our finding that such staff could *interpret* the assessment through the medium of the visual profiles.

The Picture of the Patient

The everyday living skills assessment described provides a relatively simple way of evaluating the patient's performance and a simple 'read-out', in visual form, of his assets and deficits. This assessment can then be used as the basis for programme planning. The nurse can decide, along with her colleagues, which existing skills should be developed, and which ones taught from scratch. As we have noted, the assessment also shines a strong light on those areas where the patient is prevented from engaging in certain activities, either through lack of amenities or policy restrictions. If the assessment was used solely to highlight the restrictive nature of a care setting, this might be a valuable function. Like all other assessments, it presents a limited view of the patient. Certain skills are neglected, while others might benefit from being broken down into even more component parts. For the present the package is complete, although manifestly deficient.[6]

The assessment is most often used in a case review setting. The visual profiles are pinned to a board for public display or, if the group is small, photocopies of each sheet are made for individuals to study. The nurse who completed the assessment is usually assigned the task of 'chairing' the discussion. She can review the general picture, pointing to various symbols and describing the patient's functioning in these areas. Finally she draws out of the overall picture the behaviours that might be selected as training targets. Our research shows that between one and three readings of the manual are sufficient to memorise all 86 symbols. In a study conducted with mentally handicapped children, the children learned to recognise and mime the action of ten symbols after only five hours of training.[7] A colleague also used ELSI as a self-monitoring assessment with mentally handicapped adults who had only limited reading ability. They learned to interpret their scores on the visual profiles, checking their progress every few months.[8]

One Step Beyond

ELSI provides a general overview of the patient's functioning. This is a global assessment. It may help pin-point specific problem areas, but its evaluation of individual skills is necessarily crude. In some cases you may wish to analyse these skills in finer detail, especially if your goal is to help a severely disabled patient acquire new, or develop existing, skills. ELSI gives only an outline of the complex actions that are needed to shave, put on a suit of clothes, board a bus, or order tea in a café. To assess these skills more 'absolutely' it may be necessary to detail all the steps or stages that are involved in their performance.

The Task Analysis. All the skills we have discussed involve a complex mix of cognitive processes and fine and gross motor movements. The patient who is going to dress himself must first go through the process of *selecting* the appropriate garments, laying them out *in order*, putting on each garment in the correct *sequence*, attending to other 'order' factors such as the distinction between back and front, top and bottom, inside and outside. Once the clothes have been transferred from the bed to his body he must arrange them so that they hang correctly: are all the wrinkles smoothed out? are all the loose ends tucked in? I am not suggesting that everyone dresses in this way, or pays attention to all these details. This is merely an illustration of 'perfect' dressing. It is clear that although many patients in psychiatric hospitals are able to dress, in the broadest sense of the word, they may neglect some of the niceties of 'perfect' dressing. This may explain why we view their performance as less than satisfactory.

A thorough analysis of any everyday living skill involves breaking the skill down into its component parts. This process is called *'task analysis'*. The task is analysed in terms of the actions, and their sequence, the patient needs to perform in order to complete the task. This process is used in most skills training settings. Nurses learn how to give an injection or test urine by learning each stage of the process. As they become more proficient they can link, or blend, the steps together more quickly. You may think that such a careful analysis is unnecessary for psychiatric patients whose problems are primarily emotional or experiential. However, as I noted earlier, in many cases the patient's problems *now* are the secondary handicaps which may have developed from his original problem, or as an outcome of restrictive care. Many psychiatric wards house patients who need 'constant care and attention'. Many rehabilitation settings, or even community hostels, house people who need substantial help with timetabling, recreation or simple cooking. In order to reduce such patients' dependence, or to 'actualise their potential', it may be necessary to analyse their performance of these key skills closely.

Preparing your Own Analysis

Although the kind of skill analysis featured in ELSI fits most people in most situations, clearly the right way to perform a skill varies from one setting, and one individual, to another. Rather than try to recommend standard analyses of specific skills, which would by its very nature be impossibly boring and highly inadequate, I shall discuss an example of a task analysis as a guide to preparation of your own. The procedure for conducting a task analysis is quite straightforward. We can observe a patient who is competent in the skill, or we can role play the skill using staff members. I favour the latter method. In either case the major steps in the performance of the behaviour are listed in the sequence in which they occur. Emphasis is given to separating out each discrete action from the next in the sequence.

Preparation. Some skills require the person to make some preparation prior to his performance. If we wanted to analyse eating, dressing or using the telephone, we would need to begin with selecting the food, selecting the clothes, and perhaps finding a telephone booth. In beginning our analysis the first question we must ask is: does the patient need anything, such as pieces of equipment? Does he need to collect something? What does he do if it is not available? Does he need to check or judge whether some facility is available? He may need to knock on the bathroom door, or ask if the washing machine is being used. These preparation questions involve 'setting the scene' for the action that follows.

The Action. The action involves at least three stages: opening, performing and closing. The opening steps in using a telephone involve picking up the receiver and dialling, the performing stage involves the telephone conversation, and the closing sequence involves terminating the conversation and replacing the receiver.

An example. Figure 5.7 shows a shaving assessment which was developed for a long-stay ward. All the patients were able to shave, but required a lot of prompting from staff. Invariably, parts of their faces remained unshaven. As a beard-wearer myself, I thought this irrelevant, but as both staff *and* patients thought that shaving was important, I include it as an example.

The task analysis was developed using female nurses as models. The nursing team isolated the stages during a 15-minute workshop held at the staff change-over meeting. I committed the task analysis to paper. The team then conducted the assessment with a sample of the residents, making notes on any small step they had missed, or any vagueness in the definitions. Prior to the development of this 'fine-grain' assessment the staff had used the shaving rating in the ELSI format. Their dissatisfaction with the global rating prompted the design of the task analysis. As the figure shows, the shaving process began with the patient collecting his razor and ended with its replacement. In between were a number of steps involving connecting and switching on the razor, feeling the face for the presence of stubble, and looking in the mirror, as well as the action of moving the razor across the face. This task analysis, translated

Figure 5.7

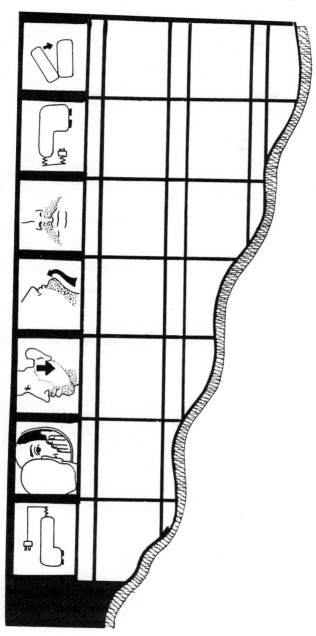

Figure 5.8

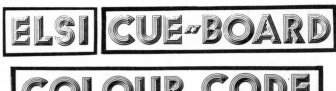

ELSI CUE-BOARD

COLOUR CODE

 Verbal prompt to begin only

 Verbal prompts during action

 Verbal/gestural only throughout action

 Minimal physical prompting mainly verbal/gestural.

 Physical prompt to begin: verbal/gestural to end

 Full physical prompt to begin and complete.

E.L.S.I. PHIL BARKER © 1978

Figure 5.9

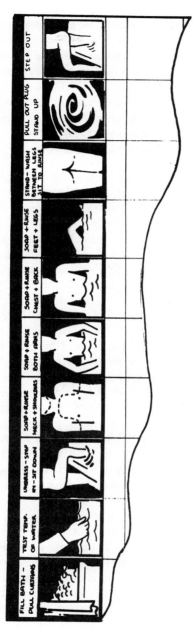

into symbolic terms, was used as a simple memory-jogger for the nurse. Each picture reminded her of the steps involved in that stage of the process. Consequently it was not necessary for her to use a lengthy checklist, and the assessment format eventually formed the 'evaluation' of the training programme.

It would be feasible to assess simply whether or not the patient performed each of the steps in the shaving chain. For the patients concerned this was thought to be inadequate. As a result, a seven-point rating scale, which is an extension of the ELSI scale, was used to judge the amount of assistance each patient required to complete each stage of the process. In common with ELSI, the higher the score, the more independent the patient. The rating is illustrated in Figure 5.8. Before beginning a shaving-skills programme each patient is assessed on two consecutive days using the format illustrated. His score is recorded as his 'baseline level', and his performance is evaluated each day thereafter, using the ratings in conjunction with the 'symbol board'. The levels of assistance that are noted in the assessment are used as the basis for deciding how much help to give the patient during the training phase. Consequently, this assessment is inextricably tied up with the treatment system.

A similar assessment system for bathing in a hospital ward is illustrated in Figure 5.9. This is a very similar format to the shaving assessment, using the same seven-point rating scale. It is worth noting that in this example a number of 'ancillary' steps are included: preparing the bath, safety, ensuring privacy, etc. The assessment is not solely concerned with washing the body. It is worth pointing out here that considerable disagreement was found between staff over the 'rights' and 'wrongs' of bathing. This illustrates the need to adapt assessments such as these to the needs of specific patients and the setting they inhabit.

A Simplified Task Analysis. An alternative to the highly detailed skill assessment described above is shown in Figure 5.10. This format was designed for a ward of elderly patients who had difficulty in dressing. The assessment includes most of the underclothes and outer clothes likely to be worn by the patient. His performance in removing and putting on each item is rated using a similar scale to those already described. This is yet another example of an *observational rating scale*: the nurse observes the patient directly and then selects the appropriate rating. This format is a much

Figure 5.10

NAME .... WARD .... AGE ....

PROCEDURE

A) Assess the subject's dressing performance with his/her <u>normal everyday clothing.</u>

B) Conduct the assessment in a quiet area which is free from major distractions.

C) Give the subject the opportunity to complete each task independently (Grade 6) if he/she does not complete within <u>1 minute</u>: give Grade 5 assistance if he/she cannot complete within <u>1 minute</u>: give <u>Grade 4</u> and <u>so on</u> until the GRADE OF ASSISTANCE NECESSARY FOR COMPLETION IS IDENTIFIED.

GRADE

6 —— completes task <u>perfectly</u> when instructed <u>once</u> to do so: requires no other assistance.

5 —— completes task without assistance but requires instruction to correct some error (e.g. garment inside out).

4 —— requires instruction to complete task (i.e. verbal directions during performance OR is shown how to perform task)

3 —— can complete <u>more</u> than half of task (requires physical assistance with other half).

2 —— can complete <u>less</u> than half of task (requires physical assistance with remainder).

1 —— co-operates as task is carried out for him (e.g. raises arms)

0 —— is unco-operative OR entirely passive.

(A) <u>BRA</u>
PUT ON
FASTEN
UNFASTEN
TAKE OFF

(B) <u>PANTS</u>
PUT ON
TAKE OFF

(C) <u>VEST/T-SHIRT/SLIP</u>
PUT ON
TAKE OFF

(D) <u>BLOUSE/SHIRT.</u>
PUT ON
BUTTON
UNBUTTON
TAKE OFF

(E) <u>TROUSERS/SKIRT.</u>
PUT ON
FASTEN
UNFASTEN
TAKE OFF

(F) <u>JUMPER/PULLOVER</u>
PUT ON
TAKE OFF

(G) <u>DRESS</u>
PUT ON
TAKE OFF
UNFASTEN
FASTEN

(H) <u>SOCKS/TIGHTS</u>
L R
PUT ON
TAKE OFF

(I) <u>SHOES</u>
L R
PUT ON
TIGHTEN LACE
TIE BOW
FASTEN BUCKLE
UNTIE LACE
UN-BUCKLE
TAKE OFF

SUB-SCORES
A
B
C
D
E
F
G
H
I

TOTAL

MAX POSS

%

SIG. ....

DATE...............

simplified task analysis: it does not describe all the steps required to move from 'undressed' to 'fully clothed'. However, it does detail all the dressing items, which allows the nurse to judge which garments the patient is competent at removing and replacing, and which present problems. The scoring is also very simple. The rating given for each garment is entered and a percentage of the 'total possible score' calculated. Using this percentage method the scale can be used for men and women, who wear different garments. In the ward where the scale was first developed the nurses were able to evaluate the progress of each resident, whilst at the same time identifying his strengths and weaknesses. By assessing all the patients on the ward they produced a ward 'norm', or average, for dressing skills. This was helpful in judging more clearly how dependent the patients were in terms of one facet of their routine care.

Aids to Care Planning

There is nothing remarkable about any of the methods described above. I would hope that their obvious simplicity would be apparent to the reader. They were designed to help nurses establish what they had already suspected, by the shortest possible route. The *method* was designed to make vague value judgements redundant and to save some time. Emphasis was given to being able to read, or interpret, the result of the assessment quickly. This was important for unsophisticated staff who are often very busy. It may be significant that these methods were designed by *clinical* nurses, for use by clinical nurses, to provide the basis for clinical care. At one level these assessments provide a practical framework for the planning of how we can help our patients to grow and develop, at least within this area of their lives. The assessments can also be used to compare one patient with another, who shares similar circumstances: either a diagnostic category (such as long-stay patient) or an environment (hostel resident). Although most of the early research with ELSI involved mentally handicapped people in hospital and the community,[9] the format has also been used with the confused elderly and has been warmly received by a range of staff working with psychiatric patients.[10] Although I make no claims for the scientific status of any of the assessments described, I believe that they represent valid and reliable measures of patient behaviour. I am also encouraged by the transfer of a system from one population to others which, traditionally, were thought to be 'different. It is apparent that although mentally handicapped people, the elderly and long-stay psychiatric patients are all different, there may be some advantage in assessing in which ways they are the same.

The Alternatives

I have discussed ways of studying everyday living skills which have been developed by nurses, for use by nurses. Before leaving this area I think it only fair to discuss briefly some of the *standard* methods of assessing everyday living skills (along with other aspects of the long-stay patient). Both of these methods have attained a high degree of respectability in the psychiatric field, and are used routinely by nurses.

The Nurse's Observational Scale for Inpatient Evaluation (NOSIE)

NOSIE has achieved a world-wide reputation as a means of assessing the *status* of the hospitalised patient. The system has also been used to evaluate change as a result of direct treatment or care. Of supreme significance is the emphasis placed upon the role of the nurse in collecting the information on the patient. First described in 1965,[11] the scale has been used across a range of clinical and research settings to judge various aspects of individual functioning. The scale covers 30 items on a single sheet, representing seven different sub-scales — irritability, personal neatness, social interest, competence, manifest psychosis, retardation and depression. Two final 'total assets' scores are also provided: here the nurse rates how 'ill' she believes the patient to be, using a seven-point scale. Using the same scale, she judges how much she thinks his *condition has changed* since admission to the ward or project.

The thirty items are framed in the form of statements: e.g. 'shows interest in activities around him' or 'keeps his clothes neat'. The nurse is asked to rate the patient's behaviour over the *three days* prior to the assessment. A five-point scale is provided for this purpose: (1) = never; (2) = sometimes; (3) = often; (4) = usually; (5) = always.

NOSIE is a well-respected and reliable method for assessing longer-term psychiatric patients. Studies have shown that similar scores are found on the sub-scales even where different age and cultural populations were studied.[12] This suggests that the scale is very valid across widely different populations. Although the scale can judge the degree of change in patients who are involved in a treatment programme,[13] the scale is of limited value to nurses in *planning* how they can help the patient. Indeed this scale is, in many ways, assessing psychiatric disorder in terms of signs of pathology or commonly occurring outcomes of chronicity, such as loss of attention to appearance, or decline of social interest. The scale pays only scant regard to the concept of assessing everyday living skills. In all fairness, however, I would emphasise that it was not designed with this goal in mind.

REHAB

One of the most interesting scales to appear in recent years is the 'Rehabilitation Evaluation of Hall and Baker'. Developed by John Hall and Roger Baker, famous for their token-economy and long-stay research, this scale is in growing use on an international scale, as a means of gaining a profile of the patient in the rehabilitation setting. The scale was not designed solely for hospital use, where it has obvious applications, but also for community settings: hostels, clinics, group homes, etc. — indeed, anywhere requiring an evaluation of the progress of the more chronic psychiatric patient. The scale was not designed specifically for nurses, but is of particular relevance to the nursing situation. Hall and Baker acknowledge that nurses, amongst a range of other professionals, *should* use their scale. As with ELSI and NOSIE, the REHAB scale acknowledges that nurses are the 'natural' assessors, in view of their up-to-date knowledge of the patient. Since they are also so close to the patient, they are also the natural evaluators of progress.

REHAB is a very broad assessment system, covering various aspects of 'disturbed' or deviant behaviour, work skills and everyday living skills. Since we are discussing only living skills in this chapter, I shall focus my attention on that aspect of the REHAB scale. A number of questions are asked about the patient's general behaviour over the week preceding the assessment. The nurse is advised to use the standard of ordinary life outside the hospital as her guide, and to give a rating for each question. Typical questions are as follows:

'How active was the patient			
	Sat or lay most of the time in one place, without moving.	Period of inactivity, but otherwise moved reasonably normally.	Normal amount of speed and activity.
'How well did the patient dress him/herself?' If not known, tick box. ☐	Made a mess of dressing. Buttons undone, clothes disarranged, items of clothing missing (if nurse dressed patient rate here).	Dressed self, but usually poor in one or two aspects (e.g. shirt or blouse not tucked in and not done up properly).	Neatly dressed self. Fit to be seen in public.

This general behaviour section of the assessment covers a range of social, self-care and community-oriented skills. The nurse rates the patient's performance by marking the point on the visual analogue scale that most closely corresponds with his performance. This mark is later translated into a score by use of a transparent sheet that awards ratings to marks on the visual analogue.

One of the important features of REHAB is its use of 'normative' data. Hall and Baker have studied large numbers of long-stay psychiatric patients over the past decade, and are consequently able to offer a comparison between the individual patient's score and those of his 'peer group'. It is possible to evaluate how far below 'normal' the patient is in terms of his general behaviour. Hall and Baker have found that such information was helpful in allocating patients to different rehabilitation, or pre-rehabilitation, settings.[14]

CAPE

The Clifton Assessment Procedures for the Elderly (CAPE) were developed by psychologists with the aim of producing a brief and simple method of assessing the mental (cognitive) and behavioural competence of elderly people. The package is recommended for elderly people in hospital or other care settings. The CAPE has been shown to be useful not only to psychologists but to 'all those professionally concerned with the care and management of the elderly'.[15]

The package consists of two measures. These can be used together or separately, depending on the needs of the situation.

The first is a Cognitive Assessment Scale (CAS), a short psychological test which, the authors state, 'can be administered with little training . . . and has the benefit of being brief [and is] not stressful to the elderly person'. The first part consists of twelve questions designed to assess current information and orientation: e.g. name, age, where he is, prime minister, American president, day, month, year, etc. The second part assesses counting, saying the alphabet, reading and writing. These simple tests also assess attention and concentration. Finally, an assessment of fine motor skill and hand-eye co-ordination is made by asking the patient to trace a path with a pencil through a spiral maze. Scores are awarded for each of the sections of the CAS and comparison with available norms allows the nurse to judge the level of 'mental impairment' on a five-point scale.

The second part of the package is the Behaviour Rating Scale (BRS). This can be completed by anyone familiar with the patient's behaviour. This might be nurses or a member of the patient's family, if still at home. Eighteen items provide measures across four main areas of functioning: physical disability, apathy, communication difficulties and social disturbance. Total scores for the 18 items, as well as for each of the four sub-areas, can be compared with available norms. This comparison allows the nurse to identify the degree of dependency present, and suggests the kind of help needed. CAPE is important in the sense that it was designed specifically for the elderly and has been closely evaluated in this setting. Its simplicity and brevity have much to commend it as a part of the nurses' assessment toolbox. I would imagine that all nurses working with the elderly would need to be well acquainted with this package in order to work with psychologists who are routinely invited to amplify our understanding of the cognitive and behavioural status of the patient.

Applications

The various scales I have described share a common interest in everyday functioning. Naturally, there are slight differences between one format and another. ELSI focuses its attention on 'living skills', whereas the other three global scales mentioned give a broader perspective, including psychiatric or cognitive function problems. It is clear that this broad perspective is gained at the expense of detail.

Many of the nurses I have worked with have been dissatisfied with these assessments. They have seen the need for a single assessment which tells them everything they want to know about the patient. At present, this is not possible. We are obliged to use a range of different methods to gain the comprehensive picture we desire, using interviews, direct observation, observational ratings, self-report methods, etc. In this chapter I have focused attention, unashamedly, on the target of everyday living skills. I do not assume, for one moment, that this represents all the patient's problems. In some circumstances they may not even be the most important problems. I have addressed simply the question, 'How can we begin to assess the patient's performance of everyday living skills?' I hope that the scales illustrated might offer some answers. It seems self-evident that the living skills assessment needs to be augmented by other systems if we are to present a fully comprehensive analysis of the patient. However, the living skills assessment may function as a good 'foundation assessment', for it is upon these fundamental activities of everyday life that the patient's overall functioning is based. As I noted earlier, if the patient has problems in everyday functioning, then other psychological, psychiatric or social adaptation problems may result. In this sense it is important that nurses recognise the relevance of everyday living skills and give them the detailed attention they deserve.

In concluding this chapter let us look briefly at some applications of the methods mentioned.

The Elderly Patient. Jackie is a 76-year-old ex-miner who has been in a 'psychogeriatric' ward for the past two years. It is a very 'busy' ward, and Jackie is one of the more able residents. He communicates well with the staff, enjoying a laugh and a joke, but at times seems confused. He has partially lost the use of his left arm following a stroke, which caused some problems with dressing and washing. Staff have now almost completely taken over the performance of these activities. Jackie moves around the ward fairly easily with the aid of a tripod walking stick. He spends a lot of time looking out of the window into the grounds.

In the typical ward for the elderly it is often wholly unrealistic to talk about 'holistic' care. The restrictions on staff time and resources often prohibit attention to anything other than the basics of care. In Jackie's case we would want to identify those areas of functioning which were a 'problem' to him, and those which — if they were developed — might enhance the quality of his remaining years. An assessment of Jackie's dressing skills, such as we have already described, can be done in a matter of a few minutes. Indeed it can be done as part of the 'dressing' routine. From this assessment the nurse might identify those areas in which Jackie is capable, and those in which he requires some help. From this assessment a plan could be devised to allow Jackie to dress alone within the limits of his competence, receiving help with the more awkward areas. The same process could be applied to his shaving and bathing. If Jackie could be assisted to engage in these activities 'to the best of his ability', it would save staff time and, more importantly, might boost his self-esteem. In such a case the CAPE would be administered as a matter of routine. If this suggested that Jackie had some severe mental impairment then the kind of reality orientation assessment discussed in Chapter 4 might be appropriate. Perhaps some of Jackie's 'confusion' relates to his disorientation within the ward environment. It may be helpful to assess this, with a view to taking some remedial action. The last area suggested by my vignette involves his recreational activity. The social and recreational sections of an assessment like ELSI might illustrate how 'under-occupied' he is, and may also suggest some of the activities which he might be helped to rediscover.

I have suggested three 'bits of assessment' here: a task analysis of dressing and shaving; a ward oriented 'reality orientation' measure; and sections of the everyday living skills inventory. If this had not been a 'busy' ward, I might have suggested more methods, or the ELSI in full. Staff would be encouraged to look at the assessment as a potentially life-enrichening exercise for the patient, and perhaps a time-saving one for them. The task analysis and reality orientation assessments might need to be repeated fortnightly, to monitor progress or regression. It would be emphasised that this will require only a minimum investment of time. The ELSI, which might take longer if several areas of functioning were to be covered, would not be repeated for at least four months.

The Hostel Resident. Tommy left hospital this year after spending 27 years there. He moved to a hostel in town where he has his own room, for the first time, sharing dining and living areas with eleven other men. He received a lot of training for community living before discharge but was in no way 'independent' when he left for the hostel. His release was due to the political pressure on psychiatric hospitals to discharge patients. A community nurse visits twice a week, discussing progress with the hostel staff. A social worker and occupational therapist also visit regularly. The team decided that many of the men still needed a lot of training if they were ever to move to a group home, which was a popular goal. The hostel officer-in-charge suggested using ELSI as a foundation assessment and undertook to complete the scale on Tommy about four months after his arrival. A meeting was then convened involving all the relevant staff to look at Tommy's profile. Although it was clear that he was fairly competent in *basic* personal hygiene, eating, dressing and socialising, he was far below the standard required for entry to the group home. He bathed and shaved only when 'badgered' by the staff, often wore inappropriate combinations of clothing, and his social behaviour at mealtimes left a lot to be desired. However, most of his problems were concentrated in the domestic skills and community living areas. He had little opportunity to develop these whilst in hospital, a fact which was graphically displayed by the expanse of blank symbols on the ELSI. The profile also showed how limited his social and recreational activities were; he did not mix with the other residents and spent most of his evenings in front of the television.

The officer-in-charge summarised these points at the case review, picking out Tommy's assets and deficits from the profile. This provided a forum for discussion within the team: how could these problems be ranked in order of priority? Which members of the team might help in their resolution? The team decided that they had the resources to mount a fairly intensive social skills training programme, and would review progress within the next three months.

The Long-Stay Ward. 'Trottick' is a fairly typical long-stay ward. Twenty-four women share far from ideal accommodation: a large open-plan living area with a toilet annexe and dining area downstairs, and a divided dormitory upstairs. The ward was formerly designated a 'disturbed area', accommodating 'chronic schizophrenics' along with a few 'organic states'. In recent years the ward has changed in function, with an increase in the number of 'young chronics' as well as an increase in the number of 'frail elderly' chronic patients. One of the problems facing staff who wished to offer a more person-centred kind of care was knowing where to begin. All the patients had a range of obvious needs. But how could they ever meet them? Last spring the charge nurse discussed with her team how they might improve the care service to the ward. She recognised that it was not possible to meet all the patients' needs. However, perhaps they could do more with the resources available to them?

At this time the team was essentially 'task-oriented': two nurses supervising bathing, another two supervising dressing, whilst two others gave out the medication. And so it went through the day. Evaluation of the patients was largely a subjective affair. At each case review the nurses gave an impressionistic overview of each patient, summarising any 'crises' recorded in the nursing Kardex. As an experiment the charge nurse suggested a trial of REHAB. Although none of the staff had any experience of using any standard form of rating scale, two 30-minute 'workshops' conducted at the staff shift change-over were enough to give each of them the rudiments of completion of the scale. Selecting a patient from the ward, the group 'ran through' the filling in of the scale. Within a month all the patients had been assessed, and profiles on each patient completed. The staff were then able to compare each patient with the rest of the ward, their relative strengths and weaknesses being compared with the norms presented by the authors. It was possible for the first time to rank-order the patients according to their 'disturbed behaviour' and their general social competence. Using the REHAB, patients were allocated to groups, representing the most dependent, the least dependent and an intermediate grouping. Finally, the team was sub-divided into three care teams, each with the responsibility of assessing, evaluating and planning care for their group. Given the size of the teams, overlapping and mutual support were essential.

One year later it is clear that a major change has occurred in the presentation of care on this unit. This can be attributed largely to the 'objective' perspective offered by the REHAB scale. Two other long-stay areas have now begun to use the scale and comparison between patients in different wards is now possible. There are plans to use this assessment in the community units where further comparisons between hospital and hostel residents will be possible. Although the nurse's clinical judgement has in no way been made redundant, it now functions as an adjunct to a wholly objective evaluation of the patient's status.

Conclusion

In this chapter I have reviewed a number of ways of looking at the patient's everyday functioning. I have also suggested that whole wards can be classified more objectively by the use of an objective assessment. Consequently there may be benefits to clinician and administrator. Each of the methods represents an alternative to clinical judgement. Although all of the scales reviewed require some subjective judgement, a framework is offered which makes it more likely that two nurses will 'see' the same performance in the same patient. These methods may not only be used to identify 'problem areas', but can be used to evaluate the development of existing assets, or the amelioration of such problems across time.

The scales reviewed here are of obvious relevance to some patients and not to others. Perhaps they are of most relevance to some elderly people and patients suffering from some 'chronic mental illness'. These groups often display a deterioration in everyday living skill function that represents either an extension of their original 'disorder' or is a function of restrictive care practices. I took the view in my introduction that our task in the assessment of independence was analogous to an architect's overview of the building of a house. It is not enough to know where each of the amenities is sited. We must be able to see each one in relation to the other — a compartmentalised whole. The same is true of patients. People do not function in isolated parts. The attention we pay to our personal hygiene and dress and the manner in which we eat at the table are linked to the kind of relationships we have with people. They influence how others evaluate us and how they act towards us. Engagement in these skills — the very basis of our lives — can also have a profound effect upon how we see ourselves, how we relate to ourselves.

Many nurses have said to me that these scales merely tell them what they already know. In some cases this is true. However, as with any assessment, there is a danger if all the data — or information — are simply stored in a person's head. What happens if they leave the ward? Or if they are off sick? How do others gain access to the 'picture of the patient'? Even if the nurse already 'knows' what the patient is like, how do I get to know what she knows? There is also an argument about cost-efficiency. All the methods described in this chapter allow some kind of summary profile of the patient to be presented. This allows a range of staff to discuss or debate the significance of the information. How long would it take one nurse to retrieve a similar quantity of information from her memory bank? Even if it could be done, the time taken would probably be greatly in excess of that taken to study one of these assessment profiles. More importantly, since her evaluation of the patient would probably take an anecdotal, story-line form, I doubt whether others would find the resultant picture easy to interpret. Perhaps the most important feature of these methods is the opportunity they offer to make comparisons between one patient and another, or between how the patient functioned last year and how he performs at present. They also offer us the chance to compare one group of patients with another. They can do this because they each rely upon a specific measure of a specific pattern of behaviour. Certainly, these tools may simply tell us what we already suspected. We suspect that the patient is dependent in some way: the method tells us in what way. In this sense these tools are very similar to some medical tools. What is a thermometer, after all, if not simply a device which confirms our suspicion that the patient is febrile. We use a thermometer as a back-up assessment, because we doubt the reliability of our clinical judgement. The same principle should prevail in the assessment of living skills. The last word on clinical judgement I leave to the English poet, Alexander Pope:

It is with our judgements as with our watches: no two
go just alike, yet each believes his own.

Notes

1. Henderson appears to have been the first to suggest a specific role for nurses in terms of provision and maintenance of activities of daily living. If she was not the first, then clearly she is the most famous in this respect. V. Henderson, *Basic Principles of Nursing Care* (ICN, Geneva, 1960).
2. Nancy Roper has developed a full account of the role of activities for daily living within nursing care. See N. Roper, *Clinical Experience in Nurse Education* (Churchill Livingstone, Edinburgh, 1976).
3. A number of clinical psychologists have begun using ELSI as an alternative to existing global assessments, especially where they are working with relatively unsophisticated staff. Dr Peter Higson of the North Wales Hospital in Denbigh comments that:

In general the comments and feedback I have received after introducing ELSI in a variety of settings have been very positive. I find this particularly encouraging given that we are dealing with a range of different staff, with quite different professional backgrounds in the different settings . . . compared to most other readily available assessment measures for use with chronic mentally ill people, ELSI has many distinct positive features and advantages, and is the most useful assessment measure I have come across in the last few years. (P. Higson, personal communication)

4. ELSI has been the subject of an extensive research project (1982–4). Readers who are interested in the findings of this study should contact the author for copies of the research report at Tayside Area Clinical Psychology Department, Royal Dundee Liff Hospital, Dundee DD2 5NF.

5. During the research project noted above, a number of centres attempted to indicate regression by (a) blotting out the shaded area with a red adhesive sticker; (b) cross-hatching the shading and (c) cross-hatching in red ink. The problem of regression appears to be a minor one. Less than 10 per cent of the subjects showed any noticeable regression. Since the scale measures skill rather than motivation, we would expect only that small proportion of the population who begin to deteriorate physically to show such regression.

6. At the time of writing (October 1984) the package has been revised again. Two versions are currently available: a modified system which is geared more towards the assessment of more severely handicapped/disabled individuals, and an extended package covering a broader range of the skill areas already described in the text. Anyone who is interested in finding out more about ELSI should write for details to the author.

7. A journalistic account of this exercise has been published in P. Barker, 'Living and Learning', *News-Link*, 3 (1981).

8. K. Kitchin, personal communication.

9. P. Barker and M. Tosh, 'Beyond the Nursing Process', a report to the Tayside Health Board Research Committee, 1984.

10. Peter Higson (see note 3) notes that ELSI has been introduced to aid individualised care planning in the following settings:

(1) a social services hostel for the mentally ill;
(2) a social services day centre for the mentally ill;
(3) an elderly persons' home (social services);
(4) a mixed-sex hospital rehabilitation unit;
(5) a hospital long-stay ward for men.

11. G. Honigfeld, R. O. Gillis and C. J. Klett, 'NOSIE-30: A Treatment Sensitive Ward Behaviour Scale', *Psychological Reports*, **19** (1966), pp. 180–2.

12. D. P. Carbonara, 'The Factorial Invariance of the Nurse's Observational Scale for the Evaluation of In-patients', *Psychological Reports*, **52**(3) (1983), pp. 843–8.

13. NOSIE was one of the measures used in the massive research programme involving long-stay patients directed by G. L. Paul and R. J. Lentz, *Psychosocial Treatment of Chronic Mental Patients* (Harvard University Press, Cambridge, Mass., 1977).

14. For details of REHAB contact Vine Publishing Company, 2a Eden Place, Aberdeen, Scotland (Tel. 0224 35333).

15. A. H. Pattie and C. J. Gilleard, *Clifton Assessment Procedures for the Elderly (CAPE)* (Hodder and Stoughton, London, 1979).

6 WALKING ON THE BRINK: THE ASSESSMENT OF ANXIETY

> Present fears are less than horrible imaginings. —
> Shakespeare

Although we tend to view anxiety as a circumscribed problem, sometimes even as a disease or illness, the experience is a natural one. We cannot afford to live without some degree of anxiety for long: we would either be flattened by the convenient passing of a truck, or consumed by the first tiger seen in our suburb for years. Clearly, there are different kinds of anxiety. Also, there are different degrees of the experience. However, anxiety always occurs when we are under threat — when we are too close to a speeding lorry or a creeping tiger — or when we interpret threat, an interpretation that may be a distortion of reality. Threat is the key. The greater the threat — perceived or actual — the greater the anxiety. We need to *feel* threatened to become anxious.

Despite the impression that anxiety is a modern phenomenon, born of our hi-tech age, it is clear that it has troubled men and women down the ages. Apart from stimulating essential fight or flight, anxiety has also served as the fuel for many a literary and artistic mind. The expression of anxiety through art is common to most 'primitive' cultures, e.g. talismen, voodoo masks and dolls, highly formalised demons and spirits. Such 'abstracted images', which draw out anxiety evoking stimuli from common objects or images, have been found in Western culture only since the beginning of the twentieth century. Abstract art, whether primitive or modern, is thought to reflect the deep anxieties at large in a society. The growth of abstract art in modern times coincided with growing preoccupations with themes of death and decay and the anxiety of living and dying in general.[1] In the world of literature such anxieties are well illustrated in the works of writers like Samuel Beckett and Harold Pinter, both from the world of the so-called 'theatre of the absurb'. Their work is assumed to reflect man's experience in a world shorn of all certainty, a world which generates a conflict between our hopes and our fears.[2] In a sense, what these writers and artists are telling us is hardly new. When people lose — or believe they have lost — the ability to control or cope with their world, they become anxious. In art such loss of control may be symbolic, similar to traditional superstitions. Such fears may have a more practical base. Our twentieth-century 'cultural anxiety' began with the ritual slaughter of the First World War. It appears to be peaking again with the insanity of the nuclear arms race and the political instability of the late twentieth century.

Much of our interest in anxiety in a psychological context will involve an unreasonable or dysfunctional fear of the unknown, or even the non-existent. Such fears appear to have plagued us through the centuries. Thomas Jefferson, the American president, complained once, 'How much have cost us the evils that never happened.' Another American statesman, Benjamin Franklin, advised us 'not to anticipate trouble or worry about what may never happen. Keep in the sunlight.' The problem seems to be, however, that is is difficult to follow Franklin's logical code. As Edmund Burke remarked, 'no passion so effectually robs the mind of all its powers of acting and reasoning as fear'. The 'fear' that our powers of logic and action were so threatened may have led Franklin Roosevelt to ask for a world which was founded upon four freedoms, one of which was freedom from fear. The man or woman who can place his fear or threat in a logical context is likely to experience a reduction of anxiety. The trick seems to involve manipulating those scarce commodities, reason and logic.

Anxiety as a Construct

A *construct* is a statement about some aspect of a person's internal state. In simple terms it is the way we describe the private events that we assume have an influence, or bearing, on the public aspects of a person's behaviour. The construct 'anxiety' is said to have been used first as a translation of Freud's use of the term *angst*. Although derived from the latin *anxietas* ('anxiety, trouble of the mind'), the term is used to denote the experience of negative affect and physiological arousal that is 'similar to the sensation of having food stuck in one's throat'.[3] Although Freud never defined specifically the important features of anxiety, it became the key component in his theory of behaviour disorders. Through time the term has grown in stature, almost achieving a status of a 'thing' in its own right. We often talk about anxiety as though it had a separate existence from the person's experience of it. It has been noted that anxiety can be viewed from a number of angles, almost like a multiple personality.[4] Sometimes we look upon it as simple *behaviour*, when we talk about a person 'appearing anxious'; or as a *personality type*, when we say that someone is an 'anxious individual'; and even as an *explanation* of the way someone behaves — she drinks 'because she is anxious', or he behaves like that as a 'defence against his anxiety'.

If one thing is clear from the vast body of research conducted over the past sixty years, it is that anxiety *is not any one thing*. It is neither an emotional state, nor a personality type, nor an underlying cause of behaviour. Perhaps the most succinct description was offered by Paul, who described anxiety as a shorthand term for a very complex pattern of behaviour, saying that anxiety 'is characterised by subjective feelings of apprehension and tension accompanied by, or associated with, physiological activity'.[5] These feelings — for clearly it is not one single feeling — can occur in response to things that happen to us (external events) or the way we think about what is happening, or has happened, or is about to happen (internal events). To some extent this may help us to appreciate how some anxiety can be seen as natural or 'normal' — for instance when we meet genuinely threatening events like a tiger in the High Street. The stereotype of 'abnormal anxiety' is perhaps the situation where people become anxious in the absence of any such obvious threat. Here, we conclude — rightly or wrongly — that the problem is all inside their heads.

Channels of Anxiety

The anxiety construct can be seen to operate through three main channels. First of all the person shows certain patterns of *motor behaviour*. He may tremble, shake, stutter, back away from a situation or try to escape or avoid the situation completely. This channel represents aspects of anxiety that are visible to the onlooker: we can pick up 'signs' of what we assume to be anxiety. This is especially the case where the person appears uncomfortable, or is manifestly 'running for his life'.

The second channel involves certain *cognitive processes*: what the person says to himself about the situation, and how he interprets his reactions to the situation overall. In this channel the person may attribute certain threatening characteristics to objects or situations that others do not interpret as threatening, or he may simply tell himself that he cannot face or cope with the situation. He may also 'report back' to himself privately, telling himself that his motor behaviour is further proof — if needed — of his inability to handle or cope with the situation. This channel is, of course, a very private channel. Access is only possible if the patient agrees to report to the nurse what he is 'reporting back' to himself. The third channel involves *physiological arousal*: the function of the sympathetic branch of the autonomic nervous system. Typically, the person reacts as though he were under serious life-threatening conditions. He may show changes in heart rate, blood pressure, respiration, muscle tension, sweating, etc. Although these are the classic features of autonomic arousal, other less commonly reported phenomena may be evident, which can often lead to patients assuming that they are going to collapse or even die, since the display of arousal is concomitant with a state of severe illness.

Although these are the three channels of anxiety that are commonly reported, all anxious people need not report all of them to the same degree. Some people may experience severe arousal and 'report back' negative thoughts about the situation *and* their performance, but may appear calm and composed on the surface. Because they manage to control their motor behaviour they manage to disguise their anxiety. A person who is frightened of cats, but who does not want to make a fool of himself, might conceal his anxiety by failing to report it to others. This does not mean that he does not experience it autonomically or does not register it cognitively. 'I felt as though I was going to collapse . . . I just couldn't stop thinking about it looking at me . . . but I couldn't let the others down by running away from it.' In other situations someone might experience arousal and some avoidance behaviour — for instance, when speaking in public for the first time. However, he might attribute this to excitement, or a 'normal state of affairs'. 'Oh, I felt terrible, couldn't stop shaking. I couldn't even look at the audience. But I guess everyone feels like that the first time.' Finally, in the classic fear situation — the dentist's chair — people commonly experience anxiety but make no attempt to avoid the situation. Presumably, the pain of any treatment is less than the discomfort of toothache. Although all three patients in these examples managed to cope with their anxiety, this does not mean that we should not assess it. These examples illustrate the need to establish what anxiety means for the person involved. What does the patient do that denotes anxiety? What does he think about what is happening to him? And how does his body react to the situation in terms of autonomic arousal?

An Unnecessary Title?

Some authorities have argued that the term 'anxiety' is a redundant construct. There has been a strong drive, especially within behaviourism, to drop the term, even as a piece of descriptive shorthand. Instead, attention is paid to the situations which give rise to anxiety, either within the environment or within the patient's own information-processing and physiological functioning. I must admit to some sympathy for this idea. As I noted earlier, there is a danger that we might attribute near 'disease' status to something that is no more than one person's way of reacting to a set of circumstances. The advantages of using the three-channel model of anxiety can be summarised as follows:

(1) It provides us with a framework for collecting information about the *manifestation* of anxiety, or what is actually happening in the case of *this* person.
(2) This framework allows us to collect details of how the three channels operate across different situations, across time, or across treatment.
(3) This information helps us to model our treatment or care plans. Careful examination should reveal the kind of behaviour, thought patterns and physiological arousal which should be the focus of any intervention.

Even is we were to accept the general construct of anxiety, and the implication that this is symptomatic of a personality type, we must question what we have gained by deploying such a label. To meet the needs of the patient we must identify the function of his anxiety. Then we must ask, 'What does the label anxiety tell us about the patient, which is not contained in the three-channel description of his problem?'

The Assessment of Anxiety

Anxiety assessment can be broken down into a number of stages. I shall begin with interviewing, making the assumption that preliminary interviews have identified anxiety as a focal problem. Then I shall discuss some of the indirect measures of anxiety in popular use. Finally, I shall discuss ways of 'observing' anxiety in the real world of the patient.

The Anxiety Analysis Interview

The anxious patient is rarely ever in any doubt about the nature of his complaint. He may be unaware of its origins, causes or other explanations. He is never ignorant of its presence. With this in mind I shall attempt to describe how the interview would try to unravel some of the mysteries of his anxiety state. Using the three-channel model described I shall illustrate a range of possible questions.

The Relationship with the Patient. Before discussing the mechanics of the interview let us acknowledge that assessment of the anxious person is rarely easy. The temptation to 'spare no blushes' and 'get straight to the point' is a tactic that may, ultimately, be to the nurse's disadvantage. Many patients may choose to discuss some trivial fear or phobia, perhaps as a cover for a more severe problem he finds difficult to disclose, especially to a relative stranger. I am not suggesting that the problems that are identified quickly should always be disregarded, in search of some deeper anxiety. Rather, I am warning against the danger of taking the patient at 'face value', especially where insufficient time has been given to establishing a positive relationship, within which the patient may feel comfortable. He already feels under threat: if we want him to disclose details about his problem and his reactions to it, we must avoid threatening him further. It is a sensible strategy to spend some time simply talking to the patient about how he feels, in fairly general terms. Give him a chance to warm up for the interview proper. Many anxious patients may feel inhibited about talking about deeply entrenched fears or worries to a complete stranger. Within this rapport-building session ask him how he feels about being questioned. Does he feel that he is under review? Is he being scrutinised? How does he feel about being interviewed repeatedly by doctors, different nurses, social worker, perhaps also a psychologist? Does he feel that this is an intrusion? How does he feel about you? Give him a chance to articulate these worries if they exist: anxiety about the process of the interview. This casual conversation will help the patient find out something important about the nurse: that she is honest, open and sincere. She is not afraid of resistance or rejection. She is also interested in the patient, rather than just his 'illness'. The nurse is trying to encourage the patient to trust her: trust her with his deepest fears, his irrational-sounding worries, the concerns that at times he thinks are no more than foolish ravings, and that cause him some embarrassment. If the patient expresses any disquiet about the interview, time can be set aside to resolve these anxieties before it begins. By offering the patient 'the first shot' — a chance to make himself heard, *before* the probing begins — the nurse may reduce his anxiety about the whole assessment significantly. The spirit of collaboration begins here, and forms the platform for the rest of the assessment. Once this rapport has been established, the nurse can begin to look *with* the patient at the nature and context of his anxiety.

Q. 'You told me earlier that you get very anxious. Can you tell me what that means to you?' The opening question is as broad as possible. The patient is given a clear field to say anything he wants about how he feels, thinks or acts when he is anxious. The nurse's task is to pick up statements asking him to elaborate, to gain more detail:

> 'You feel awful? How exactly do you feel?' (looking for 'giddy, sweating, palpitations, tense, etc.')
> 'You say that you just panic? What do you do, when you panic?'
> '. . . and what sort of thoughts are running through your mind when you feel like this?'
> 'How bad would you say this feeling is? I mean, is it always the same? Or does it vary? How long does it last? . . . I see . . . and what is "a long time"?'

In these open-ended questions the nurse tries to shape up a more detailed picture of anxiety, in the patient's own words. This might cover:

Motor behaviour: what he does. Does he fidget, get up, walk around, leave the situation, turn away, chain-smoke, talk a lot, get stuck for words?

Thought processes: what does he think? What does he imagine or visualise? 'I can't stand it. I'm going to collapse. It's getting closer. They're looking at me. I must look a fool. My heart's going to burst.'

The nurse's intention is to help the patient express himself, taking care not to put words into his mouth. Don't ask questions like 'Do you ever feel really tense?' unless the patient is finding it difficult to express himself. During the interview reinforce the joint nature of the exercise, saying things like 'OK. Let's have a look at what we have got now. You said first of all that you . . . . . . Is that right? Do you want to change that in any way? I'm just trying to see it as closely as I can from your angle. So that I can understand how you feel.' If the nurse intends to make notes this should be discussed with him at the outset, making explicit the aim of note-keeping — to act as a guide to greater understanding of the problem, for nurse *and* patient.

Q. 'When do you usually feel like this?' This second question tries to identify the situations (or conditions) under which anxiety shows itself. Again the question is open-ended. Follow-up questions will try to nudge him gently towards identifying objects, people, places, events, activities, etc. which relate directly or indirectly to his experience. His anxiety may be focused clearly: fear of dogs, heights, insects, injections, disease or confined spaces are examples of a range of a hundred or more *specific phobias*. In some cases the patient may feel anxious *only* when in the presence of this focal object, animal or situation. It is important to clarify that other situations have not been neglected, especially where one specific situation stimulates high anxiety. It is impossible to deal clearly with anxiety without relating it to the situation which 'triggers' or stimulates it. Within this question it may also be appropriate to ask further *clarification* questions: e.g. '. . . and what is it about spiders that you don't like?' or 'You feel anxious in shops? What is it about shopping — the store, the people, crowds, talking, the queues, traffic in town? Can you tell me exactly?' The patient may have slightly more generalised problems, where a number of situations trigger anxiety. Here it is important to find out which situations are more of a problem than others. For instance, what kind of people trigger anxiety? Strangers, people he knows well, crowds, close contacts? Alternatively, what sort of 'things' does the patient think might harm him? Contact with people, food, animals, toilets, dishcloths, dust? The patient may experience anxiety across a range of apparently unrelated situations such as these. Anxiety may be even more generalised than this. He might feel anxious when meeting people, when he is alone, when on buses, when in shops, when he is in his garden. Highly generalised anxiety like this is often called 'agoraphobia' or 'the agoraphobic syndrome'. Although there are common focal situations reported by a number of 'agoraphobics', all such patients need not have problems with exactly the same situations. Consequently it is important to keep an open mind on what might trigger anxiety, rather than trying to diagnose 'agoraphobia'. In this context it is worth noting that some patients report 'impressions', where their experience of the situation is more important than the situation itself. For instance, many agoraphobics describe feeling anxious in any situation where they cannot identify 'security'. This leads to anxiety in 'public' places, which diminishes when they reach some 'private' place such as home, or even up a side-street. Other patients may describe their impression of an interpersonal contact: 'My mother really stifles me.' The patient's evaluation of the 'stifling presence' of his mother is perhaps more obvious than the fact that he is in the same room as his mother. He may be aware of this 'stifling presence' even when she is not present: this impression may be stimulated by familiar objects, the room or even memories of his mother.

Finally, there is the most generalised anxiety state of all: the so-called free-floating anxiety. This appears to be unrelated to any situation. Research is beginning to show that this phenomenon may not be quite as inexplicable as we once thought.[6] It may be that the experience of anxiety is related to the patient's *perception* of events that may already have passed, may be ongoing or may be imminent. In some cases this perception may be 'subconscious', and the patient may need some assistance to detect his thoughts and beliefs about himself and his situation. Even if we accept the traditional concept of free-floating anxiety we may be able to tie this to events — such as the time of day, when awakening or falling asleep, when lying down, when in the bath, whilst eating etc. The anxiety may, however, be unrelated to any event. In such cases the nurse should attempt to establish when it is present, and when it is absent.

Although the illustrations given of possible 'related events' are fairly classic, I hope that I have indicated the potential breadth of influence. Indeed, some precipitants of anxiety are not concrete events. For some patients it may be the *thought* of doing something (or not having done something) which produces anxiety. This leads us to the next question.

Q. 'Do you ever feel anxious just thinking about something? Perhaps something which has happened, or maybe is about to happen?' This closed question aims to identify any 'anticipatory anxiety'. There are a number of situations where this is likely. The patient who has lived in hospital for a long time may feel apprehensive about living in the community again. What is it about 'living in the community' that frightens him? Many people are apprehensive about meeting people, going to formal functions, making complaints, being interviewed for a job. All of these involve the patient's *expectations* about what might happen. The patient may be painting a vividly threatening scene, which may be more threatening than the reality. To clarify the source of his anxiety the nurse should arrange for the patient to specify thoughts, images and memories which trigger anxiety. If the patient finds this difficult, he might be helped by being invited to do an action replay, re-running the situation where he last felt anxious in his imagination.

Example

I understand how difficult it is for you to answer these questions. Let's try a little experiment. Let's see if we can find out what you are thinking, whenever you get anxious. I often think that this is like an action replay — you know like we see on sports programmes. Lie back and close your eyes. Now just run through, in your mind's eye, what happened the last time you felt anxious. Let's take that incident you mentioned just now. When you started to feel tense in the dayroom, with the other patients. Imagine that you are in your seat. OK.? Try and picture what is going on around you. OK.? Who can you see? What are they doing? How are you feeling? Are you thinking anything about them? Is anyone else about? Are you thinking anything as all this is going on? That's good. Keep it going. Just try to re-live the situation. Just like an action replay.

The nurse should make notes of the comments the patient makes during this exercise. Afterwards she can clarify the relationship between what he was thinking and what was happening around him. This may reveal his 'expectation' that someone was going to say something to him, or do something. This expectation may constitute the threat.

Q. 'We have described how you feel when you are anxious, and what sorts of things appear to be related to those feelings. How do you think you handle those situations? Here the nurse is trying to help the patient to *evaluate* his problem. Although we assume that the patient is unhappy about his anxiety reactions there may be times when he feels that his reactions are acceptable, given the pressures of the situation. In this context we are trying to get a balanced evaluation of his anxiety. We want to distinguish the times when his reactions are appropriate (when he is 'under threat') from the times when his reactions are dysfunctional.

In discussing his reactions it is important to ask whether he ever contributes to the situation which leads to the anxiety experience. For instance, a man once described how he felt anxious each time his wife went out on her own. He was afraid that she might be seeing other men. It might be important to ask him whether he has ever done anything, or not done something, which might cause her to want to hurt him. He may have quarrelled unnecessarily with her, or failed to show her affection. If a person is frightened that people may be laughing at him, has he ever done anything to cause them to express this attitude? Is he socially unskilled in some way? Does he tend to make indiscreet remarks? In this context it is important to broaden out the assessment to include other possible deficiencies: things the patient has not done, errors he has made, skills he may lack, etc., that might contribute in some way to the creation of the anxiety-evoking situation.

Q. *'What happens when you get anxious? How do you cope with it? What do others do, such as members of your family?'* Here we are looking at the outcome of his anxiety. All our actions lead somewhere. They all have some outcome, however subtle. Here we are trying to find out what happened after the onset of the anxiety. Does the patient run home from the shops? Does he call his doctor, and go to bed? Does he take medication to try to calm himself? And how does he feel after taking such action? Does he feel differently after avoiding a crisis? Do his 'coping tactics' make him feel better or worse? If he feels better, does this last, or is it short-lived? What do other people do to try to help him cope? Does he approve of their actions? Does he ask for such assistance? How does he feel about being helped in this way?

By the end of the interview the nurse should have a clearer idea of what the patient calls *his* anxiety reaction. This can be summarised in terms of how he feels (physiologically), what he thinks (cognitively) and what he does (behaviourally). These three channels will be related to some situations which appear to trigger these reactions. These situations may be real, in terms of things which actually happen, or they might involve the anticipation or expectation of what might happen. Some idea of the relative severity and fluctuation of his reactions should also be possible. For example, is his anticipatory anxiety worse, the same or less than anxiety related to 'real events'? It may also be possible to open out this picture by inviting the patient to evaluate his reactions. How appropriate does he think they are? How does he compare his reactions to those of his friends, family, etc. in the same situations? Finally, we would try to gain an insight into how he copes with anxiety. What measures does he take to resolve his difficulty? What do other people do to encourage his tolerance or avoidance of stress?

Some readers may have grasped that what I have described is, unashamedly, a cognitive-behavioural analysis of anxiety. I have not entertained the alternative view of anxiety as a personality trait. I have one simple reason for taking this line. I am assuming that we are trying to assess anxiety in order to help the patient to initiate some strategy which will help him to overcome or come to terms with this problem. The personality model of anxiety is something of a dead end in this respect: change is seen either as an impossibility or very much a long-term venture. If our aim is to help the patient in the short term, this three-channel model seems to be the most straightforward way of understanding the patient's plight. More importantly, it is clear that this structure provides a comfortable working model for nurses who are unfamiliar with the analysis of complex psychological problems. One of my goals in presenting this anxiety analysis model is to allay some of the anxieties of the nurse called upon to pursue such an assessment.

The last stage of the assessment interview is simply to ask the patient for any additional comment. Is there anything he wants to add? Does he have any questions about what has taken place? In this interview the nurse has tried to encourage the patient to adopt the role of 'collaborator' rather than 'guinea pig'. It is appropriate, in winding up the interview, to invite him to comment, or perhaps make a suggestion about where the assessment might go next.

A Stage Further: Indirect Methods

A lot of valuable information can be obtained through interviewing. In some instances this can be a lengthy and arduous process. Often important points are missed. This may be due to the patient's anxiety, the pressure on time, or the nurse's lapses of memory. Various assessment questionnaires and rating scales can be used as an adjunct to the interview. These may help to amplify points raised in the interview or may yield wholly new pieces of information. Methods of indirect assessment have several advantages and only a few disadvantages. In their favour is the fact that a lot of information can be obtained for very little nursing time. The patient can be instructed briefly in the completion of the scale. The information is analysed at the nurse's convenience. The methods I shall describe have all been carefully researched to serve as useful guides to various forms of anxiety. This offers some assurance that they will provide a truly useful overall picture of various facets of the problem, covering areas which the nurse might not have considered in her interview. To some extent a 'good' rating scale looks like a godsend to the less experienced nurse, who may feel that she needs pointers or guidance. However, there are also disadvantages. These paper and pencil methods rarely tell us anything like the whole truth. Patients are often unhappy about having to answer 'true' or 'false' to questions to which they would like to answer 'Sometimes' or 'It depends on the situation.' The situation-specific nature of anxiety is one of the main arguments against the traditional personality trait theories. These assume that the patient will act in exactly the same way in any situation, because of the action of his underlying 'anxious personality'. The reality, shown in a number of studies, is that people vary enormously in their reactions across different situations. This causes some problems for the more specific kinds of anxiety rating scale. The range of situations, or examples, offered may be too limited to catch the patient's actual response. Another problem is that although patients may answer truthfully, what people *say* they would do is not always the same as their actual practice. Consequently it is important to be cautious about relying too heavily upon the patient's reported anxiety. What the patient reports on paper may be different from what he experiences in reality.

Having tried to weigh up the pros and cons of the use of these methods, I am confident that careful selection and cautious interpretation of the findings will help to broaden the picture. These scales may also provide pointers for further questioning or investigation. For example, following the first interview the nurse might choose an appropriate scale, showing the patient how to complete this. She returns later to collect and score the scale, using the findings as the basis for further discussion with the patient. These findings might lead to self-monitoring by the patient himself, or closer observation of the patient's responses by members of the staff team.

What Kind of Method shall we Use?

Many nurses use nothing other than their eyes and ears to assess patients, simply because they do not know where to start in selecting rating scales or questionnaires. Even if they had access to such methods they might not know how to use them. I can appreciate their difficulties. Most indirect methods have been developed by psychologists and psychiatrists, and are often used only in research programmes. Clearly, however, if a method of assessment has proven useful, then as many people as possible should learn to use it. Where would we be if only doctors used thermometers? The methods I shall discuss represent only the tip of an iceberg. Indeed, casual study of various journals that report the development of assessment methods shows that we are spoiled for choice. These methods are, in my view, the most appropriate for nursing use. They are, perhaps, also the most reliable methods available at present for dealing with particular facets of anxiety. I shall deal with each example in turn.

The Assessment of Specific Fears or Phobias

The Fear Survey Schedule (FSS) has been used in clinical and research settings since 1956.[7] In the intervening years a number of variations have been developed. The length of these various schedules ranges from the original 50 items to one with 122 factors listed.[8] A vast amount of research has been done in an attempt to identify the 'best' schedule. Sadly, no clear answer is available. As with many of the indirect measures discussed in this book, these studies have employed university students as the key sample population. The scores used represent, therefore, a biased sample: younger, well-educated, possibly more affluent individuals. As a result, the value of such 'norms' for comparison purposes may be limited.

The schedule does, however, have an important function. It can be used to screen fears or phobias in a patient who is manifestly anxious. One of the most popular schedules is the one developed by Wolpe.[9] This covers 91 fear situations: 'being in a strange place', 'flying insects', 'sick people', 'a lull in the conversation', etc. The patient is asked to indicate how unpleasant or upsetting he finds each situation. A five-point rating scale, ranging from 'not at all' (1) to 'very much' (5) is used for all items. Studies of students suggest that women score significantly higher than men, and report differences in their ratings of specific fears. Both men and women rate 'fear of failure' highest. However, women are more troubled by dead people and rejection by others than men, who rate looking foolish and seeing one person bullying another as more threatening. Despite my scepticism about the value of norms, it is clear that we cannot accept the patient's scores at face value. High scores need not necessarily indicate 'a problem', especially where such a fear is shared by most of the population. However, the scale can show how widespread the patient's anxieties are. The various situations on the schedule can be grouped together under categories: fear of 'noise', 'tissue damage', 'social-interpersonal situations', 'animals', 'classical fears' and a 'miscellaneous' category. This kind of screening may be helpful in identifying a class of fears, where they are evident. Often a patient presenting with a singular fear may show a range of other fears, following completion of the Fear Survey Schedule. Such findings are obviously crucial in terms of planning an appropriate anxiety reduction treatment programme.

The 'Fear Questionnaire' is a similar schedule which uses only 23 items.[10] In the first item the patient is asked to describe his 'phobia' in his own words. In the succeeding 15 items fears involving (e.g.) hospitals, being watched or stared at are rated using a nine-point scale. The patient is asked to indicate whether he would not avoid the situation (0) through to 'always avoid it' (8). A total score is gained through adding items 2–16. The patient then identifies any other situations which he might avoid, again using the same rating. Finally he is asked to rate how troublesome he finds various 'feelings', e.g. 'feeling irritable or angry'. Again a nine-point scale is used to rate the degree of disturbance by these feelings. This is a very useful schedule for distinguishing 'agoraphobic' problems from other common phobias: 'blood-illness-and injury' and 'social phobias'. The scale allows separate scoring for these three phobic areas. Apart from its cost-effectiveness in identifying the presence of various common fears and phobias, the schedule offers a simple yet effective way of monitoring the patient's progress during treatment.

The Facets of Anxiety

One of the key figures in anxiety assessment is William Zung, the American professor of psychiatry. In common with other clinicians and researchers Zung noted that although there was a wide range of methods available for anxiety assessment, either as an affect, a symptom or a disorder, there was no standard method for recording and evaluating anxiety as a clinical entity. By analysing existing scales and noting differences between one and the other, he argued that such was the disparity between different scales that no common target was evident. The rating scale he designed was intended to meet the following criteria. He wanted to devise a scale that would assess the presence or absence of all significant anxiety symptoms, but should also *quantify* the amount of anxiety present by a short and simple method. The method he finally devised is available in two formats. The first is a scale that can be completed by the patient himself, and the other is completed by a member of staff based upon his observation of the patient in an interview. Zung's scale[11] is based upon his analysis of a range of other descriptions of anxiety disorder. These commonly refer to various *affective* symptoms, e.g. apprehension, fear, dread, helplessness. They also describe a range of somatic symptoms: disturbance of the musculo-skeletal system (tension, tremors, weakness, restlessness); the cardiovascular system (palpitations, increased pulse and blood pressure); the respiratory system (dizziness, choking, constrictions in the chest, parasthesia); the gastro-intestinal system (nausea, vomiting, anorexia); the genito-urinary system (urinary frequency or urgency); the skin (flushing, sweating, pallor); the central nervous system (loss of concentration, poor memory, irritability, sleep disturbance, insomnia, nightmares). The scale which Zung finally produced reflected these common symptoms.

Two Formats. The rating scale devised for use by staff is called the Anxiety Status Inventory (ASI). This covers 5 affective and 15 somatic symptoms. A guide is given to help the clinician to interview the patient, using the same approach with each patient. For example, in relation to 'mental disintegration', on the twenty items on the scale, the patient would be asked, 'Do you ever feel that you're falling apart?' His answer would be rated on a four-point scale. This describes the *severity* of the symptom: how intense is it? How long does it last? How often does it occur? The scale awards a score of 1 if the symptom is not present at all, is very slight or does not last long. A score of 4 is given if the symptom is severe in intensity, lasts a long time, or is present most of the time. The following extract illustrates the use of the scale.

Nurse: Have you ever had times when you felt yourself shaking or trembling?

Patient. Oh yes, often.

Nurse. When was the last time you felt like that, *within the last week*?

Patient. Yesterday, when I was speaking to my daughter on the telephone.

Nurse. How bad was the trembling? (intensity)

Patient. I would say pretty bad. I could hardly get my coins into the slot.

Nurse. How long did it last? (duration)

Patient. Only a minute or so. Maybe not even that long. Till I started talking.

Nurse. Over the past week how much of the time would you say that you felt like that: having these trembling attacks? (frequency)

Patient. Oh, perhaps every other day. Sometimes twice a day.

A score (1−4) must then be given which in the *judgement of the interviewer* represents the severity of the particular symptom. This judgement should try to balance what the patient describes with what the patient observes. For instance, the patient may say that she never experiences tremors, but may be shaking visibly during the interview. In making the judgement it is clear that if the patient shows a particular symptom or describes it, or acknowledges that it is a problem, then a high score must be given. If the symptom is not shown, reported or complained of, then a low score may be given. The real difficulty lies in attributing the intermediate scores.

Each of the 20 items should be considered independently. The interviewer must finish scoring one before moving on to the next. At the end of the interview a total score can be given by adding up the scores, the maximum score being 80 and the lowest possible score 20.

The same 20 symptoms are presented on a simple rating scale for completion by the patient. This is called the 'Self-rating Anxiety Scale' (SAS). For example, the symptom 'restlessness' provides the statement, 'I feel calm and can sit still easily.' The patient must indicate one of four responses to this statement by circling 'none or a little of the time'; 'some of the time'; 'a good part of the time'; or 'most or all of the time'. This self-report method has been worded

so that some of the symptoms are phrased symptomatically positive, suggesting that 'I do not have a problem in this area.' Others
are worded negatively, suggesting that 'I do have a problem here.'
This is a safeguard against the patient detecting a trend in his
answers. A code for scoring the scale is provided in Zung's original
article. Once completed, a total score can be converted to an 'index
score' by dividing the score achieved by the total possible (80) and
multiplying by 100. The patient's score can now be compared with
those patients surveyed on Zung's original study. This can help to
judge 'how anxious' the patient under review is, compared with
other psychiatric patients. However, as I have noted earlier, there
are some difficulties in comparing patients in one country with a
sample population in another. Of paramount importance is the fact
that an evaluation of change or progress can be made using the
total scores. Also, it is possible to identify specific symptoms
clearly, evaluating how severe they are, and how they change across
time.

In my experience, this is a valuable assessment method which can
be used by nurses with limited experience. It provides a major
advance on other existing scales and, through its 20-item anxiety
analysis, provides the novice nurse with a valuable framework to
dismantle the complexity of the anxiety state.

Zung's scale can be used as a short cut to identifying exactly how
the patient feels when he is anxious. It can also be used as an
adjunct to the identification of the situations which provoke
anxiety, in these various forms. Consequently Zung's scale has
widespread applicability, from specific to more generalised
anxieties. For instance, a person who is afraid of going out of his
house can tell the nurse exactly how he feels in a variety of situations by using the Zung scale in conjunction with the fear survey
schedule. This will identify *where* he becomes anxious and how he
feels. The combination of the Zung scale and the FSS may prove
useful for a wide range of anxiety problems. However, there are
other anxiety-related disorders which are more specific, and which
require a slightly different approach.

Coping with Anxiety: the Obsessional Individual

One of the commonest maladaptive ways of coping with anxiety is
through the performance of 'obsessive-compulsive behaviour'.
Although it is traditionally viewed as a specific *neurosis*, obsessional thoughts (ruminations) and actions (compulsions) are to be

found in other psychiatric disorders. Here I want to discuss briefly how the presence of these dysfunctional strategies may be clarified. I call these patterns of behaviour 'dysfunctional coping strategies' since this seems to be the simplest possible explanation of their function: the patient engages in obsessive-compulsive behaviour in order to avoid feeling anxious. Typical examples involve taking steps to avoid contamination, avoid making mistakes, etc. In keeping with our original discussion, the patient anticipates some 'threat' and takes steps to avoid it. These coping strategies usually become more of a problem than the perceived threat is ever likely to be.

In line with my argument earlier in the book about the diagnosis of disorders, I see little value in labelling the patient as 'an obsessional'. It seems more important to describe *in what way* his behaviour reflects an obsessional state. What are the key patterns of action or thought that trouble him, or those around him? In line with the functional analysis of anxiety already described, it is appropriate to identify the situations in which 'obsessional' behaviour take place; the events which appear to make it more or less likely; and what happens as a result of these patterns of behaviour. A key question to be asked is, 'How would you feel, or what do you think would happen, if you didn't perform this behaviour?' It is also important to try to gain the patient's views on these thoughts and behaviours. Many authorities have reported that patients presenting with severe 'obsessional disorders' maintain that these behaviour patterns are not a problem to them. In this context it is crucial to assess the patient's view of the 'problem' and also his attitude towards change.

Screening Obsessional Behaviour. A number of sophisticated scales have been developed to assess obsessional behaviour. Many of these have been concerned with identifying obsessional personality traits.[12] Critics have noted that the items in such questionnaires tend to be non-specific, e.g. 'I tend to brood for a long time over a single idea.' This often means that information from such 'measures' tells us little about how the patient practises obsessional behaviour. More specific and highly complex methods have been developed, such as Cooper's Leyton Obsessional Inventory.[13] This provides information about obsessional symptoms and traits. Although different questions are asked for these two categories, some questions are simply phrased differently to try to identify traits appearing in the absence of behaviour. For example, on the subject of cleanliness the patient would be asked, 'Do you regard cleanliness as a virtue in itself?' (a trait question); and 'Do you hate dirt and dirty things?' (a symptom question). The patient is required to answer 'Yes' or 'No' to 69 questions related to thoughts, checking, dirt and contamination, dangerous objects, personal and household cleanliness, order and routine repetition, overconscientiousness, indecision, hoarding and meanness, irritability and moroseness, health and punctuality. Cooper acknowledges that the inventory has some problems, including the time it takes to complete, estimated at around 45 minutes. He also notes that, despite its rigorous appearance, the inventory is still far from comprehensive. In particular it lacks many of the more unpleasant obsessional symptoms, such as blasphemous, obscene or violent thoughts. He also notes that the patient cannot complete the inventory unaided. The person supervising the completion of the inventory must follow a detailed set of instructions in order to minimise any variations due to his participation.

From a nursing viewpoint it is clear that this method could be extremely useful in selected cases or perhaps in the hands of certain nurses. However, a more convenient method of gaining an insight into obsessional problems may be the Maudsley Obsessional Compulsive Inventory. Developed by Rachman and Hodgson,[14] their intention was to construct a simple questionnaire to assess the presence or absence of certain obsessional rituals. The inventory carries 30 questions, to which the patient has to answer 'True' or 'False', circling one or the other. They are told that there are no trick questions and that the answer should be given quickly without spending too much time thinking about the exact meaning of the questions. Typical questions include 'I frequently have to check things (e.g. gas or water taps, doors, etc.) several times.' Or 'I can use a well-kept toilet without hesitation.' The scores on the inventory can be collapsed into categories of different types of obsessional-compulsive behaviour e.g. checking, cleaning, slowness and doubting. Since the authors have published data distinguishing the scores of 100 obsessional patients and 50 'neurotic, non-obsessional' patients, it is possible to judge how obsessional the patient under review is by comparing his scores with those of the two sample populations. The nurse in the average clinical situation might wish to set her sights lower, perhaps using the inventory to pin-point the extent to which the patient complains of checking, cleaning, slowness or doubting. It should be noted, however, that this scale carries only two questions related to obsessional thoughts (ruminations) and is therefore not really appropriate for patients who present with this kind of problem.

Other Targets: Other Methods

The three assessment formats described above are probably the most useful of the available indirect methods in any nursing situation. These will reveal the nature of anxiety, the situations in which it shows itself, and the kind of avoidance tactics in which the patient engages. There are, of course, other indirect methods. The other key area for the exhibition of anxiety is the 'social situation'. As we have noted already, anxiety experienced in the presence of individuals or groups, or in anticipation of meeting people, is a common focus of anxiety. A number of important methods have been developed to assess this problem area. However, because this overlaps with the area of 'interpersonal behaviour' I have left the discussion of these methods to Chapter 8.

Closer Observation

Self-study Methods

Once the anxiety response is defined and some idea of the situations that precipitate attacks is clear, more detailed information can be collected. The patient can also participate in this exercise, providing that he is given some assistance. Two kinds of detail can be added to the picture. The patient may extend the subjective *rating* of the experience of anxiety to his everyday situation; or he may add more details of what he does, and what happens to him, in anxiety-evoking situations.

The Self-rating of Anxiety. In Figure 6.1 I have illustrated a simple anxiety rating scale which the patient can carry in his pocket, recording his anxiety at periods during the day. On the format illustrated the patient records how anxious he feels, using a ten-point scale (0–9) every two hours, from rising to going to bed. This little booklet (10 × 15 cm) fits in his pocket, and requires only a few seconds to note his reactions throughout the day. We have used this format with a wide variety of hospitalised and community-based patients with good success. Of course this format gives no

Figure 6.1

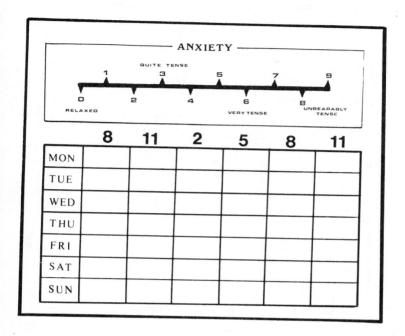

information as to the situations surrounding the anxiety experience. In general, the format is most applicable to 'free-floating anxiety' problems where no specific focal situations are evident, but fluctuations in the level of anxiety do take place. Using this format, it is possible to monitor the rise and fall of anxiety during the day and across longer periods of time. The patient requires little instruction and the method is highly cost-effective.

The Incident Diary. In Figure 6.2 I have illustrated a diary format which can be used to collect more detailed information about the situations that provoke anxiety and the way the patient responds to these situations. The record sheet is broken down into three sections: the setting, the patient's reactions, and the outcome. The patient can summarise any critical incident in which he felt anxious,

Figure 6.2

SETTING	REACTION	OUTCOME
WED - 25th DENNIS TOOK ME SHOPPING — SHOP CROWDED	FELT AS THO' I WAS GOING TO PASS OUT — CHOKING IN MY THROAT	DENNIS TOOK ME OUT — BOUGHT ME A DRINK IN PUB.
WED - 6:00 LONG QUEUES @ BUS STOP	PANICKY FEELING LEGS WOBBLY	DENNIS GOT ME A TAXI — RELIEF
THURS MORNING Mr MILLER ASKED FOR THE ACCOUNTS BY MONDAY	PANIC ++ WENT TO TOILET — CRIED	JENNY SAID SHE WOULD HELP OUT

noting where he was, what was going on around him, what he was doing. These make up the 'setting' for his anxiety reaction. Next, he notes how he felt, what he was thinking, and what he did next. These represent his 'reaction'. Finally, he notes what happened as a result of his reaction. What did other people do? What did they say? How did he feel? What did he think? This format can be filled in as soon as possible after an 'anxiety incident', or regularly each evening, as a résumé of the day's events. This format is appropriate for a wide range of anxiety situations, from the highly specific 'fear of public speaking', which might happen only once a month, to 'interpersonal anxiety', which might occur several times a day.

Self-monitoring of Behaviour. In many situations the number of times the patient does something, or the length of time he spends in that behaviour, may be an important measure of the anxiety experience. For instance, the number of cigarettes smoked, the amount of food 'binged' or the length of time spent 'concentrating' on a book or television programme might help us to appreciate the level of anxiety present. This would be an appropriate procedure for someone who reported chain-smoking, binge-eating or loss of concentration as a result of anxiety. The patient might also be asked to monitor 'avoidance' behaviour: the things he fails to do because of anxiety. A patient who feared he was going to have a heart attack each time he experienced palpitations began to avoid activities he thought physically taxing, e.g. climbing stairs, walking long distances, sexual intercourse. He was asked, therefore, to 'tick off' each time he avoided these activities on a simple checklist. Patients who are frightened of meeting people might be asked to record each time they spoke to someone, distinguishing between 'new' and 'old' acquaintances and perhaps between 'short' and 'long' interactions. Again, a simple checklist can procure this information.

Almost any kind of behaviour, either motor or cognitive, can be self-monitored. Apart from behaviours which involve 'doing' something, the patient may record each time he thinks a certain kind of thought or experiences a certain 'mental image'. Anxious patients often report 'self-defeating' thoughts or impressions. They may think, 'I've made a fool of myself' or 'I'm going to make a mess of this,' or they may imagine that 'People are laughing at me' or 'They must think I'm mad.' Where these thoughts or impressions are regularly repeated a simple checklist may be composed, and the patient asked to tick off each time he has this particular experience. A tally counter can also be used which fits in the pocket or can be attached to the wrist. The patient 'clocks' up negative thoughts or impressions as they occur. A young woman who experienced high levels of anxiety related to a fear of making mistakes recorded between 150 and 200 of these thoughts each day during the assessment stage. This information proved to be more valuable than the experience of anxiety which the thoughts accompanied.

There are some behaviours that it is not appropriate to self-monitor. Subtle 'displays' of anxiety, such as minimal eye contact, speech hesitation, facial touching or repetitive hand movements, may suggest anxiety to an onlooker, but may not be noted by the patient. Even if these are pointed out to him, their subtlety may render them too elusive for self-monitoring. In this context it is worth re-emphasising that self-monitoring can be a tedious procedure for the patient, especially where high levels of the behaviour are evident. This usually means that the activity quickly becomes aversive, and the patient gives up the exercise. This outcome can be avoided by making the exercise as attractive as possible, which is often very difficult, and by giving the patient plenty of encouragement whenever he loses interest, or especially when he completes the record.

Staff Observation

A number of different kinds of staff observation are possible, usually involving a combination of ratings and direct observation of the patient's behaviour. For simplicity's sake I shall divide these into two categories: the 'avoidance test' and observation.

The Avoidance Test. The avoidance test is a format developed by behaviourists to assess the extent to which a person is afraid to approach some feared object or situation. Although commonly used with highly specific fears, such as spiders, snakes, etc., the format can be used for almost any situation. The patient is asked to *approach* the situation he fears. He might be asked to walk across the room to a cage with a cat in it, pick up the cat and hold it to his chest. The 'measure' of his anxiety will be based upon *how far* across the room he can get, or how long he can remain within a certain distance of the feared object. The patient is advised that he can end the test at any time by simply asking for it to be stopped.

This would, of course, also provide valuable information about time tolerance. The nature of the patient's anxiety would influence the organisatio.i of the test. If he was afraid of touching an animal, then the test would include this as part of the instruction. If he couldn't stay in a room with the door closed, this situation would be arranged to assess 'how long' he could remain there. Someone who is afraid of heights might be asked to climb a ladder, counting the number of steps he climbs before coming down. The avoidance test is usually conducted under artificial conditions. This represents its major weakness. In real life the patient is under a *range* of pressures: not simply the one, single 'stress factor' we are assessing in this experimental context. The very fact that the patient is being studied, and perhaps also accompanied, makes this test markedly different from normal. Finally, the fact that the patient can terminate the painful experience makes the test wholly unrealistic. In real life he would have to tolerate the distress or risk possible social sanctions by 'escaping'. The avoidance test makes it almost 'acceptable' to take this escape route. Despite these drawbacks, this exercise can be very useful in certain cases. Providing that the same format is used all the time, it will be possible to compare the patient's performance before and after treatment. The assessment experiment may also provide useful pointers for the design of an appropriate therapy strategy. In this sense the advantages may outweigh the drawbacks.

Observation in the Natural Environment. The problems noted above regarding the 'unreality' of the avoidance test can be overcome by transferring this experiment to the patient's natural environment. The patient who becomes anxious in crowds can be assessed as the nurse accompanies him down a busy shopping precinct. The patient who experiences anxiety when confronted by any sharp object can be observed as he handles cutlery, needles and gardening tools at home. The patient who is afraid of certain animals can be assessed at the local zoo, pet shop or in the city square, which is thronged with pigeons. This approach is not without problems. The presence of the 'observer' can influence the behaviour of the patient, usually making things easier because of assumed moral support. The nurse may find it inconvenient to take one patient out on such an assessment trip. If she can afford the time she may be uncertain as to what kind of information to collect. Despite all these practical problems I think that this *in vivo* assessment technique has much to recommend it. The nurse has an opportunity to study the reactions that the patient has described. She also has an opportunity to note facets of the problem, or his coping style, that he may have omitted. It is almost impossible to recreate an anxiety-evoking scene under artifical conditions. Perhaps the simplest solution is to head straight for the real world. Many of the situations the patient describes may be near at hand, in any case. Crowds, queues, heights, animals, friends, needles, confined spaces, insects, people staring, people laughing, and being alone are all situations in which people report anxiety. These situations are either naturally available in a hospital or can be organised to look natural without much difficulty. For the hospitalised patient, assessment in the natural environment may be only a few minutes' walk away.

What kind of information should be collected in this situation? My preference lies in the direction of collecting as much information as possible. Most of the direct measures — of how close, how high, how many people, how long he remained in the situation — can be recorded fairly easily. These can be combined with ratings, by the nurse and by the patient himself, of anxiety at various points during the exercise. Finally, the nurse might make short notes on changes in the patient's behaviour in response to changes in the situation, points which may not have been noted previously. For example, I was once accompanying a man who was afraid to travel in a lift when the lift jammed. I was able to study his reaction at close range, and was able to compare his relatively cool response with my own panic reaction. This proved to be an insightful experience for both myself and the patient.

Other Direct Observational Methods. Two other ways of studying the patient's reactions are possible. Both of these involve 'artificial situations'. In the first a *role play* is arranged in which people act out the sequence of events that leads to the onset of anxiety. The patient is encouraged to imagine that he is in the real situation, requiring him to attribute 'real' status to the other performers, usually other patients or members of staff. This is usually used in social or interpersonal anxiety and will be covered in detail in the chapter on relationships. The second method involves 'representations' of the problem situation. The patient who is frightened of the sound of thunder, rushing water or traffic may be assessed by studying his reactions to such sound played on a tape recorder.

This approach may be the easiest or the only way to test the patient's reactions. This kind of 'experiment' may be much less time-consuming than taking the patient to the real-life setting. On the other hand, the sounds he is frightened by may be so unpredictable — like thunder — that planning of the assessment may be a near impossibility. Visual material, either in the form of photographs or video-tape recordings, may also be used for common fears, e.g. animals, crowds, heights, etc. In some cases these experiments may suggest that 'no anxiety' is experienced under these simulated conditions. However, even where the patient's response is 'unrealistic', these simulations can be used to help explore the kinds of feelings and thoughts the patient experiences when confronted by such scenes. In this sense, the use of such aids may be indicated where the patient is unable to explain exactly how he feels in such situations. Recordings, photographs or film material may help him to express his anxiety in a verbal manner.

Summary

Anxiety is probably the single most common clinical problem and represents an experience which is shared by highly disturbed patients and the normal public alike. Anxiety can express itself through various other disorders or may be seen as a problem in its own right. In this chapter I have tried to talk about anxiety as something which can be a problem to the autistic child as much as the disoriented adult. In between there is a range of people who may show a highly characteristic kind of anxiety, such as the obsessional individual, or who have difficulties which are remarkable in terms of their diffuseness — the free-floating anxiety. I have tried to demystify the problem by defining it in terms of the three channels of functioning that are involved. Through this understanding of anxiety we can begin to examine the relationship between the patient's world and disruptions of his physiological, cognitive or behavioural state. We can also start to understand how these aspects of the person play a part in maintaining the problem.

Notes

1. See A. Ehrenzweig, *The Hidden Order of Art* (Paladin, London, 1970), p. 292.
2. M. Esslin, *The Theatre of the Absurd* (Penguin Books, Harmondsworth, 1968).

3. T. R. Sarbin, 'Anxiety: Reification of a Metaphor', *Archives of General Psychiatry*, **10** (1964), pp. 630–3.

4. This view was expressed by T. D. Borkovec, T. C. Weerts and D. A. Bernstein, 'Assessment of anxiety' in A. R. Ciminero, K. S. Calhoun and H. E. Adams (eds.), *Handbook of Behavioural Assessment* (John Wiley, New York, 1972).

5. G. L. Paul, 'Outcome of Systematic Desensitisation I: Background, Procedures and Uncontrolled Reports of Individual Treatment' in C. M. Franks (ed.), *Behaviour Therapy: Appraisal and Status* (McGraw-Hill, New York, 1969), p. 64.

6. A. T. Beck, *Cognitive Therapy and the Emotional Disorders* (International Universities Press, New York, 1978).

7. D. A. Akutagawa appears to have been the first to develop a Fear Survey Schedule: 'A Study in Construct Validity of the Psychoanalytic Concept of Latent Anxiety and a Test of Projection Distance Hypothesis', unpublished doctoral dissertation, University of Pittsburgh, 1956.

8. For a detailed history of the development of the Fear Survey Schedule see D. L. Tasto, 'Self Report Schedules and Inventories' in Ciminero, Calhoun and Adams, *Handbook of Behavioural Assessment*.

9. J. Wolpe, *The Practice of Behaviour Therapy* (Pergamon, New York, 1973).

10. I. M. Marks and A. M. Mathews, 'Fear Questionnaire', *Behaviour Research and Therapy*, **17** (1979), p. 264.

11. W. K. Zung, 'A Rating Instrument for Anxiety Disorders', *Psychosomatics*, **12** (1971), p. 371–9.

12. J. Sandler and A. Hazari, 'The Obsessional: On the Psychological Classification of Obsessional Character Traits and Symptoms', *British Journal of Medical Psychology*, **33** (1960), pp. 113–22.

13. J. Cooper, 'The Leyton Obsessional Inventory', *Psychological Medicine*, **1** (1970), pp. 48–64.

14. R. J. Hodgson and S. Rachman, 'Obsessional Compulsive Complaints', *Behaviour Research and Therapy*, **15** (1977), pp. 389–95.

7 PLUMBING THE DEPTHS: THE ASSESSMENT OF MOOD

Yet there's no one to beat you
No one to defeat you
'Cept the thoughts of yourself feeling bad — Bob Dylan

Parallels to many of the experiences we associate with psychiatric disorder can be found in the works of the great writers, poets and artists. In many ways, the experiences associated with mental disturbance are universal: they are features that are common to nearly the whole human race. The only difference is that in true psychiatric disturbance these experiences are exaggerated or distorted far beyond the range encountered by 'normal people'. Depression is perhaps most typical of such a universal experience. Some people will never experience extreme anxiety, and many people will never experience the kind of perceptual disturbance we associate with psychotic states. How many of us, however, can pass through life without experiencing the depths of despair, or severe unhappiness, even where such an experience is short-lived and natural, as in bereavement? The answer is, probably, none of us. The inevitability of our chance encounters with despair led Homer to conclude, somewhat pessimistically, that 'twins from birth are misery and Man'.

Yet, some people can be unhappy without apparently being inconvenienced by their low spirits. We all have encountered the stereotyped pessimist, that classic 'prophet of doom' who repeatedly moans about this or that, who never deviates from his sober expression, and who can always manage to see the black side of any happy event. In principle, he is the classic depressive personality. But is he? His view of the world is undoubtedly negative. Yet this jaundiced perspective does not seem to obstruct him: he is not disabled, or handicapped in any way. He is unlikely to commit suicide, although on the surface his life appears to lack any real purpose, and is a thoroughly joyless experience. Perhaps, however, he enjoys being pessimistic. Perhaps his crusade, which involves deflating egos, demystifying wonders, collapsing dreams, and generally bringing everyone down to earth with a thump, should give us an important clue. Perhaps the whole point of his life is to make the rest of us aware of the futility and pointlessness of our life-experience. Although the pessimist shows a lot of depressive features, he is in no way disabled by these 'abnormalities'. The absence of any impairment is crucial. In this chapter we want to discuss people who not only appear despairing, unhappy or even ridiculously happy — given the circumstances — but who also are restrained, obstructed or eventually defeated by their state of apparent, or disguised, melancholy.

It is interesting to note that the term 'melancholy' is being revived in psychiatric circles.[1] This shows how many of our 'advances' involve moving in a full circle: the completion of a true revolution. Melancholy is one of the four classic humours of ancient times. In attempting to understand the role and function of 'unhappiness' in our lives, many a philosopher or poet has compared depression to *true* vision. Instead of assuming that depression is a weakness or in any way pathological, some have argued that the depressive sees the world stripped of all falsehood and superficiality. However, this may become a surreal, nightmarish vision that he cannot handle. For example, Lord Byron believed that 'melancholy is a fearful *gift*; what is it but the telescope of truth, which brings life near in utter darkness, making the cold reality too real?' This idea is reinforced in quite a different context by some of the anti-psychiatrists who viewed the 'insane' as having more insight and understanding than those who were not psychiatrically disturbed. The *contrast* between pleasuable and unhappy experiences is another common area of interest for poets. Shakespeare, among others, notes how our misery is heightened, rather than reduced, by our awareness of the happiness of others. 'Oh how bitter it is to look into happiness through another man's eyes.' The Western cultural tradition has established and maintained the idea that sorrow, struggle and unhappiness are all part of the rich tapestry of life. Seneca, the Stoic philosopher, warned us against extremes, however. 'An excess of sorrow is as foolish as profuse laughter; while on the other hand, not to mourn at all is insensibility.' From such a history of ideas has developed the traditional view that deep and sustained despair (melancholia) or extreme happiness (mania) are disturbances of our normal reactions to the world and its events. In recent years the view that depression is a 'perceptual problem' — brought about by the person's distorted view of his world — has grown in popularity. This cognitive model involves a re-working of a theme that has intrigued the poets and philosophers down the ages. La Roche-foucauld, in the seventeenth century, shared Bob Dylan's later view that thought was a crucial factor. 'No person is either so happy or unhappy as he *imagines*.' The heritage of today's cognitive theories can be traced back even further to Dante, the great thirteenth-century Italian poet. He would have had little time for the lay-person's 'Come on, cheer up' philosophy, observing that 'there is no greater grief than to recall a time of happiness when in misery'. The recognition that our thoughts, perceptions and even our memories can play a part in the construction and maintenance of the emotion of depression is an important issue, and one to which we shall return over and over again in the course of this chapter.

Affective Disturbance

The term 'mood' (or 'affect') is an umbrella expression encompassing all emotional states. Commonly, however, the term 'affective disturbance' is reserved almost exclusively for a *depression* of mood — when the person is manifestly 'low in spirits' — or *mania* — where an exaggerated happiness or excitement is evident. Since we have discussed anxiety, the other key emotional problem, already, and partly for the sake of simplicity, I shall restrict my discussion of *mood* to the presence of absence of an *adaptive* state of happiness or well-being. I shall say little about 'normal affect'. As Chateaubriand, the French author and statesman, observed, when it comes to unhappiness it is very much an individual affair:

> One can never be the judge of another's grief. That which is sorrow to one, to another is joy. Let us not dispute with anyone concerning the reality of his sufferings; it is with sorrow as with countries — each man has his own.

I shall try to stick to this person-centred philosophy, whilst at the same time acknowledging that the use of some standardised measure to judge the relative weight of despair of all sufferers can also be helpful.

The depressions — for surely these states are many and varied — are a major problem in psychiatric practice. Apart from the significant population afflicted with affective disorder,[2] there are many other groups who suffer mood disturbance as a function of some other problem of living. I have noted earlier that there is much debate over the causes and treatment of mot psychiatric disorders (see Chapter 1). However, despite these disputes there is, at least, agreement over the definition of the disorders. It would appear that this cannot be said of the depressions. We appear to be undecided as to the very nature of the problem: is it a single symptom, or is it a syndrome involving a group of disease symptoms?[3] The whole position is confused even further when we realise that writers not only disagree about the symptoms of depression,[4] but also that many of these symptoms are not peculiar to depression, existing within other disorder definitions. Traditionally, depression has been listed under a range of diagnostic headings: *psychoses* — e.g. involutional melancholia, manic-depressive illness; *psychoneuroses* — e.g. depressive neurosis; and *personality disorder* — cyclothymia. Commonly, a disturbance has been made between 'reactive' depression, where some external event — such as bereavement — is used to explain the disturbance of affect, and endogenous (or psychotic) depression, where no such obvious factors can be identified and the depression is assumed to arise from *within* the person. Recently, this distinction has fallen into disfavour. Researchers have begun to explode the myth that external factors relate to one group and not the other. Some writers have suggested that the best way to look at the problem is to use a three-way classification. In the first class we could include problems such as 'normal grief'; in the second depression which is secondary to some other problem, such as agoraphobia; reserving the third for 'primary' affective disorders, usually referred to as 'unipolar' or 'bipolar' disorder. In the first of these disorders only depression is shown. In the second, depression and mania are commonly present. Despite the practical, common-sense appearance of this classification system, it is clear that *severity* is the most commonly used way of classifying the problem. Close behind is the presence of accompanying, non-depressive symptoms, and the attitude of the clinician, especially his attitude towards the assumed 'cause' of the problem. I make these observations simply to draw the reader's attention to the fact that depression is a complex phenomenon, which can mean many different things to different clinicians. It seems clear that depression is a major problem that manifests itself in a variety of guises. Common to all these subgroups is a common group of symptoms. This depressive thread is highlighted by many of the assessment systems, which we shall discuss in a moment. In view of the confusion that appears to exist in the field at present, it is important that nurses are fairly confident about *what* they want to study, in order to understand the patient's disturbance of affect. In this chapter I shall try to offer some suggestions that might encourage just such an orientation.

The Assessment Targets

The present state of depression research has two important messages for nursing. First, we should understand that a generally accepted classification does not exist. Consequently, we should acknowledge that we may well not be dealing with a single problem. The 'depressed person' could be suffering from any one of a number of disorders, none of which are defined unequivocally. Second, the term 'depression' is a classic 'umbrella' concept, embracing a wide range of symptoms, behaviours or aspects of the patient's functioning. As we have noted already, when one person talks about depression, he need not necessarily embrace the same group of symptoms as the next person. In the light of these observations, nurses should concentrate more upon the study of 'what the patient complains of' (i.e. his behaviour), paying less attention to the study of his assumed disorder. This orientation might help them to appreciate more fully the relationship between the patient's problems of affect and other facets of his life-experience. In this sense we are trying to follow Chateaubriand's advice by accepting the patient's reality of his own suffering.

When I use the term 'target' I mean an aspect of the patient's functioning that we single out for close attention in the assessment process. Despite the disagreements over the definition of depression, there is some agreement about the kind of behaviour patterns that characterise the disorder.

Mood. Disturbance of mood (or affect) is central to the problem. The patient may complain of feelings of sadness, loss of enjoyment, loss of feeling itself. He may report losing interest in things, feeling apathetic and bored with life. He may also complain of anxiety, which can be either psychic, in terms of worrying thoughts, or physical, shown through tension, for example. Not all patients will complain of all, or indeed any, of these problems. Some patients will report feeling well, despite appearances to the contrary. Other patients may emphasise physical distress, such as pain, at the expense of reporting their mental symptoms. Such patients may only admit to feeling sad, unhappy, tense, etc. if asked directly. Indeed, some patients find it easier to report 'physical' symptoms where psychological problems either embarrass or confuse them.

Behaviour. Change in the patient's observable behaviour is commonly observed. He may show a marked reduction in activity, doing less, saying less than is habitual or routine. In parallel with these behavioural *deficits* may emerge certain excesses. He may complain more: about financial worries, problems at work, lack of affection, etc. He may also lose his temper more often, become upset more quickly, or spend more time checking pieces of work — displaying his indecisiveness. All these patterns of behaviour are observable to friends and family, and may be the first signs that 'something is wrong'.

Physical state. The patient may also complain of certain somatic problems. These are related to disruptions or dysfunctions on a biological level. Pain, tiredness, loss of appetite, urinary disturbance, sleep disruption and loss of sex drive may all be reported. Occasionally, he may report chest pains and tachycardia, similar to the experiences of the anxious patient.

Thinking. Three main kinds of cognitive, or thought, disturbance are possible. The patient may experience low self-esteem, and overall evaluation of himself may be poor; he may think that he is a failure, hopeless, inadequate or in general 'powerless' to control his situation. Second, he may have negative expectations. He may see only the gloom ahead. He may see no light at the end of the tunnel when things go wrong, thinking that things will never improve. Lastly, he may blame himself for things that are not his fault, 'accepting' blame which should be attributed to others. Or he may severely criticise himself for things he has done, perhaps in the distant past; or for things he *believes* he has done, or has failed to do.

Motivation. Finally, the patient may be unable to tackle things he 'needs' to do, or seems unwilling to try that might — in the views of others — make him feel better. The patient may see no point in doing anything, believing that he will get no enjoyment out of it; or that he hasn't got the energy; or that he couldn't do it, even if he tried.

The Assessment Interview

If the patient is depressed he may be reluctant to be interviewed. Although this is not true of all depressed patients, the withdrawn or uncommunicative patient poses the biggest problem for the nurse. I shall take this, therefore, as the model for our hypothetical interview. How does the nurse cope with a patient who appears unwilling or unable to provide the information she needs? There is no simple solution. In the following notes I merely make some suggestions about how the interview might be structured to some advantage.

The Beginning. The patient should be given some simple outline of the nurse's intentions. These should be offered in a confidential and confident manner. She should try to suggest that she is there to help the patient express how he feels: not to diagnose, judge or otherwise label him. If her aim is to help amplify a medical assessment, she should say so. If the aim is to provide guidelines for the nursing team, this should also be indicated in a simple straightforward manner. These proposals should be put forward in the form of suggestions, which the patient may reject if he so wishes. By doing so the nurse is trying to establish some *collaboration*, from the outset.

Example

Hello, John. Do you mind if I sit down and talk to you for a few minutes? I wanted to have a word with you about how you're feeling today. Do you feel up to that just now? I know that you've been quizzed quite a bit already, but I haven't got a long list of questions. I just wanted to find out how you are feeling . . . so that we can get some idea of what is bothering you . . . any problems you may have that we might be able to help you with. OK?

Labelling. I have already begun this chapter with a prejudice. I have mentioned 'depressed' people a number of times. I hope that you accept that as a convenient hunch or hypothesis, which shall be investigated in the assessment. This raises an interesting point. Often we check the patient's notes on admission or following an inter-ward transfer, to see what he 'is suffering from'. We cannot close our eyes to such diagnostic criteria. However, if we begin our assessment with some label fixed in the forefront of our minds we may only look for, and find, evidence to confirm someone else's diagnostic prejudices. If we can stick to the person-centred approach described in the early chapters, existing diagnoses may prove to be less of a filter of our experience of the patient.

Structuring the Questions. If the patient finds it difficult to answer questions, the nurse should take a more active role. At least initially, the line of questioning should be more direct, perhaps using closed questions, which are short and well punctuated, to help the patient concentrate and absorb their meaning. Where the patient fails to answer, the question should be rephrased or another topic selected. Silences should be avoided. It is now generally accepted that where the patient is passive or withdrawn the nurse should become more active to compensate for this. Silences serve only to allow the patient more time to reflect upon his inability to answer simple questions.[5] He may also attribute incorrect negative attitudes to his interviewer.

> (Thinks) I can't even answer a simple question. This just shows how far gone I am. She must think that I'm hopeless. That's it. I'm hopeless. What's the point any more.

The General Picture

Our first step is to establish an overview of the patient's problems as he sees them. We begin by asking how he feels? This can be extended to cover other facets of his experience: how is he getting on with others? How is he sleeping or eating? Can he concentrate at work, television, etc. Is he still going out or doing the sorts of things which are part of his routine? Many patients volunteer such information. They have already judged that 'something is wrong' because of changes in one or more of these areas. Where the patient is more withdrawn it may be helpful to structure the questions around the kind of 'problem list' shown in Figure 7.1. This can act as a cue, ensuring that discussion of none of the typical problem areas is omitted. The nurse should review her information at intervals, allowing the patient to add or withdraw comments as he desires. Giving feedback like this can also help ensure that the patient is 'tuned in' to the interview: is he taking part or merely 'sitting in'?

Figure 7.1

NAME .... WARD ....

DATE OF ASSESSMENT .... ASSESSMENT No. ....

PROBLEM LIST
AFFECT   Sadness
          Anger
          Anxiety
          Guilt
          Shame
          Other (specify)

MOTIVATION
          Avoidance
          Dependency
          Reduced activity
          Other (specify)

COGNITION
          Indecisiveness
          Self-criticism
          Overwhelmed
          Concentration loss
          Memory loss
          Absolutist thinking

BEHAVIOUR
          Passivity
          Coping deficits
          Social skill deficits

PHYSIOLOGY
          Sleep
          Appetite
          Sex

Example 1

From what you have said you seem to have some problems with sleeping — mainly getting off at night. Occasionally you waken early, but not every morning? You are also having trouble at home. Your eldest son has been taking drugs and you are worried about him. You also worry a lot about your husband. He isn't sleeping with you any more. You feel that this may be your fault. How do you feel about that? Is that an accurate reflection of what we have discussed so far? Have I left anything out, perhaps? Is there anything you want to change?

Example 2
We have talked a bit about your problems. How you feel about various things. Trying to get things into perspective. Do you think that you could summarise the points I have made so far? Just to see if you and I are in agreement?

In the first example the patient is given a potted summary of the interview, to check and modify if he wishes. In the second example he is asked to *evaluate* the discussion which has just taken place. If he can do this, it shows that he has been participating fully. If he gets lost, it may be an indication that the nurse needs to adapt her style slightly, perhaps asking shorter questions and summarising points as she goes along. This procedure also has a therapeutic value. By discussing, defining, clarifying and then summarising the whole conversation, the patient may begin to see his problems more clearly. This may offer him some relief.

Support and Stress

The level of support and stress is crucial in most psychiatric disorders. In depression the role of such life events may be even more significant. The nurse should ask detailed questions about the significant people in the patient's life. What role do they play in supporting him? The relationship format discussed in the next chapter may be helpful in this respect. The nurse should ask about his family, friends and other people in his life. Are they close confidants? Or are they the kind of people who avoid or resent such disclosures? This part of the interview establishes the level of support present. Who can the patient depend on, in what way and to what extent?

It is also important to establish the role of any significant stress factors. Is he in any debt? Threatened with divorce or separation? Is he experiencing any interpersonal conflict — with family, friends, employer, etc.? What about his home? Does he have problems with repairs? electricity? troublesome neighbours, etc.? Here the patient should be encouraged to identify features of his life that are causing distress, or that he perceives as distressing, as well as the existing support services he draws upon to reduce this.

Coping and Self-esteem

The patient who is depressed will find no difficulty in listing his faults and inadequacies. For this reason it is important to restore some balance. What does the other side of this 'personality coin' look like? What are the patient's assets? What sort of coping skills are still present? In order to establish this, the patient might be asked to describe how he deals with difficult situations — no matter how inadequately.

Example

You have been under a lot of strain recently. You moved house and then found that it had dry rot. Then your wife fell ill and you had to look after her when she came out of hospital. How did you cope with all of that?

The patient may be aware of no coping abilities. He may see himself as a complete write-off. Where this is the case the question may be framed in a different manner:

Example

I can appreciate how you feel. You feel that you buckled under the strain of all that upheaval and illness. Obviously you didn't cope at the end. You failed to some extent to hold your own. What made you seek help? Perhaps that was a sign that you weren't 'all washed up'? You had the presence of mind to look for assistance?

Where the patient feels defeated and hopeless he may toy with the idea of suicide. He may comment upon the pointlessness of his existence. He has no assets. He is worthless. In such cases it might be worth asking what is preventing him from committing suicide right now? This question might elicit some comment about religious beliefs, loyalty to family, or the chance that something might turn up — the Micawber syndrome. These replies may reflect the values or ideas which help him continue living, fighting or trying to avoid further descent into depression and suicide. These are also important assets in his overall self-concept.

On a similar level, what is the patient's view of himself? There is a temptation here to invite the patient to comment upon his successful job, the success of his family, his qualifications and various other 'merits', in an attempt to correct his negative view of himself. The assessment is a premature place to do this: the patient may 'accept' the argument presented simply to escape from further discussion. Instead of trying to correct his style of thinking, the patient should be engineered into admitting — however reservedly — what his assets are. Are you punctual? Do you talk about people behind their backs? Are you loyal to friends? Have you ever made anything with your hands? These questions are carefully phrased to elicit a 'Yes/No' answer, in which the chances are that 'Yes' will occur more often than 'No.' By such a line of questioning, a picture of the patient's present — or recent past — assets is possible.

Translation of Problems

The interview may produce only the vaguest of problems: 'I just can't cope any more. Life is pointless. I'm all washed up.' At the end of the interview it may be necessary to try to re-define these vague problems more clearly. *What* does the patient feel that he cannot cope with, any longer? Arguments at home? His job? His weight? The size of his overdraft? In some cases he may say *everything*. This may indeed be the way he feels. However, it is important to check that some problems are not more acute and troublesome than others. Where the patient feels that life is pointless, he may be ignoring — or minimising — the importance of some things. Does he feel that everything is pointless? Or are some things more important than others, no matter how small? In translating the problem, the nurse should try to define, using the patient's own words, the affective difficulties he is experiencing.

Presentation and Appearance

The final task in the interview is to summarise the appearance of the patient. Many of the points covered in the next chapter will be of relevance here. How is the patient dressed: is he untidy or poorly groomed? Is he smart and clean shaven? Does he appear to have made an effort with his appearance? How long does he take to answer questions? Does he appear hesitant in his replies? Does he avoid eye contact, stare or frequently close his eyes? Does he sit facing the nurse or turned away from her? Does he use gestures, making use of his hands to express himself, nodding appropriately? Or does he appear rigid, frozen, perhaps clasping himself tightly? At the end of the interview it is important to summarise the non-verbal qualities of the patient, as a back-up to the verbal information that has been collected.

At the end of the interview, or perhaps series of interviews, a picture of how the patient is functioning, across the various areas of behaviour, emotion, physical and psychological states, will be available. This will be based mainly upon what he has reported. However, the nurse's close observation of his appearance and behaviour during the interview may indicate levels of pain, discomfort, restlessness, loss of concentration, etc. that he fails to report or perhaps wishes to keep a secret.

Standardised Methods

Self-report Methods

A number of self-report methods have been developed to help depressed patients describe their experience. This allows their distress to be measured in some way.

The Beck Depression Inventory. One of the earlier self-report methods, the BDI is still viewed by many as the best available measure of the severity of depression. The scale covers 21 items, which are presented in the form of four statements. The patient is asked to read through the statements, circling the one that most closely corresponds with his present experience. The BDI covers various facets of affective disorder, e.g. feelings of sadness, shame, guilt and disappointment, as well as thoughts about appearance, decision-making, work, etc. A number of physical factors are also included, such as eating, sleeping, weight loss and sex. A typical item looks like this:

0 = I don't feel that I am worse than anybody else
1 = I am critical of myself for my weaknesses and faults
2 = I blame myself all the time for my faults
3 = I blame myself for everything bad that happens

The inventory is scored simply by totalling the scores circled by the patient in his replies. A vast amount of research has been done with this scale and Beck has published norms that allow us to judge how severely depressed the patient is by comparing the patient's score with various gradings of mild, moderate and severe depression. The BDI can be used as a screening assessment to see whether any depression exists. It may also be used as a pre- and post-treatment measure to evaluate the effect of various kinds of therapy. Where the patient is chronically depressed, the scale may be given at regular intervals to monitor changes in mood. The scale is very simple to administer and can be completed by the patient in a matter of minutes. Where the patient is more severely depressed it may be more appropriate for the nurse to read out each of the statements slowly, asking the patient to indicate which reflects how he feels.[6, 7]

The Zung Self-rating Scale. Developed in 1965, this scale is made up of 20 self-statements.[8] The patient is required to rate each one using a four-point rating scale. Two of the items deal with affect, 8 with physiological and 10 with psychological equivalents of affect. Typical examples are:

I get tired for no reason (physiological)
I still enjoy the things I used to (psychological)

Each of the statements is rated on a scale ranging from 1 — 'a little of the time' to 4 — 'most of the time'. The statements are balanced between negative and positive expressions. This is shown in the two examples: the first is negative, the second positive. This format is used to avoid sterotyped answers where the patient simply scores each statement in the same way. Because of this positive/negative balance the scores run 1–4 for negative items and 4–1 for positive items. The higher the final score, the more depressed the patient. Zung designed this scale to provide a quick and short assessment. He felt that existing scales were too long or time-consuming for the patient, especially if he was having psychomotor problems. The scale has gained some popularity as a convenient tool for assessing the general level of depression. However, some concern has been expressed about its lack of sophistication in a psychometric sense.

The Visual Analogue. A number of studies have used a simple visual analogue scale to measure the general feeling of depression. A line 100 mm long has been used to gauge the severity of depression: the patient simply puts a mark on the line to indicate his perceived level of depression. It has been argued that this method is sufficient for most clinical purposes and is almost as accurate as much more detailed and sophisticated interview methods.[9] In our research with depressed women my colleagues and I have developed

Figure 7.2

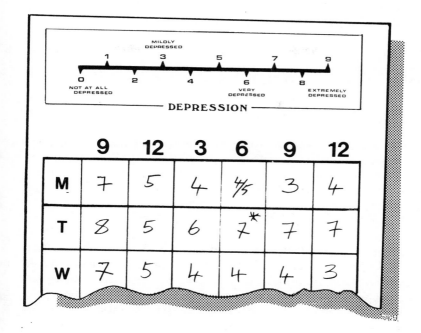

a similar format where the patient selects a rating from a visual analogue (see Figure 7.2). This little booklet can be carried in the patient's pocket and allows regular monitoring of mood levels throughout the day.

The Value of Self-reports

As I have noted previously, some concern may be expressed over the value of self-report data. There is a concern that what the patient 'says' on such paper and pencil tests may not reflect the truth. For instance, a patient may record that he finds great difficulty in sleeping. Staff may report that this is not the case — he sleeps soundly every night. Surely this illustrates the weakness of the scale? However, this is not really the problem it appears to be. Depression involves a distortion of the patient's experience. The very fact that the patient *complains* of sleep disruption, which he *thinks* is a problem, qualifies this as of interest to us. The problem involves the patient's perception of his sleeping behaviour, not the behaviour itself. I emphasise this point since there may be a temptation to conclude that because reports on a scale like the BDI do not correspond to the staff's observations, either the patient is being dishonest or the scale is faulty. These two self-report methods only assess the problem of depression from the patient's side of the fence. They are not 'objective' measures of reality.

Interview Methods

A number of scales exist to help us assess the depth of depression during an interview with the patient. The BDI was designed originally for this purpose. Here I shall briefly discuss two of the more popular methods.

The Hamilton Rating Scale[10]

This scale can be completed during the course of an ordinary interview, although supplementary information is often required from staff or relatives. Since it aims to assess the patient's condition over one or two weeks prior to the interview, it cannot be completed any more frequently than this. The scale consists of 17 items covering the commoner symptoms of depression. Each of these is rated on a three- or a five-point scale. Cognitive, behavioural and physiological symptoms are included along with less usual symptoms such as depersonalisation, derealisation, paranoid and obsessional symptoms. Designed first in 1960, it was revised slightly in 1967. It is thought that, although popular, the scale has some psychometric weaknesses. It has been noted, for instance, that items often mix what the patient thinks and says with his actual behaviour. The suicidal intent item mixes 'feels that life is worth living' (a cognitive-verbal expression) with 'attempts at suicide' (which denotes actual behaviour). For this reason the scale, although a helpful guide, may be structurally weak.

MADRS

The Montgomery and Asberg Depression Rating Scale[11] has attracted considerable attention of late. This scale covers ten items related to: sadness — apparent and reported, tension, sleep disruption, appetite, concentration, lassitude, loss of feeling and pessimistic and suicidal thoughts. All the items are rated on a 0−6 scale:

'not apparent or in keeping with present circumstances' to 'extreme, continuous or highly explicit'. Each of the items carries a guidance note on how to rate the presence or absence of the factor.

Example: Inner Tension

Representing feelings of ill-defined discomfort, edginess, inner turmoil, mental tension, mounting to either panic, dread or anguish. Rate according to intensity, frequency, duration and the extent of reassurance called for.

0 = Placid. Only fleeting inner tension
1
2 = Occasional feelings of edginess and ill-defined discomfort
3
4 = Continuous feelings of inner tension or intermittent panic which the patient can only master with some difficulty
5
6 = Unrelenting dread or anguish. Overwhelming panic

Although this scale is specifically designed to be sensitive to change, especially as an evaluation of treatment, more research is required to demonstrate its effectiveness. However, the scale appears to provide a useful assessment of the various facets of depressed behaviour.

Comment

Interviewer rating scales are used where the information cannot be collected by any other means. In some cases these ratings will be completed only by doctors. In other settings nurses may apply such measures routinely. The interview rating may be used where the patient is unable to complete a self-report scale. Where this is the case it may be more appropriate to interview the patient using the BDI or Zung as a guide, rather than switch to the interview format. It is often argued that self-report methods are unreliable. We have discussed this point already. Even where the patient's ability to answer the self-report is in question, or the patient is unable to answer the self-report, his family might be able to rate him using the BDI or Zung as their guide. In the case of the hospitalised patient, the nursing staff could do this. It could be argued that these people can draw on a wide experience of the patient, and may offer a more valid rating than is possible during a brief clinical interview. Self-report methods are best suited to evaluate the patient's thoughts and perceptions, his verbal-cognitive behaviour. Where other aspects of his functioning are thought to be important, such as overt behaviour, perhaps these are best measured directly, through observation. The value of the interview rating scale is probably restricted to situations where the patient cannot be observed closely in his natural habitat. Of course there are some patients who may respond to neither. I am thinking here of the withdrawn, perhaps mute, depressed patient.

Closer Observation

General Activity Measures

The Behaviour Rating Scale. Where the patient is hospitalised there is an opportunity to study his behaviour directly. This kind of closer observation may be most appropriate for withdrawn patients, such as the one mentioned above. One of the few standardised methods described in the literature is the Behaviour Rating Scale, developed in the early 1970s.[12] This scale looks only at observable behaviour, ignoring all subtle behaviours, speech and estimates of affect. The four areas defined on the scale are as follows:

(1) Talking: verbal behaviour towards another person.
(2) Smiling: facial movements in which the corners of the mouth turn up. The teeth may not show.
(3) Motor activity: the following are activities —
  A. Patient in room with visitor.
  B. Patient at card table talking, reading or sewing, dressing, taking a shower, watching TV, playing cards, drinking coffee. *N.B. Behaviour such as lying down or looking out of the window is not counted as an activity.*
(4) Patient out of the room.

Using these operational — or working — definitions nurses observe the patient at random intervals, on average every 30 minutes. The observations are taken between 8 a.m. and 4 p.m., resulting in 16 observations over this eight-hour period. In the original study of this scale comparisons were made between the scores of the patients on the BDI and the Hamilton, with scores obtained from these behavioural observations. The authors concluded that these behavioural samples were one way of verifying self-report ratings or interview ratings. A small follow-up study suggested that the changes in overt behaviour were a more reliable way of predicting improvement once the patient had left hospital. The advantages of this method can be summarised as follows:

(1) Since the behaviours are defined precisely, staff need not make complicated decisions. The patient either is or is not *engaged* in the behaviour.
(2) Staff require little training to make the observations.
(3) The observation format does not interfere with patient care.
(4) This kind of careful observation may increase the quality of nursing care.
(5) Interview scales, such as the Hamilton, are usually done by a doctor. This is not only a more expensive method, but describes the patient only at a certain time of day, in a certain situation. If these are done repeatedly, they may interfere with the patient's care routine.
(6) Behavioural measures overcome the problem of patients who cannot or will not complete self-report methods.
(7) Taken over a period of time, behavioural measures provide an accurate record of behaviour change during the course of depression. Such day-to-day observations can identify crises, and may be compared with biochemical measures.

For the reasons stated, and because it focuses attention on the role of the nurse as 'assessor', I would recommend this format as an effective way of monitoring the patient's progress.

The Pleasant Events Schedule. Most depressed patients report a lack, or a loss, of pleasure or satisfaction. They may have lost friends, pets or treasures. Or they may simply see their lives as being low in satisfaction. The behavioural treatment model of depression emphasises the role of reinforcing or pleasurable events, planned as part of the patient's life. Even if we do not accept this theory it is clear that nurses do try to engage patients in activities of a therapeutic nature. We might improve this procedure if the activities selected were the ones which the patient used to enjoy, or which still offered some satisfaction. The Pleasant Events Schedule[13] is a 320-item rating scale that lists a range of activities, from walking around naked to talking with friends. The patient is asked to read through the statements, indicating how often he has engaged in each activity over the past 30 days. A three-point scale is used for this purpose. He then goes through the scale again, indicating how pleasurable he finds, or found, each of the activities.

Although this schedule, with its 320 items, may appear a little exhaustive, American nurses have been using it routinely with patients in Oregon, where it was developed, for many years. However, British nurses intending to use the schedule may need to translate some of the American phraseology for the British market.

The Activity Questionnaire. A number of authors have pointed out that depressed people tend to be slow and confused in their thinking. For this reason the lengthy Pleasant Events Schedule may prove to be arduous, although it is important to try to find out which kinds of activity might help to restore their mood to something near its normal level. The following questionnaire is used by my colleagues in work with depressed women, as part of the plan for nursing care.[14]

Introduction: You're feeling pretty depressed at the moment. You feel that you can't be bothered doing anything. Nothing gives you any satisfaction any longer. You don't see the point of trying to do anything. Maybe we could spend a few minutes talking about the kind of things *you used to enjoy doing?*

(1)   What sorts of things did you use to enjoy doing before you became depressed?

(2)   Did you enjoy learning new things — like new sports or crafts — before you became depressed? What sort of things?

(3)   Did you enjoy going places? Where did you used to like going? To the beach? Up into the hills? Visiting stately homes?

(4)   What sorts of things did you enjoy doing on your own? Reading? Playing solitaire? Doing jigsaws?

(5)   What sorts of things did you enjoy doing with other people? Playing sports? Playing cards, dominoes, talking, gossiping on the phone, having a drink?

(6)   What sorts of things did you use to do that didn't cost anything? Going to the library? Watching pigeons in the square? Walking the dog?

(7) What sorts of things did you enjoy doing that didn't cost much — let's say less than £3. Having a few drinks with friends? Having a snack in a café? Going to the cinema? Buying a glossy magazine?

(8) What sorts of things did you use to enjoy at different times of the year? (Sunbathing in summer; walking in the woods in autumn; feeding the birds in winter; watching bulbs grow in the spring?)

(9) What sorts of things did you use to enjoy at different times of day? Reading the newspaper in the morning? Listening to the lunchtime news? Watching the sun set?

(10) What sorts of things do you think you could enjoy if you didn't have inhibitions about doing them? Learning to paint? Jogging? Going dancing?

In addition to identifying the sorts of activities which the patient *might* enjoy doing again, some record of his present activity is also necessary — if only to serve as a comparison. In Figure 7.3 I have illustrated a typical activity schedule belonging to a depressed patient in hospital. The patient is asked to make a brief note of what he is doing at each hour of the day. If the patient is unable to do this, staff may sample his behaviour every hour, noting the prevailing activity.'

Comment

These three methods all look at activity, but have diffrent functions. The BRS provides a specific measure of the patient's behaviour from random samples throughout the day. High levels of activity may suggest that he is 'less depressed', low activity levels that he is 'more depressed'. Although I have noted the usefulness of this measure, it should be clear that such a method would tell us little about the 'masked depressive', who may appear happy, smiling and active but he may be deeply depressed. The Activity Questionnaire is designed simply to help the nurse draw up a list of activities that might be included in the patient's care programme. Such a list is also possible from the Pleasant Events Schedule, but this can also tell us something about his present activity level and his potential for gaining satisfaction in the future. The assessment of activity may not only tell us something about the patient's current affective state, but may help us plan how to raise this by arranging the occurrence of more pleasurable activities.

Figure 7.3

ACTIVITY SCHEDULE   Name Jennifer Wilkinson   Week beg. 2nd Feb.

	MONDAY	TUESDAY	WEDNESDAY	THURSDAY	FRIDAY	SATURDAY	SUNDAY
8 – 9	In bed		POSTMAN WOKE ME				
9 – 10	"		READ LETTER				
10 – 11	Coffee		RANG DICK.				
11 – 12	Washed	Group @ 11	WALKING				
12 – 1	Peeled pot.	Shopping	/				
1 – 2	Sat	/	CAME HOME @ 2.00				
2 – 3	/	/					
3 – 4	/	Coffee in town					
4 – 5	Woke up 4.30	Met Dick					
5 – 6	Made sandwich	/					
6 – 7	Watch. TV	Home 6.30					
7 – 8	"	Dinner					
8 – 9	"	TV					
9 – 10	Bed.	Bed					

Figure 7.4

DATE	EMOTIONS How did you feel? How bad was it?	SITUATION Where were you? What were you doing or thinking about?	AUTOMATIC THOUGHTS What thoughts just popped into your head? How far did you believe them?
Monday 25/Oct.	Angry 80 Jealous 80	Walking down street. Thinking about going to job centre. Saw neighbour in flashy new car.	Why does he have all the luck 95 My whole life's been a disaster 75 I'll never get out of this rut 90

The Patient's Thinking

We have discussed ways of assessing the patient's emotional state through self-reports and a few days of assessing his behaviour patterns. The patient's thinking style is the next key area to which we need to turn our attention. We need to collect information about how the patient thinks about events in his life, and how these thoughts might relate to his affective level.

The Triple-column Technique. Aaron Beck has popularised a method known as the triple-column technique. The patient is asked to identify a situation that occurred recently and was related to some unpleasant feeling. This is written down in the first column. The patient is then asked to do a 'mental replay' of the scene, noting the events that led up to the unpleasant feeling. If nothing of any consequence happened, what sorts of thoughts were in his head just before the feeling occurred? These events, or his 'stream of consciousness' are written down in the first column. He is then asked to specify the emotion. How did he feel? Angry? Hurt? Jealous? He is also asked to rate — on a 0–100 scale — how unpleasant the feeling was. Finally, he is asked to try to pick out the kind of thoughts that occurred to him at the time of the incident, or within his daydream. These are called 'automatic thoughts' because they simply 'pop' into the patient's head. These are also written down in the form that they 'appeared' to the patient: e.g. 'I'm all washed up; everyone's against me; there's no point in trying.' The exercise is completed by asking the patient to rate the extent to which he believes the automatic thoughts, again using the 0–100 scale. Figures 7.4 and 7.5 illustrate the use of the triple-column method, along with a simpler questionnaire method, both aimed at identifying these thinking styles.

Thinking Errors

A wide range of *cognitive distortions* have been described by some of the important figures in depression research.[15, 16] Their view is that certain thinking errors play a large part in triggering, or maintaining, painful affect. Among the thinking errors described by Beck are the following:

— *all-or-nothing thinking:* the person sees things only in terms of black and white, rather than shades of grey. 'You're either a total success or a complete failure.'

Figure 7.5

<u>IDENTIFYING YOUR NEGATIVE AUTOMATIC THOUGHTS</u>

We have discussed how the way you feel is influenced by the way you <u>think</u>. I want you now to practise finding out what sort of thoughts you have when you feel bad. Think about the last time you felt bad; you might have felt sad, or angry; guilty or frightened. Try to remember how you felt and what was happening around you and answer the following questions.

<u>Feelings</u>

How did you feel? _Angry / Jealous_

How bad was the feeling - measure it by using a scale of 0 - 100 (100 is the very worst)

Score _80_

<u>Situation</u>

Where were you? _In town_

What were you doing? _Walking down street_

What was going on around you? _Saw neighbour with new car_

Were you thinking about anything in particular? _whether I should_
go to the job centre, or not

<u>Automatic Thoughts</u>

What thoughts just "popped into your mind" at that time?

Why does he have all the luck?
My whole life's been a disaster.
I'll never get out of this rut.

Did you <u>believe</u> these thoughts? Measure to what extent you believed them using a scale 0 - 100. (0 means you did <u>not</u> believe them at all; 100 means you believed them <u>completely</u>).

Score _95_

— *over-generalising:* assuming that because a bad experience happened once, it will always happen in similar circumstances. 'I was unhappy the last time I saw him. It will be the same this weekend.'

— *exaggeration:* reacting to a difficult situation as though it were a major disaster: blowing events out of proportion.

— *catastrophising:* assuming that something terrible will happen as a result of the way he coped with a difficult situation, e.g. fearing that because he has had a row with his wife she will leave him; he will lose contact with his family; and his whole life will be in ruins.

— *discounting the positive:* overlooking the positive aspects of any situation; assuming that they 'don't count' for some reason. Thinking that he is all weaknesses and failings, with no positive qualities.

— *jumping to conclusions:* coming to a conclusion without recourse to any obvious facts to support this view, e.g. deciding that someone doesn't like him because he has not come over to introduce himself. Often called 'crystal ball gazing'.

— *shoulds and musts:* the person feels extremely anxious if he does not live up to some very high standard of social or ethical behaviour: 'I must always be nice to people, or they won't like me; I should always be on time or people will think that I am lazy.'

Although there is some dispute as to the significance of these thoughts in the production of mood disorder, it is often easier to understand the patient's state if his major thinking errors are identified. The idea that these thinking styles are a barrier to effective problem solving or coping is a very plausible one. By asking the patient to make a note of the kind of automatic thoughts he has in 'depressing' situations, we can draw up a list of his typical thinking errors. This may help us understand at least one of the reasons *why* he becomes depressed.

I have developed a simple visual aid (see Figures 7.6 and 7.7) to help the patient recognise these thinking errors. The nurse selects one of the 'automatic thoughts' described by the patient from the record sheet. She then tries to identify the kind of error involved. Once she has identified the thinking error, she relates this to one of the illustrations on the visual aid. She then asks the patient to explain to her why the particular thought is called a thinking error.

Figure 7.6

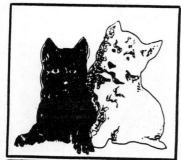

BLACK + WHITE THINKING

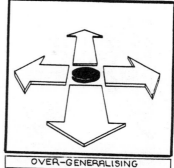

OVER-GENERALISING

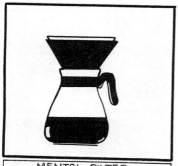

MENTAL FILTER

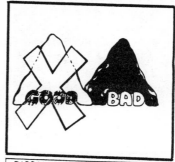

DISCOUNTING THE POSITIVE

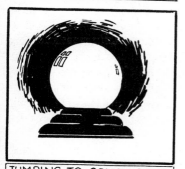

JUMPING TO CONCLUSIONS

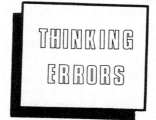

THINKING ERRORS

Figure 7.7

CATASTROPHISING

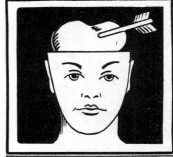

EMOTIONAL REASONING

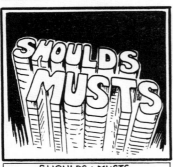

SHOULDS + MUSTS

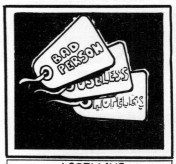

LABELLING

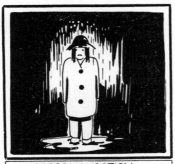

PERSONALISATION

Example

Last week you had a pretty bad week. You tried a number of times to get involved in some activities on the ward, but had to give up most times because you couldn't concentrate. When you couldn't concentrate you thought to yourself, 'I'm no use. I'm a total failure.' (producing the visual aid) Here are some pictures which we use to illustrate different kinds of thinking styles. The way people think about things. Now when you couldn't concentrate, you thought that you were a 'total failure'. Not just 'a bit of a failure' but a *complete* failure. The fact that you had stuck at the activity for ten minutes or so didn't count. Because you didn't stay there for a long time you were a 'total failure'. That sounds a bit like black-and-white thinking to me. Either you are perfect *or* you're hopeless, there is nothing in between. You don't accept that you can do something quite well, or a little bit. You either do it brilliantly, with no problems, or you have failed *completely*. The two little dogs from the whisky bottle should remind you of that error: they are black and white as well. There are no shades of grey. Do you think that you could explain to me what those two little dogs represent?

This part of the assessment would not be done until much later. By this time the patient will be receiving different kinds of help and his depression may be beginning to lift a little. However, the assessment is not restricted to the beginning of the patient's stay in hospital, or the acute phase of his illness. Assessment should be continuous, opening out new facets on the patient's functioning, or enlarging upon existing pieces of information. This process is most evident in the assessment of depression, where the investigation of the patient is carefully graded to suit his presentation.

Suicide

It has been estimated that more than 1,000 people in the world commit suicide each day. In Britain there are over 3,000 deaths each year from suicide with attempts — or parasuicide — being ten times as common. Suicide is a highly emotionally charged subject. It is also one surrounded by myths. There are well-established beliefs, even in professional circles, that suicide happens most often without warning; that those who threaten suicide rarely carry it through; that all attempted suicide is attention-seeking or trivial; and that all people who kill themselves must be mentally ill. *All these beliefs are false.*

Suicide is the situation where someone brings about his own death, the assumption being that he did so knowingly. This separates it from accidental death: death by misadventure. Where someone makes a *non-fatal* suicide attempt — parasuicide — this usually involves drug overdose. I mention parasuicide here because there is evidence that 1 per cent of those admitted to hospital after parasuicide will commit suicide within one year. It is also known that 20 per cent of parasuicides will make another attempt within one year. This risk factor remains at a high level for about ten years, with the result that about one half of the people who commit suicide have made earlier attempts.[17] These findings slay the myth that suicide is always unexpected, or that parasuicide is a trivial issue, which never leads to the real thing. It is also clear that many people kill themselves when in a highly rational frame of mind. We do such people a grave disservice by suggesting that everyone who kills himself is unbalanced. Suicidal thoughts are commonly expressed by depressed patients and, as the figures show, may be crucial signals of a potential death threat. For this reason the assessment of suicidal intent is a crucial issue in the assessment of the depressed patient.

Talking to the Patient

Staff often avoid talking to patients about suicide. A commonly expressed fear is that this will put the idea of killing themselves 'into their heads'. Most authorities believe that nothing could be further from the truth.[18] By asking about suicidal thoughts, or even past attempts, we may offer a degree of relief, providing that the subject is handled in a non-threatening or non-judgemental manner. In this sense the suicidal intent assessment can be therapeutic. It is clear that many nurses are alarmed, however, by the prospect of talking to patients *at any length* about suicide. The skill and courage needed are often only acquired through painstaking training and experience.

Choosing the Moment. Information about suicide is often collected when the patient is communicative or when an attempt has just been made. In the former he may not feel suicidal. In the latter his faculties may be blunted by the emotional or physical effects of the attempt. The best time to discuss suicide is when he is highly suicidal. This is, of course, the most difficult time. The threat to the nurse is greatest here, especially if she fears she may make matters worse. Yet this is perhaps the only time when a realistic picture of his depair or commitment to dying can be assessed. Here we can find out what is motivating him to take this action, how he might go about it, and what might be deterring him, even temporarily. When the patient does not feel suicidal his views may be more carefully judged, even academic. When he is toying seriously with his 'final solution' a more accurate evaluation of his position may be possible. Contrary to popular myth, many suicidal patients plan their exit down to the last detail. In many senses it is an affront to their integrity to classify all suicides as of unsound mind. The interview with a suicidal patient can be a chilling affair. It is not for the faint-hearted and clearly is not the job for the novice.

We should be aware of other factors that might influence the patient's report on his feelings. He may exaggerate the seriousness of his intent to increase staff or family support. Although we may suspect this, we may not dare risk doubting the patient's word. In other cases the patient may reduce the emphasis of his true feelings. He may have high moral principles or may feel guilty about harbouring such thoughts. In some cases he may simply fear being labelled as a suicide risk, perhaps resulting in compulsory detention. On the other hand he may not wish to lose the respect of staff for whom he has some affection. Any of these factors may encourage him to conceal his intentions, or inflate or play down the seriousness of his feelings.

Suicidal Intent

By assessing the patient at the height of his suicidal risk we may identify the factors of most significance. This information may also be 'news' to the patient. He may get a chance to look more objectively at what is driving him to his death. Paradoxically, this may help him come to terms with his situation. The assessment may have therapeutic value. Discussion with the patient at other times is also important. Where the patient is thought to be a suicide risk, persistent monitoring is indicated, increasing this at times of obvious crisis. Like many of the other problems we have discussed, suicide is a continuum. At one extreme is the strong desire to go on living; at the other, the intention to kill oneself. Attitudes towards living and dying change as one progresses towards either end. In the simplest form of assessment the patient might be asked to indicate where he thinks he is at present on this line. Even a simple line drawn in pencil on the back of a notebook, with the poles of living and dying noted, can be used for this purpose.

Parasuicide. The patient who jumps from a high-rise building, or leaps into a deep river, is taking an irreversible course of action. Other death games may carry risks but may be less absolute. Russian roulette is an experiment in mathematical probabilities. An overdose, taken in the knowledge that someone will find him, is also an experiment in the schedules of fate. In both cases, if the experiment is done often enough, the odds will eventually be loaded against the patient. Even if the patient 'expects' to be found, the risk remains, and will increase with each attempt. We have to ask the question, 'Why should he take such a risk?' It is well known that certain life events — like bereavement — can decide the patient in favour of suicide. Other events, such as the arrival of a friend, or the anticipated forfeiture of his wife's insurance claim, may act as a deterrent, at least temporarily. Let us now consider two factors that play a part in the creation of suicide, factors that need to be identified in the assessment.

The Escape Solution. Suicide can be seen as a means of escape. It can solve what is seen as intractable distress. This distress may be real, as in bankruptcy, or bereavement; or perceptual, where the patient *feels* that something is insoluble,though others might not agree. Either way the patient feels hopeless in the face of adversity. He may even show a disturbingly calm acceptance of the pointlessness of his existence. The 'best' solution may be to commit suicide. He may even suggest that this is the best solution for all concerned, reducing the burden on family, friends and even staff. Often the action taken may be absolute. Although rare, violent means may be used by the patient who feels hopeless, and wishes to guarantee his escape.

The Change Effect. The patient may try using suicide as a problem-solver in a less dramatic fashion. He may try to make others realise how desperate he is, or may try to force them to give him more support. This is often called the 'cry for help'. It has been suggested that more than half the patients hospitalised for suicidal attempts tried to kill themselves to escape what they saw as intolerable situations. A smaller proportion tried to manipulate others in the way described here, and a third had mixed motives.[19] Those who take the escape route may be much more seriously depressed than those who are trying to influence others. The 'escapers' feel hopeless. The 'influencers' are by definition hopeful of some change.

Clues and Cues. A number of factors may make suicide more or less successful. In the assessment we should try to identify these, to reduce the risk. Patients who talk a lot about death or dying, even obliquely, may be signalling their future actions. They may be fairly explicit: 'I don't see the point in carrying on any longer' or 'This is the only way out for me.' In other cases the message may be less clear: 'Things aren't going to get any better' or 'I know that I'm just a burden on everyone.' Some patients may let slip their intention to kill themselves by saying 'Goodbye' instead of 'Goodnight'; or when saying, 'I don't suppose that I'll see you again.' These 'slips' are not always indicative of suicide intent. The rule is, however, 'Better safe than sorry.' All such comments should be recorded verbatim, as part of the overall assessment of the patient.

The dicovery of stockpiles of drugs or potentially harmful objects may also be important clues, which should be noted. The same is true of sudden decisions, such as changing a will or getting rid of pets. Where the patient is extremely agitated, he may become very calm before committing suicide. This calm may be interpreted as a sign of progress and may lead to a slackening of observation. Although these 'clues' may lead to nothing, there is no harm in being suspicious.

Significant Features. Our assessment should attempt to judge the risk involved. As I have noted already, there is always some risk. In time all attempts, no matter how abortive, may acquire significance. However, positive answers to the following questions may help identify attempts that already indicate seriousness, and which might herald a fatal attempt.

(1) Did the patient commit the act in isolation, where he was unlikely to be found?
(2) Did he fail to make any attempt to summon help?
(3) Did he develop a pattern of missed appointments or general 'unreliability' before the attempt? Did he apologise for his lateness or bad organisation?

(4) Did he make any 'final acts': making a will, arranging insurance cover for his family, or settling finances?
(5) Did he ensure that he had ample means to commit the suicide?
(6) Did he leave a suicide note?

The Assessment

In assessing suicidal intent we must try to see his situation and his actions from his perspective. Staff and families are often stunned by suicide. They cannot understand why he should want to die. 'He had everything to live for — a lovely family, nice home, good job.' Although apparent to us, such 'realities' may not be so clear to the patient. He has his own way of construing reality. Alternatively, he may appreciate that he is fortunate, but may believe that he does not deserve such good fortune. His unworthiness, coupled with his well-endowed status, may be the provocation for his suicide.

We need to see things through the patient's eyes. We must be open to what he sees as missing from his life, and why he feels that life is not worth living. Both viewpoints may illustrate his distorted vision. They may illustrate how he evaluates his own worth or his life in general. We should try to see his problems as he sees them, *at least at first*. It is very tempting to reassure the patient: 'Don't worry, you'll get over this. Lots of people feel like you do. They get over it.' This temptation should be resisted until it has been established *why he thinks that he won't get over this*. The nurse needs to find out what kind of beliefs might serve as the basis for killing himself. Alternatively, he may not face any tangible problem, but may find his life a vacuum — devoid of any pleasure or meaning. Again it is important to establish why he thinks this is so, instead of trying to point out all the things he might do to restore his reason for living.

In some cases the patient may have real problems. He may be in financial difficulties; he may live in bad housing; he may have terminal illness. He should be given the opportunity to express his feeling about these 'trials' before any attempt is made to soothe his distress, or to help him adjust to these problems. We try to see his problems through the patient's eyes. At the same time we try to retain our objectivity. Where the patient has experienced major trauma or is massively disadvantaged it is difficult to avoid feeling for him. This is to be avoided wherever possible. The patient may interpret such emotion — especially sympathy — as further indication of the hopelessness of his situation. So how should the nurse respond to the patient who has much to be suicidal about? She should show concern, empathy and a willingness to allow the patient to express his feelings to the full — at least for the moment. I suppose I am advocating a sensitive, controlled show of grave concern. Grave enough to show the patient that he is being taken seriously, yet not so grave that he interprets this as a sign of the futility of his situation.

The Hopelessness Scale. Although much of the information we need about suicidal intent can be obtained from interviews and observations, a specific scale has been developed to help enhance the assessment of this key area.[20] In Beck's view the patient's confessed 'hopelessness' is a better predictor of suicide than his level of depression. The Hopelessness Scale tales only minutes to complete and may be given to the patient at regular intervals to monitor the risk of suicide. Hopelessness is defined as the patient's negative attitude towards himself and the future: he does not *expect* any change. The scale carries 20 items which are scored in a straightforward true or false format. Although of special relevance to suicide and depression, it has been suggested that this scale is relevant to other forms of psychological disorder, such as psychosis, physical illness and drug abuse.

A Case Illustration

Marion is a 28-year-old dentist. She is unmarried and lives alone. She was admitted to hospital after a drug overdose. This is her fourth admission, the first occurring when she was a student. On admission she is withdrawn and uncommunicative. Staff feel that she is unable to complete the BDI, which is routine after 3 days on the ward. The registrar completes the Hamilton. Marion is thin and pale in appearance. Her eyes are dark, adding to the gauntness of her appearance. She is weighed on admission and daily thereafter. Staff begin the Behaviour Rating Scale observation on the third day, following a case conference. Ratings of her sleep are also kept by night staff. Over the first few days these observations are monotonous: Marion rarely stirs from her chair where she sits, curled up, only occasionally getting up to look out of the window. She comes for meals when encouraged by staff, but eats little. On day 4 a food and fluid intake record is started. On the same day a nurse completes the BDI by reading out the statements. Marion simply answers 'the first one' or 'that one'. Her voice is weak and thready. She avoids eye contact and sits turned away from the nurse during any interaction. The nurse notes these features and draws up a short checklist covering these key verbal and non-verbal behaviours. On day 5 the staff rate the level of appropriate eye contact, orientation to the nurse, gestures, volume and tone of voice during each interaction. Staff also note her predominant activity on the activity schedule, hour by hour. At the end of the day they total the number of hours spent in different activities.

By the middle of the second week Marion has become a little more active. However, she does not volunteer any information or start any interaction with staff or patients. Staff hold regular short conversations with her to try to gain a more detailed history of the events leading up to her admission. All the questions are 'closed', eliciting only 'Yes/No' answers. Her mother is interviewed on day 8, having flown from Australia. On day 10 Marion is able to complete the BDI with a little help from the nurse. On day 12 she begins to talk a little to the nurse who handled her admission. This nurse is identified as the 'keyworker' and begins to extend the range of the short interviews to cover Marion's thoughts about work, friendships and her overdose. On day 19 she completes the Activity Questionnaire interview, and a list of preferred activities is drawn up. On day 21 she begins to keep her own activity schedule. By day 25 the interviews with the nurse have progressed to analysing her thoughts about some of the unpleasant events in her recent past, using the triple-column technique.

Conclusion

Marion's assessment is a fairly typical example of the assessment of a depressed patient. Initially, various physical observations are made — weight, pallor, etc. In some settings these might include various blood analyses. Close observation of her behaviour begins early on and is maintained for the duration of her stay, expressed through the Behaviour Rating Scale, activity schedules and sleep record. Close observation is also maintained on her food intake due to her wasted and undernourished appearance. Her affective level appears to be very low on admission, but can only be assessed indirectly through the Hamilton. Later the BDI gives a rough estimate of her actual mood state, and is eventually done weekly through to discharge. The nurses use a range of interviews — some formal, others less so — to monitor her verbal and non-verbal behaviour and also to collect some information about her expressed emotions and beliefs. As her depression appears to lift, the intensity of the assessment increases. She begins to monitor her own activity, draws up a list of possible 'pleasurable' activities, and starts to evaluate her thinking style. By this stage treatment is well established, but the assessment is ongoing.

This kind of assessment is typical because it reflects the need for assessment to build up gradually. It should be geared to the actual presentation of the patient. By closely observing the patient, the nurse will know when she might be ready to move on to a new 'level' of assessment. In this sense assessment and treatment run together, although it is to be hoped that the assessment done at the beginning will influence the choice of care and treatment methods. In some situations it is possible to arrange that all the assessment takes place at the beginning, using this information to plan the treatment, then following up with evaluations of progress. In this example we should see the need for 'staging' assessment, building it up, layer upon layer, in order to collect more *elaborate* descriptions of the patient's state or information about different aspects of his problem.

Notes

1. The term 'melancholy' is experiencing something of a revival, in an attempt to distinguish severe depression from other affective disorders. See J. Mendels, *Concepts of Depression* (John Wiley, New York, 1970).
2. A. T. Beck, *Depressions: Causes and Treatment* (University of Pennsylvania Press, Philadelphia, 1972).
3. See Mendels, *Concepts of Depression*.
4. M. Hamilton, 'Symptoms and Assessment of Depression' in S. Paykel (ed.), *Handbook of Affective Disorders* (Churchill Livingstone, Edinburgh, 1982).
5. See A. T. Beck, A. J. Rush, B. F. Shaw and G. Emery, *Cognitive Therapy of Depression* (John Wiley, New York, 1979).
6. A. T. Beck, C. H. Ward, M. Mendelsohn, J. Mock and J. Erbaugh, 'An Inventory for Measuring Depression', *Archives of General Psychiatry*, 4 (1961), pp. 561–71. Beck has since developed a further version of this inventory, which is illustrated in Beck *et al.*, *Cognitive Therapy of Depression*.
7. See Beck, *Depressions*.
8. W. K. Zung, 'A Self-rating Depression Scale', *Archives of General Psychiatry*, 12 (1965), pp. 63–70.
9. A. C. B. Aitken, 'Measures of Feeling Using Analogue Scales', *Proceedings of the Royal Society of Medicine*, 62 (1969), pp. 989–93.
10. M. Hamilton, 'Development of a Rating Scale for Primary Depressive Illness', *British Journal of Social and Clinical Psychology*, 6 (1967), pp. 278–96.

11. S. A. Montgomery and M. Asberg, 'A New Depression Scale Designed to be Sensitive to Change', *British Journal of Psychiatry*, *134* (1979), pp. 382−9.

12. J. C. Williams, D. H. Barlow and W. S. Agras, 'Behavioural Measurement of Depression', *Archives of General Psychiatry*, **27** (1972), pp. 330−3.

13. D. MacPhillamy and P. M. Lewinsohn, 'The Pleasant Events Schedule', unpublished manuscript, University of Oregon, 1971. This schedule is available from Peter Lewinsohn at the University of Oregon. See also D. Macphillamy and P. Lewinsohn, 'Depression as Function of Levels of Desired and Observed Pleasure', *Journal of Abnormal Psychology*, **83** (1974), pp. 651−7.

14. This questionnaire is heavily influenced by the work of Beck *et al.*, *Cognitive Therapy of Depression*.

15. Beck, *Depressions*.

16. A. Ellis, *Reason and Emotion in Psychotherapy* (Lyle Stuart Press, New York, 1961).

17. N. Kreitman and J. A. T. Dyer, 'Suicide and Parasuicide', *Nursing*, **30** (1981), pp. 1310−11.

18. Beck *et al.*, *Cognitive Therapy of Depression*.

19. M. Kovacs, A. T. Beck and A. Weissman, 'The Use of Suicidal Motives in the Psychotherapy of Attempted Suicides', *American Journal of Psychotherapy*, **29** (1975), pp. 363−8.

20. A. T. Beck, A. Weissman, D. Lester and L. Trexler, 'The Measurement of Pessimism: The Hopelessness Scale', *Journal of Consulting and Clinical Psychology*, **42** (1974), pp. 861−5.

8 HERE COMES EVERYBODY: THE ASSESSMENT OF RELATIONSHIP PROBLEMS

Tell me with whom you live and I will tell you who you are.
— Spanish proverb

Modern psychiatry has paid much attention to the issue of relationships. The psychoanalytic model of mental disorder suggests that the patient's distress arises from dysfunctional relationships with significant others in his environment, either past or present. These relationships often feature, although at times obliquely, in the therapeutic process. In this chapter I do not wish to talk about relationships in this rather specialised way. I accept that our relationships play a central role in shaping the direction of our lives. However, this constitutes a vast canvas, too great for either the space available or my own experience to do justice. Instead I shall discuss the role that relationships play in our lives at present: the relationships we have with people in general, from our intimate contacts through to the more general context of our place in society.

It is a cliché to acknowledge that man is a social animal. Yet this is where we must begin: at the banal end of the spectrum, looking at the individual's place in a highly complex society. If he can fit into that society we call him adaptive or adaptable. If he does not, history tells us that he will be labelled a deviant, a misfit, an eccentric or some kind of inadequate personality. There is great pressure to conform to society's rules and regulations. Those who decide to flaunt them must be brave indeed; or may simply be incapable of keeping up with the standard. One of these rules is that we should have relationships. The man or woman who has no friends or acquaintances is viewed with suspicion. 'What is he hiding? Why do people not want to know him?' Apart from the convention expressed by relationships, it is clear that they serve important functions. As Aristotle noted, 'in poverty and other misfortunes of life, true friends are a sure refuge'. The characteristics of a true relationship were echoed by Oliver Cromwell when he said that 'the light of friendship is like the light of phosphorous, seen plainest when all around is dark'. And from Plato we derive the idea of a relationship which is genuine because it is freed of passion and instinct, a relationship which Plato thought would be longer-lasting since it was based upon more elevated forms of choice. The 'Platonic' relationship would help each person aspire to new heights, rather than simply meet basic needs. The idea of an elevating relationship was expressed also by Confucius: 'never contract friendship with a man who is not better than thyself'. Here also is found the idea that relationships can be a means to an end: the enrichment of the individual through positive association with others. However, not anyone can provide this growth function for us. As the old saying goes, 'Never become the fourth friend of a man who has had three before but lost them.' We all know the pitfalls, as well as the heady heights of the relationship game. Perhaps the most significant comment I can find on the subject comes again from Doctor Johnson: 'A man should keep his friendships in good repair.' When we come to consider the relationship problems of the psychiatric patient, the need for repair is often all too obvious.

I said at the start that I would also try to cover (wo)man's place in society. This is a vast topic which I shall not do the injustice of considering here. What I mean is that through our discussion of certain kinds of interpersonal difficulty, I hope to shine some light on our wider role as members of a society: a society which indirectly fabricates the interpersonal rules and regulations which people find awkward. In this sense we are citizens first and individuals second. This can present a significant conflict for many of us, a conflict which we often cannot resolve.

Relationship Problems

In order to simplify matters a little, I shall classify relationship problems under five main headings:

(1) The person who experiences social anxiety.
(2) The person who is unable to assert himself.
(3) The person who finds the mechanics of interaction difficult.
(4) The person who believes that he is isolated or alienated.
(5) The person who is isolated or alienated.

These are rather simple, non-exclusive categories. A person with 'relationship problems' may show two, three or perhaps all of these problems. However, in terms of the assessment it is important

Figure 8.1

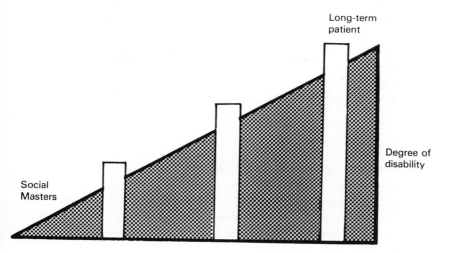

that we identify in which way these subgroups of relationship problems may be evident in the case of the patient concerned.

In Figure 8.1 I have tried to illustrate how relationship problems might mirror varying degrees of social incompetence. At one end of this figure we have the 'social masters': those people who are active in a wide range of social arenas, and who cope successfully with all manner of social problems. Because of their 'master' status, making and maintaining friends present no problem. As we move further along the base of the figure, we encounter people who are progressively less masterful. At first we meet people with singular problems: teachers who find it difficult to 'relate' to large classes; party-goers who find it difficult to relate to strangers. Then we meet people with a few such problems: the worker who cannot keep his emotions under control when in conflict with colleagues, especially if they are relative strangers to him. Or the young man who finds large groups of people threatening *and* is uncomfortable when required to discuss personal material in a 'one-to-one' interaction. As we progress further along the figure, the nature and scale of people's social interaction problems increase, making them more and more socially incompetent. At the furthest end of the figure we would probably meet some of the very withdrawn patients in our long-stay wards: people who avoid almost any kind of relationship. This model of social competence can be misleading. A person might have a single relationship problem which differs according to his situation. A 'shy' person in a small community might be liked and respected for his sensitive nature. In a bustling metropolis he may be ignored or alienated by people used only to the pressures of the concrete jungle. Although the person is the same in both situations, the problem can vary enormously.

Assessing Social Skills

The Relationships Interview

Most people discuss their relationship problems in terms of their reactions to others: feelings of depression, agitation, embarrassment, anxiety, etc. Many people who complain of these problems may, in effect, be complaining about their relationships. The first task is to gain some idea of how the patient developed his social skills; how he formed relationships with people as he was growing up. Was he a shy child? Did he have many friends? Did he tend to fight or get bullied? When did he have his first girlfriend? From this brief review the nurse might move on to look at some of the typical problems which can cause us all some discomfort.

(1)   How do you find starting conversations with people? Do you find it easier to talk to strangers, acquaintances, individuals or groups? Why is this?

(2)   How do you feel about asking favours of people? Do you do this often?

(3)   Are you able to express your opinions to people? Can you disagree with people, e.g. at work, or with someone who is teaching you something?

(4)   Can you refuse what you think are unreasonable demands? Does it make any difference if they are friends, stangers or family?

(5)   Can you pay someone a compliment? How difficult or easy is that?

(6)   How easy do you find it to make appointments with people? What about making 'dates' with women (men)?

(7)   Can you negotiate with people: give and take, show some compromise (e.g.) with family or friends?

(8) Can you ask people for help when you are stuck? Do you ever back out of that? Why?

(9) How do you feel about applying for jobs? How do you feel about being interviewed or asking for a transfer at work?

(10) Can you make a complaint without losing your temper?

(11) Can you resist people who are trying to get you to do things against your better judgement or beliefs? Like drink, take drugs, have sex or give information about people?

(12) Are you able to tell someone how you feel about her/him? How does that make you feel?

A General Social Skills Questionnaire. In Figure 8.2 I have illustrated a short questionnaire which may help identify the areas of the patient's life which are a problem to him. This covers many of the areas we have already covered in the relationships interview. However, here there is an opportunity for the patient to decide for himself, at his leisure, which are the most or least problematic. The results of this scale might help the nurse identify some of the 'kinds' of relationship problem discussed in this chapter. Although it could be used as a measurement tool, its main purpose is to point towards more specific areas of assessment.

Following on. Once we have some idea of the situations which cause the patient some difficulty, we need to establish more clearly what these situations mean to the patient. He might complain of anxiety in public. What does he do in such situations? Does he feel unable to speak? Does he talk incessantly or excitedly? Does he stammer or stutter? Does he feel deficient in some way, but is unable to specify this clearly? Why are any of these things a problem to him? How does he think he should behave? What does he think is wrong with his performance?

The Person Who Can't

The person who can't presumably *could* if something wasn't stopping him. The question is, what? In this first class of relationship problems we are dealing with people who know what they would like to do, but are prevented from carrying this out for *fear of what might happen*. This fear may have some history. The patient may have had a bad experience with people in the past. Or it

Figure 8.2

NAME .... DATE.....................

Please read each of the following statements. Rate how you handle each of these situations using the scale below:

> 1 = I have NO DIFFICULTY doing this
> 2 = I have a SLIGHT DIFFICULTY doing this
> 3 = I have QUITE A BIT OF DIFFICULTY doing this
> 4 = I have GREAT DIFFICULTY doing this
> 5 = I NEVER do this or would AVOID the situation

CIRCLE THE NUMBER WHICH MOST CLOSELY REFLECTS YOUR REACTION

TALKING TO PEOPLE

1. When I meet people I can start a conversation with them.   1 2 3 4 5

2. I can start talking about something and carry on a conversation.   1 2 3 4 5

3. When others are talking I can join in.   1 2 3 4 5

4. When someone is talking to me I can appear interested.   1 2 3 4 5

SAYING HOW I FEEL

1. When a person has done well I can compliment them.   1 2 3 4 5

2. If someone does something for me I can thank them.   1 2 3 4 5

3. I am able to encourage others.   1 2 3 4 5

4. If I care about someone I can show them how I feel.   1 2 3 4 5

5. I can tell someone that I am angry without losing control.   1 2 3 4 5

EXPRESSING MY NEEDS

1. I can put my point of view in an argument without losing control.   1 2 3 4 5

2. I can give people instructions without feeling embarrassed.   1 2 3 4 5

3. I can ask to see the person in charge if I am making a complaint.   1 2 3 4 5

4. I can tell people exactly what I want (e.g. in shops)   1 2 3 4 5

DEALING WITH OTHERS

1. I am able to understand how other people are feeling.   1 2 3 4 5

2. I can listen to what a person has to say.   1 2 3 4 5

3. If I fall out with someone I can work out what went wrong.   1 2 3 4 5

4. I can deal with someone who is angry without becoming upset.   1 2 3 4 5

Figure 8.2 *(continued)*

FRIENDSHIP

1. I can talk to people I have met for the first time.		1 2 3 4 5
2. I can talk to people in a group.		1 2 3 4 5
3. I can make dates to see people.		1 2 3 4 5
4. I can take the initiative to make a friendship.		1 2 3 4 5
5. I can go to a new place in order to meet new people.		1 2 3 4 5

DEALING WITH MYSELF

1. If I am upset I can calm myself down.		1 2 3 4 5
2. I can control my temper before it gets out of hand.		1 2 3 4 5
3. I can make plans and stick to them.		1 2 3 4 5
4. I can negotiate with people.		1 2 3 4 5
5. I can work out how I feel and how I should deal with it.		1 2 3 4 5

GOALS

Read over the scale again and pick out the situations which you would like to be able to deal with better. Make a list of these below.

1. _____

2. _____

3. _____

4. _____

5. _____

6. _____

---

may be based entirely in his imagination. Either way, this fear hinders the creation of effective relationships. In some cases this may be made worse by friends telling the patient that 'It's all in your mind, you only think that you've got a problem.'

This interpersonal anxiety is a variant of the generalised anxiety discussed in Chapter 6. Here the patient feels distressed whenever he *plans* or is *required* to meet with people. In some cases he may have no problem with strangers. In others, he may be comfortable with friends but awkward with everyone else. He may say that he 'doesn't know what to say' when meeting people for the first time, or feels uncomfortable 'talking about myself'. He is rarely ever unskilled. He may doubt his ability, but he does know what to say.

He is prevented from putting this knowledge into practice by his anticipation of what might go wrong. This leads to an avoidance of social contact, or very superficial relationships. In some cases he may break the contact in mid-sentence to escape from his distress.

The social skills we are discussing here are far more complex than the basics reviewed in Chapter 5. The ability to communicate information, show interest in others, establish rapport, take risks in self-disclosure, and say and do the 'right things' are complex interpersonal skills. For many people this is a tall order. Situations play an important part in deciding what constitutes appropriate skills. For example, appropriate behaviour on a first date, when making a complaint, or when paying a compliment are all variations on a theme. They all require the use of gestures, speech, facial expression and the use of what actors call 'timing'. However, if the way these actions are performed didn't vary from one situation to another, we would not be able to tell a complaint or a compliment from hesitant love-making. Those who are 'social masters' often find it difficult to imagine how complex such interpersonal behaviour can appear to the socially anxious. The person who finds such interactions threatening may be overwhelmed by their inherent complexity. It appears so complicated that he can never imagine himself getting it right.

Who Experiences Interpersonal Anxiety? Most of us have felt uncomfortable in the presence of someone, at some time. This may be someone of high status, such as a supervisor, or dignitary, or someone to whom we attribute importance, such as a bank manager or a 'blind date'. In such situations our anxiety centres upon our ability to handle the situation correctly or successfully. The person with interpersonal anxiety feels much the same. He is apprehensive about the situations we all take for granted. He might be the 'shy young man' who fails to grow out of his adolescent lack of confidence. He might be the older person who has never felt comfortable with people. Such people lack the social contacts most of us use as the base for our lives. Or they may be unable to use such contacts to their satisfaction. People who are interpersonally isolated — lacking friends and 'confidants' — are psychologically vulnerable. Their interpersonal anxiety may be a harbinger of more serious psychological distress. In other cases it may coexist with an established psychiatric disorder, where it is difficult to say which came first.

Case Examples. Roger works in a small electronics firm on an assembly line. He is in his early thirites, unmarried and living with two friends in a flat in a large town. He used to be a drummer with a rock band that split up some years ago. Despite his experience 'on the road' Roger has always had difficulties in dealing with people. He appears 'normal' but confesses to considerable inner anxiety. He has several friends and regular relationships with women. He retains a great fear of meeting new people, entering new situations and talking to women. Surprisingly, he has no problem with sexual relationships. His anxiety centres upon simpler things like eating in restaurants, holding hands in public and expressing his feelings.

Harry is 50 and is diagnosed as a schizophrenic. He lives with his wife in a council flat and attends hospital each day for 'day care'. As a young man he was an art teacher and retains an interest in cultural pursuits. His wife says he was a quiet young man, who mixed well and played the organ in church. He was also secretary of the local art club. Harry confesses that he finds any interaction with people difficult. 'I've lost all of my confidence. All those years in hospital have just chipped away at me.'

Roger and Harry have similar problems. Their ability to socialise is limited by anxiety. Both men have grown up acquiring at least a modicum of social skills. However, Roger does not appear to have gained the confidence to be himself. Harry once had this to some degree, but has lost it with the passage of time. Both men could do the things they would like to do, but their faith in themselves does not match their technical ability. As a result they become the 'people who can't'.

Assessment of Interpersonal Anxiety

The social anxiety shown by our two patients can lead to avoidance of almost any kind of social contact. The patient may feel that he will make a fool of himself; embarrass others; lose control or 'go mad'. 'Spectatoring' is another problem where he scrutinises himself closely during each and every social interaction. This preoccupation with his performance reduces his chances of behaving normally, and leads to further avoidance. The general approach to anxiety is discussed in Chapter 6. The same format may be used here, stressing interpersonal relationships.

The Social Anxiety and Distress Scale (SAD)

Developed in 1969 by Watson and Friend,[1] this scale measures the tendency to avoid or feel anxious in social situations. The question-naire deals directly with *individual interactions*, for instance 'I usually feel relaxed when I meet someone for the first time'; and with *groups* — 'even though a room is full of strangers, I may enter it anyway.' The scale carries 28 items which are scored true or false. Some of the statements are worded positively, such as those above. Others are negative, such as 'I try to avoid people unless I know them well.' After completion the scale is scored by counting the number of times the patient gave a negative reply to either positive or negative statements.

The scale has been well researched and shown to be reliable and consistent in a number of studies. Although helpful in assessing general social anxiety, it does not deal specifically with hetero-sexual situations. Despite this, some studies have shown that people with high scores tend to be 'minimal daters' with few heterosexual relationships. This is a popular scale in work with patients showing social anxiety of an interpersonal nature. The patient needs little preparation. The scale can be completed in a few minutes and scored just as quickly. Studies indicate that changes in the level of interpersonal anxiety and distress are reflected in a change in the total score. This emphasises its value as an evaluation tool.

The Social Situations Questionnaire

This method was developed and published by Trower, Bryant and Argyle.[2] It comes in two parts. The first part deals with the patient's feelings in various situations. He is asked to rate his degree of diff-culty on a five-point scale. He rates how difficult he finds the situa-tion *now* and how he felt approximately *one year ago*. The scale includes general social situations, e.g. 'going into shops', as well as the more specific 'being in a group containing both men and women of roughly the same age as you'. It also includes some highly specific social behaviours, such as 'looking at people directly in the eyes'. The first part includes 30 such statements. In the second part the patient is asked to rate *how often* he has performed various social activities, this time using a seven-point scale, ranging from 'almost every day' to 'never'. In this section there are 22 items, including once again 'going into shops' as well as more specific items such as 'making the first move in a relationship'. The patient is asked to rate the relative frequency of each action over the last three months, and a similar period a year ago.

Although this scale covers many more areas of behaviour it is no more difficult to complete than the SAD. The statements are clearly presented and clear instructions are given in the use of the ratings. The scale has obvious uses in the evaluation of progress. It may also prove very helpful in selecting specific treatment goals, such as 'anxiety in groups' or 'talking to people'.

The Person Who Doesn't

The person who doesn't is a variant of the person who can't. He fails to do things he knows are appropriate and regrets this for a long time afterwards. The man who would like to pay his wife a compliment, or tell the office grouch to stop complaining, but who 'chickens out', is a typical example. We might call him *unassertive*. The unassertive person has become almost a vogue problem ever since Alberti and Emmons highlighted various methods for solving such problems in 1970.[3] Often seen as a branch of the West Coast American obsession with 'personal growth', assertion deficit is often a bigger probem than we care to admit. Often it is overlooked because such people merge into the background. They make few demands. Society even encourages unassertiveness as a way of maintaining control, or resisting political change.

The unassertive person is often described as lacking in spontaneity, emotionally inadequate, inhibited or otherwise constricted. Some people have argued that assertiveness is the open expression of practically all feelings with the exception of anxiety. Anxiety seems to inhibit the show of other emotions. However, there is some dispute over the definition. I feel that it is my responsibility to try to draw together some of the key descriptions in the pursuit of simplicity.

Dictionary definitions are often conflicting. Some define assertiveness as 'imposing one's proper authority' and would include 'domineering'. Perhaps it can be defined simply in terms of 'standing up for one's rights; exercising the right to say no, to tell the truth, to stand one's ground, to refuse to be manipulated'. The assertive person carries out these various actions without infringing the rights of others. Assertion may be seen as the mid-point between aggression and passivity. The assertive person won't allow himself to become downtrodden: neither does he trample on others.

Assertive Behaviour. Contrary to popular belief, assertiveness is not a personality trait. It is a skill that may be exercised in some situations but not in others. The managing director of a large firm may be a forthright leader in the boardroom, but a hen-pecked husband at home. A small number of people are unable to assert themselves anywhere. More commonly the problem is situation specific. For instance, men find it easier to be assertive towards women; and both men and women can be assertive with people they know well rather than with strangers. This tells us that we should avoid looking at assertiveness as a global construct. It is a facet of individual functioning which can vary from one situation to another. All unassertive people do not always appear meek and downtrodden. In some cases the patient may be a mixture of very passive and highly aggressive reactions. The two cases here illustrate this dichotomy.

Case Examples. Sally is a clerk in the civil service. She is in her late twenties and has just returned to her old job after a period in a travel agency. Attractive, intelligent and sociable, she was the picture of health when she married Dick, a self-employed printer. She began to feel the pressure at work about two years ago. Her office is very hierarchical. She is still a junior clerk, because she broke her service, and as a result she gets most of the work to do. Most of the staff feel overworked, but don't complain for fear of recrimination. Sally began to dread going to the office. She hated the pressure, the fear of making mistakes, the deadlines. One Sunday night she resolved to resign. She told Dick, who at first supported her. They would manage. She felt a wave of relief. By the end of the night Dick had confessed that the business wasn't going too well and would she reconsider? In a fit of depair she locked herself in the bathroom and took an overdose of sleeping pills.

Alex is 25 and is married with a young daughter. For the past two years his GP has been treating him for depression. He complains of headaches, listlessness and anxiety about going out. He has a long record of convictions for assault and has been in prison several times. His record of violence dates back to his youth. He has had a number of psychiatric admissions, all involving overdoses or mild self-injury. Each admission relates the catalogue of violence and ends pessimistically with the diagnosis 'severe personality disorder'. Alex is very soft spoken, almost inaudible at times. Although heavily tattooed, and with a scar across his cheek, he appears shy and retiring. He tells his story with much embarrassment. He describes all his 'outbursts' as situations where he gets frustrated or annoyed or when people disagree with him. He simply 'flies off the handle' and feels better for this release of emotion, but suffers regrets later when he sees what he has done.

These two people could hardly be more different. Different classes, different capabilities and different presentation. Yet they represent the same core problem. They are unable to solve their interpersonal problems without using some maladaptive coping tactic. Sally plays the 'neurotic female' and Alex the 'aggressive male'. Although Sally is a 'doormat' at work, at other times she is seen as witty and strong-minded and certainly no 'loser'. Alex is at the other extreme. He swings markedly from being shy and retiring to violent, almost homicidal, behaviour. He can also be tender, especially with his family. Like Sally, his problem is situation specific.

To assess these problems we need to study the patient's behaviour and the situations in which it takes place. We need also to ask the question, 'What is appropriate behaviour for these situations?' How should Sally have dealt with the pressure at work? How should Alex have dealt with his frustration?

The Assessment of Assertion

A number of methods have developed to study assertiveness. Most follow similar lines to that developed by Rathus, the designer of one of the best-known scales. The Rathus Assertiveness Scale[4] covers 30 items. The patient is asked to rate how characteristic these are of his behaviour in various interpersonal situations. A six-point scale is used which ranges from $+1$ ('somewhat characteristic of me') to $+3$ ('very characteristic of me'). Negative ratings of -1 to -3 are used to suggest how 'uncharacteristic' of the patient is each statement. Two typical examples are as follows:

I am careful to avoid hurting other people's feelings, even when I feel I have been injured *and*
If someone has been spreading false and bad stories about me, I see him as soon as possible to have a talk about it.

All 30 statements reflect these negative and positive qualities and are arranged randomly to reduce the risk that the patient will answer in the same way to each statement.

Norms developed by Rathus show that men do score more highly than women. Using these norms it is possible to judge, crudely, how assertive the patient is. However, I would again recommend caution against assuming that American and European patterns of behaviour are exactly the same. It has been reported, for instance, that there are differences between 'white' and 'coloured' populations. The key role of this scale is to offer a standardised format for evaluating the progress of the patient.

The Assertiveness Inventory. Another popular self-report method is the Assertiveness Inventory.[5] This covers 40 items on which the patient is asked to judge how *anxious* he would feel in the situations, and the extent to which he would *perform* the behaviour. A five-point scale is used in each case, with 'none' (1) and 'very much' (5) used for the anxiety rating; and 'always do it' (1) to 'never do it' (5) for the probability rating. Two typical examples are:

> give a friend a compliment
> cut short a telephone call when you are busy

This scale has the advantage that it judges what the person *might do*, as well as how he *might feel*. This is usually important in the evaluation of treatment. Does the change in the patient's level of anxiety influence his behaviour, or vice versa? This scale also helps pin-point areas in which the patient thinks that he needs some help. Once he has scored the scale he is asked to go through it again, circling those statements which represent areas in which he would like to change. As we have noted earlier, to try to cover all of these 40 areas in an interview would be boring and lengthy. The self-report methods have an obvious cost-effectiveness feature, but would only be appropriate for certain patients, such as the two illustrated. A patient who is poorly educated may feel threatened by the scoring system. In this case the nurse might help him complete the scoring.

The Person Who Doesn't Know How To

In this category the problem is one of a skills deficit. The patient has not acquired the ability to handle certain social situations, or his skills may be limited in some way. Social behaviour is a complex activity, combining speech pattern and content with body language. Some people fail to develop these skills beyond a basic level. If they are not painfully aware of their shortcomings, we can be sure that their gaucheness will not escape the notice of their peers.

We usually pick up our social skills from our parents, or whoever rears us. We look to these early 'role models' for guidance in the art of growing up. Peers at school or play influence further development. We learn to express ourselves at a primitive level in the home. We then use these skills to adapt ourselves to a variety of social situations. Where children grow up alone, or in an isolated area or separated from their parents, their social development may be impaired. Often such children fail to repair such damage as adults.

The role of social skills in mental health has been neatly summarised by my colleague, Calum McFee. Using a motorway analogy, he compares the influences of parents, brothers, sisters and friends to the slip roads feeding the motorway. The person who is socially proficient can handle any situation with self-assurance. He may have had good role models and a wealth of experience as a child. He merely needs to acclerate a little to respond to any new challenges. His sophisticated abilities make the fast lane his natural place on this motorway, where he speeds past those who are less proficient. The less sophisticated person may have had poor role models, lack of practice or a learning disability. As a result he is ill-equipped to face the stresses of the road ahead. He is suffering from a 'primary handicap', which is like driving a car with poor brakes or faulty steering. At the first hazard a crash is likely. People with underdeveloped skills often fail to deal with the pressures of the world. Such failures may herald the onset of a psychiatric disorder.

Another group of people on this motorway once had social skills but have lost them. The best example is the long-stay patient whose social functioning has been eroded by years of hospitalisation. This is often called a 'secondary handicap'. It follows, rather than precedes, the psychiatric disorder. His lack of social skills may be much greater than the person with a primary handicap. He may have lost the ability to communicate altogether. This patient has moved into the deceleration lane, or the hard shoulder. He is leaving the motorway to look for some assistance.

I do not want to misrepresent social skills as cocktail party behaviour. The ability to establish a social identity and to cope in society, however, does involve us in playing roles. To assess social skills we need to study the way the person uses his body and his voice to project an image: to play a part. When people are required to be sympathetic or assertive, to handle a drunk or pay a compliment, they need to play special roles. Our assessment of their social skills focuses upon the specifics of their ability to play these roles.

Case Examples. Jill is 20 with a history of manic-depressive disorder dating back to the age of 14. She is also mildly mentally handicapped. She is outstanding for her indiscretion and lack of tact. She is overtly explicit when discussing personal material and openly gives away family secrets. Her awkwardness extends to a rather wooden posture: she is slightly stooped and she rarely gestures. She smiles all of the time, even when telling a sad story.

Derek has been in hospital for more than 20 years. He works in the stores department. He was a civil servant before his admission with a severe depressive disorder. He rarely mixes with other patients and spends most of his free time walking in the gounds. He is quietly spoken, but tends to be rather verbose, taking a long time to explain what he wants to say. He rarely looks at others when in conversation, rarely smiles or shows any emotional expression.

Derek and Jill are both ill-equipped for their role in wider society. Within the shelter of the hospital they have few problems. In society at large they are manifestly handicapped, although perhaps for different reasons. Jill has failed to develop her skills to the full; Derek's may have been eroded. The distinction is largely academic. Their present difficulties are our main concern. We need to know *in what way* they are unable to fulfil some of the commoner social roles. Most relationships depend on three features:

(1) Each party is able to be direct — to say what he thinks and feels.
(2) Each party is able to be honest.
(3) Each party knows when and where such directness and honesty are appropriate.

We have noted already that Derek tends to be rather verbose. This lack of directness may be annoying, especially if the other person is impatient. Jill, on the other hand, tends to be too direct, often failing to allow conversations to 'warm up' before she starts to become intimate. In the same vein she is too honest about what she thinks and feels, which earns her the label of being indiscreet. In her case she does not know whether this is appropriate. Derek seems to have similar problems. He treats everyone much the same; he doesn't discriminate between friends and workmates and rarely lets people know how he feels or what he thinks. This is a kind of dishonesty.

Assessing the Mechanics

The assessment of social skills can be done in the natural setting, but is perhaps easiest under role-play conditions. Here the patient is asked to act out a scene from his life: standing at a bus stop, making a complaint to the ward sister or telling someone that he likes her. The situations selected must be relevant to the problem in hand, and the people who would accompany the patient should also be appropriate: e.g. staff or patients; friends or workmates. The idea of this role play is to evaluate some of the mechanics of social interaction, knowing full well that the patient's behaviour under these artificial conditions may be better or worse than in real life.

Verbal Behaviour

The following four areas seem to be of general importance.

Volume. Does he speak too loudly or too softly? In some situations a soft voice is appropriate (confidentiality). In others a louder voice is appropriate (making a complaint).

Tone. The resonance of the voice communicates a lot. If it is too sharp he may sound helpless or frightened. If it is flat, he may sound bored or depressed. Where his voice sounds 'thin' he may appear weak or submissive. If it sounds 'cracked' — breaking between fullness and threadiness — this may be interpreted as anxiety.

Rate. The speed at which the person speaks may suggest that he is anxious, angry or excited (too fast); or depressed or disgusted (too slow). Again appropriateness varies with situations. A person telling a story in a fast, breathless manner may sound excited or happy, which may be seen as appropriate. A person telling a workmate how to work a piece of machinery in the same fashion may sound impatient or anxious.

Interruptions. Any breaks in speech may also be significant. Some people 'um' and 'er' incessantly, as though they are uncertain of what they are trying to say, or are a trifle bored. Where long pauses occur between sentences, this may be interpreted as anger or irritation. In this category we might also include stammering and stuttering, which tend to reflect anxiety, although all three could reflect this.

Body Language

Among the various patterns of non-verbal behaviour that can occur, the following are most important.

Eye Contact. The extent to which people look at each other during conversation varies. It is even influenced by the sex of the speakers. It has been suggested that people might spend as much as 75 per cent of the time looking at the other person when *listening*, but only 40 per cent of the time when doing the talking.[6] Here we are anxious to judge marked absence of eye contact, which might be interpreted as embarrassment or lack of confidence; or staring, which might suggest hostility or confrontation.

Interpersonal Distance. The space between speakers is important. In a confidential exchange closeness is appropriate. Where conflict exists, the parties will be wider apart. In assessing this we need to ask, is he standing too close or too far away for this situation?

Gestures. The patient might use gestures which are *descriptive*, nodding his head to indicate 'over there', opening his arms to suggest 'this big'. He might also use gesture to add emphasis to what he is saying, nodding or shaking his head in agreement or disagreement; pointing in an aggressive display; putting his hands up to suggest 'no way'. He might also give away signs of emotion: touching or scratching his face — self-doubt; tapping his feet or picking at his clothing — impatience; picking or biting his fingernails, moving around in his seat — anxiety.

Facial Expression. Usually we 'accompany' the words we are saying with different facial expressions. If something is said to be disgusting, we screw our face up; if something is said to be funny, our face creases in smiles; if something is deadly serious, we hold a deadpan expression. Of particular importance here is the need for appropriate partnering of speech and facial expression. Does the patient's face communicate the same thing as his words?

The Content

We have looked at the *way* in which the patient might communicate. Now let us consider the nature of what he says.

Length. The length of any communication says a lot about the person. Too short and it may suggest lack of interest, anxiety or depression. Too long and it suggests dominance or aggression.

Appropriateness. The appropriateness of his speech depends very much on the situation. Does he disclose too little, or too much, about his personal life? Does he answer the questions asked? Does he talk about relevant material?

Quality. Finally, we might wish to evaluate the quality of the content. Does it contain appropriate humour? Is the content varied and interesting? or boring and monotonous? Is the material too vague or too specific?

Rating the Role Play

Various ratings of the role play are possible. The amount of detail included depends upon the skill of the observer, the time at her disposal and the problems of the patient. In Figure 8.3 I have illustrated a format which my colleagues and I have used for many years. It covers eight facets of social behaviour, some of which have already been mentioned, plus additional items such as posture, fluency of speech and spontaneity. This format is often most appropriate for evaluating the social behaviour of the longer-term patient. Short role plays are held covering (e.g.) holding casual conversations, asking for help, accepting a compliment, disagreeing with people, making a complaint. The role play is described briefly on the form and ratings are given for the patient's performance of each of the eight facets. A number of short role plays can be done one after another, including any appropriate comments.

In the second format (Figure 8.4) the observer collects much more detailed information and needs to be much more skilled.[7] Again, an appropriate situation is selected and noted on the front of the form, along with details of the patient and the observer.

Figure 8.3

Social Interaction Assessment

Name Bobby Buchanan

Rating

1. Poor: serious difficulty – disturbing to others.
2. Fair: needs a lot of improvement – interferes with social interaction.
3. Average: needs some improvement
4. Good: needs polishing – generally appropriate.
5. Excellent: little room for improvement – definite asset.

Date	Eye contact	Gestures	Facial expression	Posture	Volume	Fluency	Content	Spontaneity	ROLE PLAY	COMMENTS
10/4/82	3	1	1	4	5	2	3	2	Asking for directions	Smiling too much – big grin. Too stiff + upright.
"	2	2	1	3	4	2	4	4	Introducing self to stranger	Contact good! Too rigid. Hands by side all time.
"	1	3	1	2	1	1	4	4	Complaining about being kept waiting	Too aggressive!
11/4/82										

The format has four sections. In part A observations are made on the *presentation* of the patient at the beginning, middle and near the end of the role play. These are noted on the form *in pencil* and an average is calculated at the end of the role play. In the other three sections ratings are made, again in pencil, as the patient answers questions, introduces new material, etc. An average of these ratings is calculated at the end of the role play. On completion, any item on the scale that was not shown is deleted, to show that the observer did not simply forget to score it. Although this scale can be used in direct observation, it may be best suited to the analysis of video tapes.[8]

The Person Who Doesn't Think He Can

In the three examples above all the problems are visible. In this sense we could say that they are real problems. In this category the problem is more ephemeral, but no less disabling. The patient *believes* that he cannot or does not function effectively. This may be wholly at odds with the evidence that meets our eyes and ears. Here, the assessment of the patient's behaviour is only part of our concern. We are interested mainly in his thoughts, beliefs and perceptions.

Case Example. Dick is an architect with the local council. He is married with two children. He is a member of the Rotary, plays squash and does a lot of charity work. He is a member of the golf club, where he goes each weekend with his wife. Over the past two years Dick has been having an 'identity crisis':

> I have been looking at myself and I don't like what I see. I am weak, ineffectual and superficial. Sure, I go out a lot, but I don't seem to communicate with people. I'm so boring, going on and on about the same old things. I just seem to struggle to be with it all the time.

Dick is feeling depressed, but hides this from family and friends, who find little to fault in him.

Although Dick's problems are still focused on his interactions with others, they involve the way he interprets these relationships. They are a product of his perception and judgement of his own

Figure 8.4

SOCIAL SKILLS RATING SCALE

NAME _____   AGE _____

SITUATION _____

RATER_____   DATE _____

INSTRUCTIONS

— Rate each item by circling the description which most accurately describes the subject's behaviour.

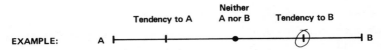

EXAMPLE:

— In section A rate the subject's overall presentation;
Notes should be made at the beginning, mid-way and towards the end of the session — and an <u>Average</u> Rating given for each item in this section.

— In sections B, C & D notes on 'Delivery', 'Content' and 'Interaction' can be made in pencil as the subject answers questions; Introduces new material; Takes turns or discusses/argues with others.   At the end of the session an <u>Average</u> Rating may be given, based upon these notes.

— If any item is not present during the session — e.g. 'Opinion' or 'Assertion' requires a discussion or confrontation setting — draw a wavy line through the scale viz:

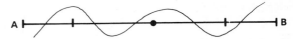

Figure 8.4 *(continued)*

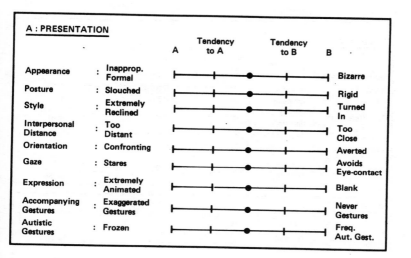

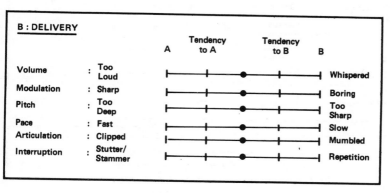

Figure 8.4 *(continued)*

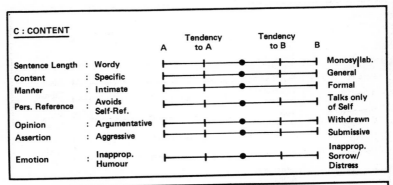

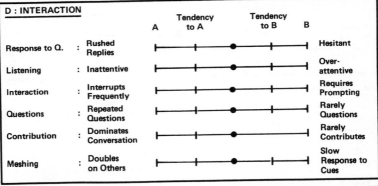

behaviour, seen against the background of his 'perfect self'. The assessment needs to compare Dick's actual performance with the way he thinks he functions.

The Interview

Dick's interpersonal alienation could stem from a range of thoughts he has about himself. His fears may be more tightly focused than the vague social anxieties we have already discussed. We might want to ask him:

(1) Do you ever fear that people will reject you?
(2) How do you feel about being criticised?
(3) Would you say that you are close to people?
(4) How do feel when other people get emotional — angry or tender, maybe?

If he has any fears in this area these may well block the establishment of open relationships. Perhaps he is constantly setting rules, restricting his relationships, blocking his contact with others. He may also be unable to discriminate between the way he *should* act towards one group of people or another. He appears to be something of a politician, always showing a friendly face, which may not reflect his true feelings. He may be dissatisfied with his life because of this lack of *genuine* closeness.

(5) Are you able to trust people with your worries or anxieties?
(6) Do you feel that you must smile and be happy with everyone?
(7) What part do you think other people play in the creation of your problems?
(8) If you disagreed with someone, or they obstructed you in some way, whose fault would that be?

Finally we need to consider Dick's *expectations* regarding his social relationships.

(9) What are you looking for in your relationships?
(10) Tell me how you see yourself?
(11) Can you describe someone who is the kind of person you would like to be?
(12) When you are dealing with people do you think that you can guarantee that it should turn out well?

Fear of Negative Evaluation

The patient who feels isolated from others may lack genuineness. He may hold distorted beliefs about his own ability, and may be uncertain about the kind of relationships he wants to have. A typical problem faced by this person is apprehension about meeting and dealing with people. They may appear, like Dick, to operate effectively, but may be troubled greatly. Watson and Friend[9] have developed a questionnaire which is a partner to the SAD scale mentioned earlier. The Fear of Negative Evaluation scale is a 30-item, true/false inventory which assesses the extent to which the patient fears a hostile reaction in some social setting. This anxiety is different from that experienced *in* the situation. A typical item is 'I am usually worried about the kind of impression I make.' People who score highly on the FNE tend to become nervous in situations where they think that their behaviour will be evaluated in some way. As a result they work harder to avoid disapproval or to gain recognition.

Looking at Thoughts

We have assumed that many of Dick's problems lie in his perception of his own behaviour. We need to look more closely at what he *thinks* about the situations in his life. In Figure 8.5 I have illustrated a format which I developed from Beck's cognitive assessment format.[10] The patient is encouraged to try to identify his bad feelings and to relate these to things which happen to him, or the thoughts he has about himself in certain situations. The patient begins by identifying a situation which occurred recently in which he felt bad. By answering the various questions he sketches out an impression of what was happening, how he felt and what his thoughts were at this time. The format also tries to evaluate the extent to which he believed what he was thinking.

Video-tape Recording. Although video-tape recording can be used as an assessment aid with any problem, it may be especially important for Dick. If our assumption that his fault lies in his perceptions is correct, recording a role play on video-tape may provide a useful basis for a discussion about how he thinks he functioned in the scene. Perhaps just seeing this recording will change his attitude towards himself. More likely, it will serve as a useful piece of evidence later on to challenge his thoughts about himself.

Figure 8.5

IDENTIFYING YOUR NEGATIVE AUTOMATIC THOUGHTS

We have discussed how the way you feel is influenced by the way you *think*. I want you now to practise finding out what sort of thoughts you have when you feel bad. Think about the last time you felt bad; you might have felt sad, or angry; guilty or frightened. Try to remember how you felt and what was happening around you and answer the following questions.

Feelings

How did you feel? _____

How bad was the feeling — measure it by using a scale of 0−100 (100 is the very worst)

                                              Score _____

Situation

Where were you? _____

What were you doing? _____

What was going on around you?_____

Were you thinking about anything in particular? _____

_____

Automatic Thoughts

What thoughts just 'popped into your mind' at that time?

_____

_____

_____

_____

_____

_____

_____

Did you *believe* those thoughts? Measure to what extent you believed them using a scale 0−100. (0 means you did *not* believe them at all; 100 means you believed them *completely*).

                                              Score _____

The Person Who Doesn't Have a Chance To

This last group covers a range of people. Here we have a person who has few relationships of a casual or meaningful nature. He has no supportive contacts, no one to share his troubles with. He may even have little contact with 'secondary groups': the news vendor on the corner or the assistant in the corner shop. Why he avoids even these non-threatening contacts is not clear.

The person who doesn't have a chance may be everyone we have already met rolled into one. He becomes anxious in any contact situation and resolves this by avoiding meeting people. When he can't avoid them he may feel that he can't communicate his feelings adequately. Such unassertiveness may be made worse by a lack of social skills. He may also be afraid that others will notice his awkwardness. Finally, he may exaggerate the importance of all of these factors. He may believe that he is worse than he really is. Others may find his company acceptable, even enjoyable. Due to his distorted perceptions he may be unable to appreciate this. If we ask the patient why he has so few friends he might proffer the old cliché: 'Who would want me as a friend?' This may be an accurate reflection of his predicament. If he is unaware of his problems, this may be an obstacle to forming new relationships. If he is aware of his shortcomings, he may predict his own repeated failure. The person who thinks that no one wants to know him will be unlikely to make an effort to establish new, or rekindle old, relationships.

The Social Context

In all the examples considered so far we need to see the patient against the social backcloth of his life. We need to quantify the number of contacts he has and their role in his life. Sociologists split such associations into two groups. Primary groups are those relationships with family or friends where we can disclose intimate details, gain support and encouragement: the fulfilling relationship. Secondary groups are more fleeting and superficial: people we speak to on the bus, staff who serve us in shops, colleagues we chat to idly in the lunch queue. These relationships rarely extend to anything beyond superficial conversation. In assessing the patient's social context we need to know who his primary and secondary group contacts are.

Case Example. Mark is a lecturer in English at a polytechnic. He has published a number of books of poetry and is working on his first novel. He is of a classically asthenic build, with a beard and close-cropped hair. He is slow and methodical in his speech, as though considering every word. Neighbours find him 'a bit strange'. He lives alone, following the break-up of a long-standing relationship. He occasionally has a lunchtime drink with colleagues from his department, and dinner with the departmental head every month. Beyond this he sees no one. Mark is the classic 'garret artist', eking out a painfully remote life-style. Others see him as a highly committed individual who has settled for a private life devoted to his work. The impression is deceptive. Mark has begun drinking heavily in secret. He ruminates constantly about his social isolation, but feels unable to change it. He blames himself for his lack of social contact: he is painfully uninteresting.

The effects of loneliness can hardly be overstated. People with inadequate or unsatisfactory relationships are prone to psychological disorder, which often ends in suicide. The abuse of drugs and alcohol is among the other common solutions used to blunt the pain of absent friends. Not everyone with poor relationships will become similarly afflicted. Some people enjoy isolation. However, the absence of confiding relationships can play an important part in the generation of psychiatric disorder.[11]

Some of the people we are considering here may never have had satisfactory relationships. In others the person may be responding to what has been called an unresolved relationship problem. He may have had an involvement with a girl-friend, family, etc. that went wrong in some way. This failure is taken as an indication that he should not, indeed cannot, get involved with others for fear of a similar ending. This is a reflection of the old adage 'Once bitten, twice shy.' Another group is those who interpret the breakdown of a previous relationship as a weakness on their part, or an illustration of their unattractiveness or unsuitability to others. This may lead to a succession of transient relationships. Contacts are made, often on an intimate level, but without any commitment. The patient may be waiting for the relationship to collapse again, as others have in the past. Consequently he is unprepared for anything other than a brief contact.[12]

Assessing the Social Network. Our first task is to assess Mark's social network. What relationships does he have at present? What do they mean to him? An important goal of assessment is to try to establish where he is socially at present. We might also retrace his steps to a time when his relationships were healthier. This might offset some of the gloom generated by a blank record sheet. The assessment of the social network should take a highly graded line. The person is questioned about close contacts first, perhaps with old friends and family, moving towards newer contacts with individuals or groups.

Example

I'd like to discuss your situation in more detail now. We have discussed how you feel isolated and alienated from everyone? (Mark nods) OK. Now I'd like to look closely at your relationships — as they are now, and how they were in the past. Let's talk about your family first. Do you have any brothers or sisters? (Mark nods) Tell me a bit about them. How did you get on together as children? Do you see them often now? Just tell me how you feel about them?

Mark is given *carte blanche* to discuss his family relationships. The nurse prompts him with the odd word or phrase to give details about 'how often' he sees them? or what sort of 'things' they do together? How does he *feel* about them? Does he trust them? feel affection? animosity? or jealousy? Does he get any support from them? Do they look to him for anything? Finally, a distinction is drawn between 'the relationship' as it is now and how it was in the past.

You and your brother have drifted apart, then? So you were close once, were you? In what way was the relationship different then?

Using the same format, the following areas would then be investigated:

— old acquaintances
— friends from the past
— neighbours or regular casual contacts
— organisations to which he belongs: clubs, church, etc.
— recent friends or acquaintances: at work or in the neighbourhood
— recent acquaintances gained through associations: clubs, societies, etc.

Figure 8.6

	CHARLOTTE	ERIC		
BEGAN	AUGUST '83	? '69		
HOW	MET @ CND	AT SCHOOL		
TIME TOGETHER	4	2		
SHARING	3	1		
TRUST	3	3		
PHYSICAL INTIMACY	. O	/		
CLOSENESS	3	3		
ENDED	JAN '84	STILL FRIENDS		
EXPLANATION	MOVED AWAY			
FEELINGS	FELT BITTER			
	SHE DIDN'T TELL ME SHE WAS GOING			

In taking this history it is important to detail the *people* and their *role relationship* to the patient. This can be used to plot ways of re-opening such relationships, or using the experience gained to develop new ones. It might also be used as 'evidence' to show that once he had relationships which were, at least, mildly satisfying. In Figure 8.6 I have illustrated a format for collecting this kind of information in a more organised manner.[13] The patient is asked to detail all his contacts, whether brief or long-lasting, beginning with the most recent. He is asked to name the person, using an alias if he wishes. The relationship is then examined as follows.

Example
(1) When did you first meet Charlotte?

(2) How did you come to meet her?

(3) Did you spend a lot of time together? (A scale is used to rate this: 0 = not at all; 1 = once a month; 2 = fortnightly; 3 = weekly; 4 = several times a week; 5 = lived together.)

(4) Did you find that you could share your feelings with Charlotte? (A similar scale is used here: 0 = not at all; 1 = rarely/superficially; 2 = a little; 3 = to some extent; 4 = a lot; 5 = to a great extent.)

(5) To what extent do (did) you think you can (could) trust Charlotte? Especially when you need support or help? (same scale as above)

(6) Did you have a physical relationship? To what extent is (was) that satisfying? (same scale as (4) above)

(7) Would you describe this as a close relationship? How close? (A scale is used as follows; 0 = extremely casual; 1 = barely friends; 2 = a friend; 3 = a good friend; 4 = a close friend; 5 = inseparable.)

(8) When did the relationship end?

(9) Why did it come to an end?

(10) How did you feel about that?

Using this format, it is possible to note down all the significant details of the relationship. We may then know how long the relationship lasted, how it began and ended and the patient's perception of the nature of that relationship.

The Spectre of Loneliness

Loneliness has been described as the 'absence, or perceived absence of satisfying social relationships, accompanied by symptoms of psychological distress'. Some people might admit to being lonely and might visibly be lacking in social contacts. Others might complain of loneliness but be seen by others to be sociable. Finally, there is a group that appears to have relationship problems but does not admit or complain of being lonely. Young has developed a self-rating scale that assesses some of the aspects of social relationships. His Loneliness Scale[14] studies the patient's attitude towards his relationships. This looks at the presence or absence of someone who cares for, or understands, the patient, someone to whom he can disclose important feelings and share problems. It also looks at membership of groups, the availability of people to share values, interests, love and activities, as well as the availability of trust, enjoyment and physical intimacy. The scale carries 18 items, each of which covers four points: for example, item 12:

0 = I can usually talk freely to close friends about my thoughts and feelings.
1 = I have some difficulty talking to close friends about my thoughts and feelings.
2 = I feel like my thoughts and feelings are bottled up inside me.
3 = I cannot seem to communicate with anyone.

The patient circles the number which best describes his feelings or situation at that time. Young has collected norms to help classify different levels of loneliness. However, the main use of this scale is to monitor any change in the overall loneliness score, during treatment or rehabilitation. A score obtained on admission might be compared with scores at discharge or following some specific relationship-forming therapy. Gains on the scale, though hardly concrete illustration of actual change, would serve as indication of progress.

The Pros and Cons of Indirect Measures

The methods of assessment discussed here rely either upon self-report or ratings by staff under role-play conditions. Both approaches have disadvantages, but the self-report methods may present more problems. Self-report scales are very economical, as they do not take long to fill in and the nurse need not be present. Most of the methods can be scored objectively, allowing meaningful comparison between people sharing similar problems. They can also help prepare for further assessment. Finally, since these methods produce a total score, progress across time can be evaluated.

However, the patient may be unwilling to fill in such scales. He may feel threatened by questions about his relationships and may also find it difficult to distinguish different aspects of his behaviour. Even the simplest social interaction involves a complex of responses. Faced with this complexity, the patient may be unable to distinguish (e.g.) his aggression from assertiveness. Some others may have little awareness of the effect of their behaviour on others. To use a term very loosely, they may lack insight. Similarly, he may be unable to judge or evaluate the behaviour of the person with whom he is interacting. When a person is 'justifiably angry' he has to be able to judge his partner's behaviour. What did he do to justify his anger? The final problem is a technical one. Many of the scales mentioned are scored true/false or with some scale of relative frequency. Most people do not behave, or feel, the same across all situations. Therefore, their score is a kind of 'flattened average'. Not only do the scales lack specificity in describing the situation that the patient finds difficult, but they also give an unrealistic report on his behaviour overall.

Direct Observation

The best assessment of most problems takes place in the real world. In Jill's case we arranged a role play to look at her social skills. Ideally, we would have liked to be a 'fly on the wall' when she talked to her neighbours in the corner shop. In Dick's case we would have liked to monitor his thoughts as he arranged seating at one of his charity functions. The information collected in role play, or drawn from memory, can be misleading. Yet, fly on the wall observations are often impossible. We may study the interaction of patients on a ward or at a day hospital, but in most other situations direct observation is contra-indicated. However, some patients may be able to collect information about their own functioning, the value of which can never be overemphasised.

Self-monitoring

Most of the methods discussed in Chapter 4 can be used here. Roger has a basic fear of dealing with people, especially where he is required to be himself. The fact that he is competent when playing the role of 'the lover' seems to reinforce this. Although it is not mentioned in our brief sketch, we might expect him to avoid situations where his fear might overwhelm him. He could be asked to *log* in his diary, in a notebook or even on a scrap of paper each time he 'opts out' of meeting someone. Over weeks or months this would give us valuable information about his avoidance behaviour. He could also rate his anxiety, using the kind of scale shown in Chapter 4, making a note of the situation and its demands upon him. On the positive side, he might count the number of times he talks to people at work, goes out into company, meets someone new.

Similar measures might be taken by Sally: how often was she

frightened of making a mistake? How often *did* she make a mistake? How often was she afraid of not meeting a deadline? or failed to complete work in time? We could extend these frequency counts to include the number of times she did speak up for herself, stood her ground, responded to criticism without tears. Ratings similar to Roger's would also be important here. Again there is no need for fancy record forms, providing that the information is collected consistently and the patient knows what he is meant to be monitoring.

In Alex's case measures of the number of times he loses his temper are obviously important. We also need to know what triggers this. He could simply write down in a notebook 'what happened', 'how I reacted' and 'what happened next'. In Dick's case the scene changes from overt behaviour and emotions to a focus on his thinking. He could count the number of times he has a certain 'negative thought' in the course of a day: 'I'm no use; I'm a bore; people must be fed up with me.' He could record these in the little notebook illustrated in Chapter 4, or even by tallying these up in his diary, or on the back of a cigarette packet. It would also be important to ask him to make a note of the things he does, such as organising meetings, taking his wife out for a meal. The kind of activity schedule illustrated in Chapter 7 might be useful here. Although this activity is not a problem, such information may be helpful later to act as a mirror to his perception of his self.

In Mark's case the frequency measure could be refined a great deal. Instead of just counting the number of times he meets people he might distinguish different kinds of conservation. He could count the number of *casual remarks* he made — 'Hello, good morning'; *asking questions* — 'Can you tell me the way to Tannadice?' and *expressing opinions* or talking about himself — 'I really admire the women at Greenham'; or 'I used to play truant when I was at school.' Mark's casual conversations with colleagues in the bar or at dinner might be monitored. Although difficult to record during these situations, he might be able to clock up at least one of these by carrying a tally counter in his pocket.

Time Measures. Some of these aspects of the patient's life could be studied in terms of time. It is unrealistic to expect him to carry a stop-watch to work or dinner parties. However, we might ask him to rate conversations in terms of length: brief (only a few words); short (one or two sentences); medium (giving a short commentary);

long (speaking for several minutes).

Quality. The content of the interactions might also be self-monitored. To ease the strain, and embarrassment, of analysing social behaviour I have often asked patients to award themselves points — or stars — for different patterns of interaction. Different weightings can be attached to asking a question, giving an opinion, offering instructions, speaking in public, etc.

Most, if not all, of these methods may be used by other people, such as staff or members of his family, to help add to the assessment of the patient.

Conclusion

Relationships have always played an important part in the explanation of psychiatric disorder. However, 'relationships' in psychiatric nursing are often thought to be bound up in the rather vague dynamics of the therapeutic community, or the magical interaction that takes place between nurse and patient, which neither can explain. I have not dealt with these rather ephemeral aspects of relationship formation. As I noted at the beginning, these broader issues were not my concern and may be beyond my comprehension. Instead I have taken a fairly direct line, trying to collapse a wealth of relationship problems into a few categories. I would emphasise that these are in no way mutually exclusive. Some patients may have two or more of these problem areas. Although these problem areas may be very disabling when they occur at great intensity, what is most interesting is that we can see ourselves in all of them. For me, this is an encouraging sign. Even where the patient is allegedly 'different' from me — suffering from some alleged mental illness — we have something in common: a difficulty in maintaining our social competence.

In this chapter I have tried to emphasise a number of points. First of all, by focusing attention on specific aspects of the patient's functioning we can help see his strengths and weaknesses through *lists* of different patterns of behaviour, emotions or thought processes. This takes him at least one stage forward from his rather vague 'relationship problem'. By specifying the different aspects of social functioning clearly, we can help him learn to distinguish his different roles, one from another. He is able to discover that he has several 'selves', some which might be useful to him and others which are less so. In this sense the assessment provides an educational facility. By trying to measure his social functioning we begin to understand a little of what the problem means to the patient or those who interact with him. By studying his thoughts and beliefs — where appropriate — we can extend his understanding of *how* he functions and how he relates to others in terms of his own value-system. Finally, the various strands of information drawn together from self-reports, casual observation, notes made on the back of cigarette packets, or detailed ratings taken from video-tapes all add up to a multi-faceted picture of a social animal. In some cases that picture needs to be complex, drawn from painstaking observation and thoughtful evaluation. In most others the information can be collected simply, using simple materials, most often of a 'home-made' nature. Either way, the picture should enlighten staff and patient about the nature of his relationship problem and should open the door towards its resolution.

Notes

1. D. Watson and R. Friend, 'Measurement of Social-evaluative Anxiety', *Journal of Consulting and Clinical Psychology*, **33** (1969), pp. 448–51.

2. P. Trower, B. Bryant and M. Argyle, *Social Skills and Mental Health* (Methuen, London, 1978).

3. R. E. Alberti and M. L. Emmons, *Your Perfect Right* (Impact, San Luis, Calif., 1970).

4. S. A. Rathus, 'A 30-item Schedule for Assessing Assertive Behaviour', *Behaviour Therapy*, **4** (1973), pp. 398–406.

5. E. D. Gambrill and C. A. Richey, 'An Assertion Inventory for Use in Assessment and Research', *Behaviour Therapy*, **6** (1975), pp. 550–61.

6. Trower *et al.*, *Social Skills and Mental Health*.

7. This format is influenced strongly by the writings of Trower *et al.*, (ibid.).

8. Further information on the use and application of this format is available from the author at Tayside Area Clinical Psychology Department, Royal Dundee Liff Hospital, Dundee DD2 5NF.

9. Watson and Friend, 'Measurement of Social-evaluative Anxiety'.

10. A. T. Beck, A. J. Rush, B. F. Shaw and G. Emery, *Cognitive Therapy of Depression* (John Wiley, New York, 1979).

11. See J. E. Young, 'Cognitive Therapy and Loneliness' in G. Emery, S. D. Hollon and R. C. Bedrosian (eds.), *New Directions in Cognitive Therapy* (Guildford Press, New York, 1981), Ch. 8.

12. See ibid.

13. This format is influenced strongly by the work of Young (ibid.).

14. Young (ibid.).

9 ON THE EDGE OF EXPERIENCE: THE PATIENT WITH A PSYCHOTIC DISORDER

All are lunatics, but he who can analyse his delusion is a philosopher. — Ambrose Bierce

In this book I have tried to discuss ways of looking at people who behave in some disordered way. I have tried to keep as open a format as possible, eschewing where possible the labels which might lead us merely to confirm our prejudices about 'what is wrong with the patient'. In this chapter I am faced with a dilemma. I wish to discuss people who have extraordinary experiences, and who appear to be affected by these in the longer term. These people are commonly referred to as 'psychotics'. I am reluctant to use the term since it might suggest that before beginning the assessment I have already made up my mind as to the nature of the patient's condition. This is not the case. I simply cannot think of an alternative way to discuss such phenomena, and their resultant problems of living. This is an illustration of my own deficiency; no more, no less.

In this chapter I want to discuss the kinds of experience which are called psychotic and the patterns of behaviour commonly associated with psychotic patients. I shall not attempt to discuss the diagnosis of psychotic disturbance. I shall, however, return to the issue of diagnosis in the penultimate chapter. The kind of personal maladaption which we call psychosis might be categorised in two ways. First, we might study the behaviour — or reported experience — of the patient. Second, we might classify the patient on the basis of the cause of his disorder, its prognosis and recommended treatment. Since the first option involves simple assessment, and the second diagnosis, I shall emphasise the former. I recognise that such information as we collect may be used at a later stage to arrive at a diagnostic classification.

In this chapter we are again looking at the way the patient perceives himself and the world around him. In the case of the psychotic individual the kinds of experience we can expect to find will be of a different form or content from other problems of living. In some cases the content may be bizarre or unusual. Or it might take a more extreme or sustained form of usual experience.

Taken together, the kinds of experiences we shall discuss represent the more outstanding, outrageous and disturbing kind of psychological disturbance. In the second part of the chapter we shall look at ways of measuring such phenomena, as well as the general behaviour patterns of people who have progressed into a chronic stage of their disorder.

Lunacy

Although the layperson has little idea of what mental illness is, he is likely to proclaim that he knows one (i.e. a madman) when he sees one. The psychotic is the caricature of psychiatric disturbance: the person who is out of touch with reality, believing perhaps that he is answering his mother's instructions to kill (as in Hitchcock's classic film *Psycho*). At a less sophisticated but no less influential level, the lunatic appeared regularly in children's comics, harmlessly proclaiming his belief that he was Napoleon before being carted back off to the asylum. The layperson might be forgiven for believing that all psychiatric patients are homicidal maniacs or immersed in some delusion. Traditional media often proclaims this in dangerous isolation from reality. The reader will be well aware that not all psychiatric patients are madmen in the sense depicted above. They may also be aware that not all psychotics are wholly out of touch with reality.

It is commonly accepted that the psychotic has experienced some loss of his reasoning power. Dr Johnson believed that 'all power of fancy over reason is a degree of insanity'. The traditional association between insanity and the function of the brain is depicted in the novelist George Moore's observation that his 'wretched brain gave way, and I became a wreck at random driven, without one glimpse of reason or of heaven'. The traditional failure to discriminate between the inability to reason, which might be shown by the intellectually impaired, and real madness was pointed out by the philosopher John Locke. 'A fool from right principles draws wrong conclusions, while the insane person draws a just inference from wrong principles.' There was great reluctance to acknowledge that mental disorder was in any way simply an exaggeration of normal behaviour. The nearest we get to this historically is a recognition that great men are close to madness. Shakespeare observed that 'the lunatic, the lover and the poet are of imagination all compact', whereas in terms of greatness John Dryden remarked that 'great wits are sure to madness near allied, and thin partitions do their bounds divide'.

An Incomprehensible Problem

In keeping with the other chapters I shall try to look at the reasons *why* we identify certain patterns of behaviour as deviant, unacceptable or pathological. I shall also consider ways of measuring what is clearly a complex problem. Before beginning to discuss these two concerns I should say what I do not intend to cover. I have expressed an interest in trying to understand the meaning of the patient's behaviour. However, there is clearly much dispute as to *anyone's* ability to explain psychotic phenomena, far less mine. R. D. Laing was fond of pointing out that there is as yet no 'fact' of psychosis (or rather schizophrenia — the commonest form of such disturbance). He argues that to explain the incomprehensible behaviour of people we might call schizophrenic by suggesting that this is due to some psychological deficit is akin to saying that a man standing on a tightrope 100 feet up in the air is suffering from an inability to stand on his own two feet.[1] Laing believed that in order to understand psychotic behaviour we need to ask why such people are obliged to make themselves often brilliantly elusive. It is not my intention to explore anything like Laing's territory of interest. I shall merely try to remind the reader of the criteria by which we arrive at the assessment of personal maladaption. I shall leave the reader to explore the available literature in her attempt to understand what the term 'psychosis' means.

The Interview

The format of the interview was discussed in Chapters 2 and 3 where some of the kinds of unusual behaviour we might associate with psychosis were also mentioned. In this section I want only to amplify some of the points made in Chapter 3.

Three major areas are the focus of our attention in the interview: reports of distortions of general experience; distortions of perception; and disturbed or disturbing beliefs or value systems. In interviewing the patient it is crucial that we do not lead him unduly. It would be inappropriate, for example, to use a checklist of all the possible hallucinatory, delusional or experiential problems he might experience, as this might distress the patient or represent a threat to him. Or it might lead him to consider or report experiences he might otherwise have ignored. Perhaps the simplest approach is to follow the kind of general 'life history' interview format, described in Chapter 3, leading on where appropriate to the kind of 'problem-oriented' interview illustrated, inviting the patient to discuss the aspects of his life, in general, that are a problem to him at present. These topics will allow the patient the opportunity to report whether he has ever felt strange; whether he has ever thought that people were conspiring against him; or has ever heard voices; etc. The nurse's task here is to encourage the patient to specify any such experiences more clearly, without appearing to be in collusion with him. In the sections below I shall try to suggest the sort of phenomena we might be interested in reporting, phenomena that are commonly associated with psychotic disorder.

Anomalies of Experience

Being ourselves is something we take for granted. We need to be ourselves in order to relate to the outside world: to attend, register and memorise information, and to use this store of experience to determine our emotional relations to the world and its relationship to ourselves. We cannot be aware of these various functions of the self. Such awareness might be more of a hindrance than a help. As long as we are untroubled by our awareness of ourselves we have no real difficulty. Many people do experience different kinds of self-awareness which they find disturbing. I shall attempt to summarise some of these difficulties below. In interviewing the psychotic patient we are collecting information, or evidence, that all is not well in his relationship with himself.

The Experience of Self

Reed describes four main disorders of experience involving the 'self'.[2]

(1) The Self and the Outside World. Some people are unable to distinguish between themselves and their outside world. The patient may report that people or objects are inside him, or that he is a part of them. He may suggest that things which are happening to the environment — such as walls being painted or carpets beaten — are happening to him. He may report feeling the effects of these environmental experiences on or in his body. The patient's self-

concept is faulty here: he appears unable to separate himself from the outside world. Often this is referred to as the *blurring of ego boundaries*. Although it can occur in a number of illnesses (such as delirium) or in drug-induced states, where it occurs in a person whose consciousness is clear and unimpaired it is often seen as a separate disorder. Comparisons have been made between such psychotic experiences and psychedelic experience. However, the two are different for the reason given. Indeed such psychotic experiences are more like self-induced mystical states, where consciousness is not impaired. Yet the person experiences a blurring of his own boundaries and a merging with the world or the infinite. Flying in the face of traditional psychiatric opinion, Reed suggests that such ego boundary blurring is not of itself pathological. It is determined by the cognitive labels that are applied by the person. A person who is delirious or suffering some pre-epileptic aura may describe such experiences as frightening. The psychotic patient may also be frightened by his experience. However, where such experiences occur in a religious or mystical context they may be viewed as blissful or wonderful. Such reports may also be made by people of an artistic or poetic nature. In interviewing the patient who reports such an experience it appears to be more helpful to ask him how he feels about the *content* of his experience than to spend too much time concentrating upon the form of the experience — how it happened.

(2) Personal Attribution. Concern with the influence of the outside world is often extended to cover the belief that the patient's actions are controlled by some outside agency. Normally, we cannot divorce our thoughts and behaviour from 'ourselves'. Although we might appreciate how a person who was controlled or manipulated in such a way might act — like a puppet or a zombie — we have little idea of how he would *feel*. Where the patient confesses to such a loss of personal control, this is often thought to be indicative of schizophrenia.[3]

There are a number of variations of this experience. The patient might report that his thoughts are *alien* to him. At a very simple level he may feel that his thoughts are not really his own. At a more complex level he might explain this away by attributing influence to some outside agency: secret police, communists, religious groups, etc. He may describe how such groups exert their influence: through hypnosis, telepathy, X-rays, etc.

The patient may also believe that his thoughts are drained away by this outside power. This is often associated with *thought blocking*: the patient appears to stop thinking, shows a lapse of concentration, and suddenly stops talking or working. In other patients *thought broadcasting* may be described: people are allegedly able to tune in, or listen to, his thoughts. Often such listening implies a criticism of what he is thinking.

In all these examples the patient is apparently *passive*, controlled by some outside force. He may specify the nature of this influence, as in the power of the secret police or Venusians. This is often called *delusional passivity*. Where no specific mention is made of the nature of the external influence, it is simply called a passivity experience. The patient may report motor and emotional passivity, as well as thoughts, believing that his actions and feelings are similarly controlled.

We must question the nature of these experiences. Why or in what way are they pathological? The answer is a complex one. Unlike the disorder of self-concept these passivity experiences are not unusual or pathological in their *content*: it is their form which makes them so unusual. Many people report situations where they believe that their thoughts are controlled, or that they are the agent of some superior or supernatural force. This is true of those who profess to contact much more bizarre characters than those cited by the psychotic — establishing links with Red Indian chiefs or ancient Egyptians. Other people have had revelations: a divine insight of a religious nature, which is allegedly put into their minds by God.[4] The same is true of all those who believe that they have had some kind of 'extra-sensory' experience: the increasingly popular ESP movement. If we wanted to be pedantic, all these people are suffering from delusions of passivity, but the *form* of their experience is quite different. It occurs only in certain situations, may be fleeting or of short duration, or occurs under some form of stress. In the interview with the psychotic patient we want to know how often they have had such experiences? How long do they last? And to what extent do they occupy their everyday thinking? Such questions about the form of the experience are much more important than a detailed description of the content.

(3) The United Self. The two experiences listed above are unusual, and tend to reflect serious mental disturbance. The next two, although reported by patients, also occur in the normal population.

Under normal stress conditions people usually experience emotional disturbance: an exaggeration of anxiety to panic proportions, or a depressing despair. In some situations this emotional exaggeration does not take place, being replaced by an eerie sense of calm. Reed suggests that this can take place in a variety of situations: e.g. in fierce wartime combat or when being ravaged by a tiger. Instead of the manifest fear we would expect, a slow-motion, blunted calm occurs. Where such experiences occur in everyday life, this is called a *dissociation of affect*. The person is cut off from his feelings. In many settings we can see how useful this might be as a biological defence against overwhelming emotion, as in bereavement. Where no obvious stress is evident, or there is a general background of disturbance, the phenomenon assumes quite different proportions. It can extend under some situations to what is called ego-splitting, where the person feels as though he is physically outside of himself. Again this is common in bereavement or severe depressed states. In the interview it is important to find out whether such experiences are generalised, occurring in a wide variety of situations, or specific to certain stressful events. In the former they may suggest a highly unusual state of affairs, whereas in the latter this may be a natural defence against major emotional disturbance.

(4) Contact with Reality. We take reality for granted. We do not analyse it or note any change in it except under the influence of some drug. However, some people report unusual experiences of reality without any obvious influence. They may, also, be bemused by the experience. Two distinct forms are possible. In the first the person may feel some change has occurred within himself. This may heighten his awareness of reality. Commonly this is called *depersonalisation*. He may detect some change in his total self or in a part only. He may believe that his bowels are rotting away, or that his body is swelling to an enormous size. One particular experience that Reed recounts appears to be peculiar to Chinese males: they fear that their genitals are shrivelling away into nonexistence, by disappearing inside themselves. At the most extreme the patient may harbour the nihilistic delusion that he no longer exists. In the second form (*derealisation*) the person remains the same but detects some change in the world around him. The world may become flattened, vague or misty. Reed suggests that the root of these experiences may have something to do with the acute focus or emphasis of the patient's thoughts. Typically we are a global

whole: we function as a co-ordinated whole. Where the person begins to focus closely upon himself, or a part of himself, some breakdown in the usual mechanics of self-concept may occur. In interviewing the patient information about *what* he experiences is obviously crucial. It may also be helpful to find out whether he has a tendency to be introspective, analysing himself, ruminating on his 'self' or some specific aspect of his experience. It will also be necessary to establish whether such experiences are continuous or related to any specific situations. Here the interviewer is interested in establishing not only the content of the patient's experience of reality, but also the form it takes.

Judgements and Beliefs

The assessment of the patient's values and belief systems is a tricky area, for we are obliged to judge the significance of the patient's faith or conviction in a certain set of ideas. Although we tend to discriminate between real and false beliefs (delusions), the situation is slightly more complex than this. Two main classes of ideas may be evident. We shall discuss these in turn.

(1) Over-valued Ideas. Where a person has a firm, perhaps extreme, conviction, which is based upon personal experience, we call this an over-valued idea. The road safety campaigner or the political activist are typical examples: both hold views which society might view as extreme. The value aspect of this title illustrates how our view of any belief system is influenced by normative considerations. An over-valued idea is one which is not greatly appreciated by the majority of the population, or some subculture of the population. Indeed the person who holds such 'extreme' views may be perceived quite differently by separate clinicians, who will be influenced by their own values and beliefs. Someone with conservative views may find the patient extreme, whereas someone else with more radical leanings may find him 'almost normal'. The normal standard that is being used to evaluate the patient is the standard of the individual clinician. In general, over-valued ideas are seen as a problem only when they tend to dominate the person's life. In the interview we should be interested again in the form that the value system takes: to what extent do the person's beliefs influence the day-to-day running of his life?

(2) Delusions. Although we commonly refer to a delusion as a false belief, this is woefully inadequate as a definition. What we refer to as 'fact' is no more than a convention. Many primitive cultures believe that rocks and trees possess spirits. Many contemporary religions hold similar views about the existence of souls, heaven or the coming of Christ. These are all 'facts' to them. In this sense it may be more appropriate to relate delusions to faith rather than belief. Delusions have much in common with religious faith, since both are often incontrovertible despite the lack of any evidence. Delusions have been defined as beliefs which are not shared by the patient's society or culture, and which are maintained despite all evidence to the contrary. However, the emphasis upon conviction (or incorrigibility) is misleading. For instance, I tend to believe that there is some good in everyone. I might be called naïve or idealistic for holding this belief, but I am unlikely to be called deluded. Even where people hold unusual religious beliefs, they will merely be labelled 'eccentric'. The incorrigibility of the deluded person can, however, be important, where for instance he refuses to change his mind even under extreme torture. But religious or political idealists would behave in the same way, so we are no further forward. Although psychiatrists have often emphasised the highly personal nature of delusions, this seems a little unfair. Any belief, held long enough, becomes part of that person's psychological make-up. What does seem more significant is that the person may ruminate or be otherwise preoccupied with the belief, much more so than the person with strong moral convictions. Here again the key charac- teristic of the delusion seems to be the way it functions, rather than its content. Does it tend to dominate the patient's thinking? Does it distract him from concentrating on other things? In general, does it interfere with the workings of his life?

The major classes of delusion are commonly described as follows.

Persecution. The patient believes that someone, or more often an organisation, is threatening his life. The organisation may be of a religious or political nature, but may also be a group of friends or neighbours. This delusion is often associated with hallucinations of taste and smell: poison in food or gas. The patient may also report *ideas of reference*, where he interprets hidden meanings in people's behaviour. For instance, he may believe that a cough represents a signal to begin some threatening action.

Jealousy. The patient believes that his wife has been unfaithful and identifies virtually anything as possible signs or clues to this effect. His wife's fervent denial may be interpreted as a sign of guilt. When she tires of resisting, this is taken as an admission or confession.

Grandeur. The patient believes that his abilities are wildly superior to their actual level of competence. This idea may even extend to the belief that the patient is someone famous, either living or dead.

Poverty. The patient believes that he and his family are poverty-stricken. This is less common now than it was in the days before state support.

Ill Health. The patient believes that he has some deadly disease, which he may have passed on via infection or contagion to his children. He may identify rotting organs or decaying bones. To a large extent this delusion is influenced by the patient's knowledge of anatomy and medicine.

Guilt. The patient experiences massive self-reproach for crimes, sins or past misdeeds. He may demand punishment for these errors. This demand is often represented by sexual misdemeanours. At its most extreme the patient will reject his own existence: *nihilism.*

In the assessment of delusions it is important to be scrupulous in recording what the patient *says*, avoiding interpretation or premature labelling. Many authorities have argued that there are two classes of delusion. Secondary delusions arise from some other abnormality, such as affective disorder. Here the patient may believe that he has committed an unforgivable sin for which he is being punished. This delusion is secondary to the lowering of mood. A primary delusion is usually characterised by a *lack of content.* The patient may note that the world is behaving strangely. He may feel eerie sensations (delusional perceptions). He may have delusional ideas or memories, remembering that the look in some-one's eyes was the cause of some recent affliction. Finally, he may have a 'delusional awareness': he knows something — e.g. that the end of the world is nigh. The assessment of delusions should attempt to capture the nature of what the patient experiences, since this may help us understand, at some later stage, the significance of his experience.

Perception

Hallucinations have been described as false perceptions that are in no way distortions of real perceptions. They arise as something new alongside *real* perception. Contrary to an illusion, a common occurrence which disturbs us sufficiently to question its reality, a hallucination is felt by the patient to have an external reality. Despite any obvious objectivity, he feels that it is real. The range of possible hallucinations is virtually limitless, but commonly they are categorised according to the sensory modality involved.

Hallucinations involving *sight* can range from simple lights and flashes to sightings of people, who may be named or merely classified. Such hallucinations may occur in organic disorders, where often the 'sightings' are of huge animals (the delirious patient's 'pink elephants'). In general hallucinations have real substance, using the environment, walking through doorways and casting shadows.

Hallucinations involving *hearing* may range from simple noises, bangs and whistles to intelligible speech of one or more people. Where people speak to the patient they may be known or unknown and may have a relationship with some persecutory delusion. A voice of criticism is common. This may be heard speaking clearly or in hushed whispers. In echo de pensées the patient thinks that he hears his own thoughts aloud and fears that others might be listening in.

Hallucinations involving *smell* might involve gas, especially where the person feels persecuted. Or he might smell an offensive odour from his body, especially where he is depressed. Hallucinations of this sort are also prevalent in organic states such as the epileptic aura.

Hallucinations of *touch* often take the form of wind blowing across the person, the sensation of vibrations or electric shocks. Often there is a strong sexual connection. The patient may feel that he is being fondled or penetrated by some invisible other.

Hallucinations of *taste* are usually focused on food, again with the persecuted individual most evident along with the epileptic with his experience of aura.

Finally, the patient may experience general *somatic* sensations of a hallucinatory nature. He may feel that his body is being twisted or torn or even disembowelled. In some cases he may report invasion by animals, snakes in his stomach or frogs in his rectum; or the feeling that his flesh is decomposing.

A further four classes of hallucination may also occur.

The patient may fail to perceive something that is evident to everyone else. This is commonly called a *negative hallucination*.

The *doppelgänger* phenomenon involves meeting an exact double who is recognised as an absolute likeness. In German folklore this is believed to be a portent of death. It is a favourite theme in literature, often reported by writers like Edgar Allan Poe, who was seen as unstable, and Dostoevsky, who was epileptic. Reed notes, however, that Goethe, the German poet, met his *doppelgänger* despite a reputation for momentous psychological stability.

Pseudo-hallucinations are the subject of much controversy, but seem to involve seeing something which even the observer recognises to be unobservable to others. He recognises that it is a subjective phenomenon. It is very similar to the experiences of visionaries, mystics and mediums who recognise that others cannot see their vision.

Finally, there is a group of *functional hallucinations* that appear to be related to the workings of the environment. Voices may be heard when taps are turned on: they stop when the taps are turned off again. Shapes and objects may appear and disappear with the turn of a light switch.

It should be readily apparent that the assessment of these experiential problems is a virtual minefield. In the case of grossly disturbed patients it may be easy to spot what appears to be a classic phenomenon. In less disturbed patients, or those who are already undergoing treatment, the picture may be subtler. This may make 'symptom spotting' more difficult. I have attempted in this brief summary to introduce the novice nurse to some of the categories of experiential disturbance that she may encounter during the interview of the psychotic patient. I have not listed these various phenomena in order to help in the classification of the patient's disorder. Rather, this sketch is intended to introduce the nurse to the lie of the land in perceptual and experiential disturbance. Her responsibility, in the interview, is to collect a detailed picture of the patient's description of these phenomena. By using my guidelines regarding probing the form or the content of various experiences this picture may emerge a little more quickly than through straightforward questioning. The key to a 'good assessment interview' with the psychotic patient is, once again, keen and impartial observation and recording. By sharpening our pencils *and* our perceptions we may be able to gain a clear account of the patient's experience through his own verbal account. If we need a rubber, it will be only for erasing any unnecessary interpretation of the patient's report.

Observing the Patient

Within the Interview

In addition to collecting information from the patient's verbal report, the interview gives us a chance to observe his behaviour under structured conditions. As we discussed in Chapter 3, there is a need to make short notes on the patient's appearance at the interview; how he interacted with the nurse; the speed of his answers; the use of gestures; any strange mannerisms; the presence of eye contact; signs of agitation or anxiety (e.g. getting up and pacing around the room). A 'good' assessment of the patient's non-verbal behaviour should be modelled on a naturalists' observation of birds: using brief, yet detailed, descriptions of behaviour to paint a verbal picture of what took place. These notes should not be translated into diagnostic labels: e.g. if the patient 'only looked up from time to time. Sat turned away and was very brief with his answers', this should not be translated into 'Patient appeared paranoid/depressed/or hostile.' The notes collected here may provide suggestions for further, more detailed, observations under different conditions. For example, observations may be taken of the behaviour of the patient in the ward, at occupational therapy, or when in a group, to evaluate whether or not the presentation noted during the interview was maintained under these conditions. In one sense the interview provides a valuable opportunity to study the patient, with the minimum of distraction. However, the very artificiality of the setting may produce a wholly unrepresentative picture of his behaviour. The main value of the interview may be in helping the nurse decide which aspects of the patient's behaviour or experience she should try to assess or measure further.

The Assessment of General Behaviour

Where the patient is hospitalised it will be possible to study his overall behaviour using one of the available 'global assessment' methods. These are of greatest value in the care of long-stay, or 'chronic', patients where problems may exist on a number of fronts. These global methods rarely provide a satisfactory amount of detail. Instead they pick out the patient's major strengths and weaknesses, and may provide pointers for further — more refined — observation.

The NOSIE

The Nurse's Observation Scale for In-patient Evaluation[5] has already been discussed in Chapter 5. This scale was developed to help nurses participate in the assessment of hospitalised patients. This and similar instruments recognised the crucial role played by nurses in the planning of health care. Since they spent all day with the patients, they were in the best position to comment on the presence or absence of specific patterns of behaviour associated with mental disorder. A number of versions of the scale have been produced, ending up with 30 items which make up six separate scales: Social Competence, Social Interest, Personal Neatness, Irritability, Manifest Psychosis and Retardation. In studies conducted in America and the UK[6] the scale has been found to be a reliable, brief and unambiguous tool for the assessment of long-stay patients. Where the patient is not chronically psychotic it has been found to be of less value as a measure of 'in-patient behaviour'. Due to the limited number of factors covered by the scale NOSIE is ideally suited for settings where staff feel that they have insufficient time to complete more extensive scales. Although the scale is short, and can be completed in only a few minutes, comparison between patients pre- and post-treatment is possible, as well as comparison between patients in different areas. This latter comparison may help in deciding upon inter-ward transfers.

The PIP

The Psychotic In-patient Profile was developed in the early 1960s in an attempt to develop a scale that would provide a more inclusive picture of the psychotic patient than was then currently available.[7] Lorr and Vestre had studied existing scales and found that none of them measured more than six or seven of the syndromes reported in the psychotic literature. Their eventual scale[8] studied eight behaviour constructs and four self-report syndromes.

Behaviour　　　　　　　　　　　*Self-report*
Excitement　　　　　　　　　　　Grandiosity
Hostile belligerence　　　　　　　Perceptual distortion
Paranoid projection　　　　　　　Depressive mood
Anxious depression　　　　　　　Disorientation
Retardation
Seclusiveness
Care needed
Psychotic disorganisation

The inventory consists of 96 separate items, 74 of which involve behavioural factors which the nurse rates on a four-point 'frequency' scale:

    0 = not at all
    1 = occasionally
    2 = fairly often
    3 = nearly always

Typical of the statements which would be rated are the following:

    Acts as if moving required a special effort (retardation)
    Complains about the food and care he receives
        (paranoid projection)
    Loses temper when dealing with other patients
        (hostile belligerence)

The nurse is required to observe the patient for a three-day period, after which she may rate his behaviour over this period. If she is uncertain of the appropriate rating she is advised to record the rating that is 'mostly true' of his behaviour over the three days. The four self-report syndromes are completed following a brief inter-action between nurse and patient. The nurse is instructed to talk to the patient in fairly general terms. She then records the presence or absence of grandiosity, perceptual disorganisation, depressive mood or disorientation, by recording 'true' or 'false' to statements such as:

    claims he has a divine mission (grandiosity)
    feels hopeless and despairing, beyond help (depressive mood)

Lorr and Vestre note that their eight behavioural categories are especially appropriate for the assessment of patients who are withdrawn, mute or otherwise inaccessible to interviewing. The format is also highly appropriate for the study of excited or aggressive patients. It was designed to provide quantitative measures that might prove helpful in evaluating the effect of different treatments, and in deciding upon appropriate ward placement or even discharge. In keeping with the rigorous research basis used to develop the profile, Lorr and Vestre provide simple norms that can be used to compare the patient being assessed with those patients who took part in their various studies. Such norms may be a little inaccurate if an attempt is made, for example, to compare Scottish with American patients. However, as a general guide such norms are extremely useful, allowing the nurse to gauge how severely disturbed the patient is on any of the twelve factors.

My colleagues and I have found the PIP to be a useful and reliable assessment tool. It is very easy to use and provides a pleasing graphic representation of the scores. The nurse rater needs only to place the rating score in the box indicated beside each statement on the scale. The scores are easily totalled to provide specific scores for each of the twelve syndromes. These can then be plotted on a simple graph on the back of the profile, which allows easy comparison between one patient and another, or between the patient and the normative sample who participated in the original studies. Like the NOSIE, the PIP focuses attention on diagnostic symptoms. It provides little information that would be of use in planning nursing interventions. However, this was not its aim. Ideally, this profile should be used to evaluate progress or regression, or to decide on placement. As with other global scales, it may also provide pointers to further forms of direct observation. I would recommend this format to nurses in the long-stay area as a simple, cost-effective instrument.

The REHAB

The Rehabilitation Evaluation of Hall and Baker consists of two main parts: part two focuses on adaptive behaviour — the everyday living skills that were discussed briefly in Chapter 5. Part one deals with disturbed or maladaptive behaviour and the scale concentrates upon a limited range of behaviours that are typical of long-stay patients. The nurse is required to indicate approximately how often the following behaviours occur:

Incontinence
Absconding
Violence
Stealing
Self-injury
Sexual offensiveness

These are all rated on a three-point scale: more than once a week; once a week; within the past year.

Three other behaviours are also monitored in a similar fashion:

Collecting rubbish
Verbal aggression
Talking to self

These are rated on the basis of: more than once a day; once a day; within the past year.

The REHAB format has recently been revised and is now available in a very attractive package comprising various record sheets, scoring manual and a guide for use of the scale, as well as individual and group profiles.[9] As I noted in Chapter 5, Hall and Baker developed the scale following extensive experience in research and clinical work with long-stay patients in Britain. Norms are available from their research that allow meaningful comparisons to be made between any individual or group of patients with the sample population from their various research programmes. Hall and Baker have also published details of their psychometric analysis of REHAB, which adds further support to its use as a reliable and valid instrument for the assessment of long-stay patients. I would recommend it to all nurses interested in this population.

The Use of Global Ratings. The three global rating scales described above are examples of rational, logical use of nursing staff in the assessment process. Traditionally, the assessment of patients has been left to the psychiatrist, who spent little time with the patient, in a highly structured and artificial interview situation. Any complementary role which nurses played was highly unsystematic and usually took the form of offering advice or information from memory during a case conference. Although I use the past tense, many nurses and doctors continue to use the 'How-is-the-patient-this-week-Sister?' method. Although by no means answering all our needs, the three scales are definite improvements as a means of patient evaluation. Each scale tries to structure the nurse's observation and knowledge of the patient into a form that everyone can 'plug into'. Nurses spend most of their working day in contact with patients, collecting valuable information. Each of these scales provides a means of reducing this wealth of observation to a workable format. All three are useful additions to the running of any case conference. Indeed, I find it difficult to imagine how one can review a long-stay patient without such guidance. If these measures are taken routinely — for instance every six months — it is possible to plot the patient's progress or regression. Where samples of a complete hospital rehabilitation and long-stay population are taken, it is possible to make meaningful comparisons between 'Joe Bloggs' and the 144 other patients in this area. Such a comparison is a useful hedge against prejudiced assessment. Finally, these scales provide a useful introduction to the selection of the more detailed methods I shall discuss below. These global methods give us an indication of where we ought to begin looking in greater detail. The 'whole patient' is unlikely to be problematic. The PIP might point out his 'hostility and belligerence', which can be monitored in a more precise fashion. The REHAB might point out the patient's deficiencies in community living skills, combined with a tendency to hoard rubbish. Again specific measures might be developed as a preliminary to establishing a treatment programme for these two problems. In many areas staff begin to assess the first problem that grabs them by the throat. In some cases this *will* be the major problem. In others, more careful consideration of the overall picture of the patient might help us select more appropriate assessment and treatment targets.

More Specific Measures

The Definition of Behaviour

In any assessment procedure the definition of the assessment 'target' is crucial. If we are not clear about *what* we are looking at, then the information collected may be meaningless. To ensure accurate recording of patient behaviour Ayllon and Azrin proposed the following rule: 'Describe the behaviour in specific terms that require a minimum of interpretation.'[10] The less the nurse has to interpret, the less the likelihood of error. This rule can present problems. If the definition is too long-winded staff may find it cumbersome, and may revert back to their original 'impressions'. If a number of different behaviours are to be studied, the nurse may end up carrying pages and pages of 'definitions' to guide her observations. For some behaviours there are simple solutions.

Where the behaviour can be monitored by an automatic device, the need for such definitions is avoided completely. Incontinence can be monitored by providing the patient — or his chair — with a sensitive alarm that signals each time urine is passed (the device does not react to tea, water, etc.). The patient who is withdrawn and speaks in hushed or inaudible tones may be assessed using a device which reacts to different levels of sound. A light will signal each time his voice reaches a certain volume. Pedometers may be attached to the waistband of the manic patient, to measure 'overactivity' in terms of miles travelled each day. However, although these methods resolve the problem of definition, they are appropriate for only a small number of patient problems, where these devices are an adjunct to other means of recording and observation.

Where the patient's behaviour leaves a *product*, the outcome of the behaviour may be studied, rather than the performance of the action. Incontinent behaviour leaves a 'wet patch' on clothing or sheets; work behaviour leaves a number of 'labels applied', or 'toys painted'; study behaviour leaves 'pages of notes written'; shaving behaviour leaves the amount of 'hair removed'; bizarre behaviour leaves the number of 'extra garments worn' or the number of 'magazines hoarded'. This approach, which again is appropriate only for certain behaviours, eliminates the need for the nurse to observe the patient *during* the action. She can check up at any time in the day to record the outcome of his behaviour.

For most other behaviour patterns it is possible to simplify the definition of everyday activities, such as living skills, to simple 'appropriate' or 'inappropriate' categories. Therefore, appropriate *washing* might be defined simply as follows:

applying soap and water to most of face and drying with towel.

Eating appropriately might be defined as follows:

uses utensils to cut and scoop foods without spilling: spoon for 'spoon foods'; knife/fork for meat course.

An assessment of the patient's everyday routines of eating, washing, grooming, dressing (etc.) might comprise a simple check-list with a column for each of the *activities*: rising on time; dressing;

washing, etc. Beside each activity the nurse could check 'appropriate' or 'inappropriate', using the kind of definitions described above. The assessment of these routines would thus be reduced to a simple three-column entry.

The patient's patterns of disturbed behaviour could be defined and monitored in a similar fashion. *Hallucinating* might be defined as 'speaking or gesturing in absence of any other person in near vicinity'. *Delusional speech* might be defined as 'supplying incorrect questions in response to questions, or discussing material of a bizarre nature'. At face value this definition seems appropriate. However, it assumes that every nurse agrees on the meaning of 'correct' and 'bizarre'. It would be necessary to draw up a list of examples as a guide to the use of this definition, but both these definitions would allow every nurse to check the presence or absence of these behaviours.

Specific Targets

Once we have defined what we wish to study we can decide *how* best to collect the information. In the rest of the chapter I shall discuss a few of the methods which can be used to study the three major areas of psychotic behaviour that are of concern in the hospital setting: self-care, social skills and 'psychotic behaviour'.

Self-care

Some attention has already been paid to this area in Chapter 5. I shall recap briefly on the assessment of skill deficits, before moving on to some of the self-care *excesses* which can be found in this population.

Checklist Methods. As I have noted already, providing that a definition of appropriate or inappropriate behaviour is available, the observation of self-care skills is a relatively straightforward procedure. The format that has already been described is a 'black-and-white' measure. We record simply whether or not the behaviour has been performed. This may be appropriate where the patient is able to perform the behaviour, but appears unmotivated. When he does do it, we can expect him to do it 'appropriately'. However, with many patients the problem involves their *ability*. The patient may rise and shave and wash and dress *every morning* without fail. However, the quality of his performance may be poor. If the goal of the assessment is to evaluate the quality of the patient's behaviour, then some kind of rating scale should be used, e.g.:

0 = complete assitance required to complete
1 = physical *and* verbal prompting needed to complete
2 = verbal prompting *only* required to complete
3 = completes unaided

This fairly crude measure may be more appropriate than simply recording whether or not he performed the behaviour. The 'checklist' may contain any number of different behaviour, which can be observed in any setting. The nurse simply accompanies the patient; observes his peformance; and notes his level of performance using the kind of scale indicated. For the assessment of routines, nothing could be simpler. The nurse is able to supervise the patient, offer help as required and can then record her observation on the checklist she may have pinned to the wall, or folded in her pocket.

Frequency Measures. The psychotic patient may also show a number of strange or repetitive behaviours associated with self-care. He may undress, wash his hands, drink water or consume food or other material at regular intervals. These behaviour patterns may be counted using the frequency record format. Providing that staff are in a position to observe the patient throughout the day, a simple count may be taken each time he engages in the defined behaviour. Various possibilities for recording exist. Staff might go to the duty station each time the behaviour occurs, making a brief anecdotal report on a special form, e.g. 'washed hands — 11.00 a.m.' or 'removed shirt and vest, then replaced — 2.00 p.m.' These incident records can be tallied each day or week to give an overall frequency for different behaviour patterns. Where the patient moves from one part of the ward or hospital to another, but remains in the sight of at least one nurse, each nurse might carry a card indicating 'morning', 'afternoon' and 'evening'. If the nurse witnesses the performance of the behaviour, she would place a tick under the appropriate heading. This format, which is only really suitable for single behaviours, will allow the frequency of the behaviour across the week — and periods of the day — to be carefully evaluated. Alternatively, the staff might carry tally counters, clocking up incidents as they occur, passing the counter on to another nurse at the shift change-over, and writing down the daily total at the end of the day. This approach is only suitable for single behaviours, and gives no indication of how the frequency is distributed across the day. However, where the behaviour occurs frequently — e.g. dressing and undressing or washing his hands up to 30 times a day — the tally counter may be the easiest method.

Freqency within Sessions. Similar methods can be used to record unusual behaviour at mealtimes, such as the number of times a patient licks his plate. One of my colleagues used a tally counter to record the number of times a patient licked plates after each course. The totals, in the region of 100–200 licks per meal, justified the use of the counter. Where similar repetitive acts occur during washing, e.g. repetitive stroking of the face or rubbing with the towel, a measure of the frequency for a limited time period (e.g. 5 minutes) may provide valuable information about the strength of the behaviour. Where such measures are taken, the length of the session — e.g. grooming, bathing, eating — should be clearly specified.

Task Completion. Where a behaviour comprises a number of steps, the performance of each step may be monitored. In Figure 9.1 I have subdivided the face into a number of areas. At the end of the sesion the nurse can record how many of the areas were completely shaven. Dressing might be broken down into the following stages:

(1) Clothes on in correct order
(2) Buttons and fastening done up
(3) All loose ends tucked in
(4) Tights/socks pulled up
(5) No torn or soiled clothing worn

Permanent Products. The measures noted above could be called products. The nurse does not observe the patient performing the behaviour: she merely checks the outcome. Similar measures of the amount of food spilled on the table or on clothing during meals are possible. A rating could be used to indicate:

Figure 9.1: Shaving Analysis

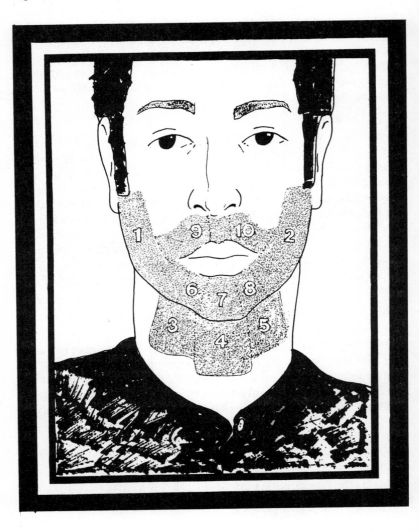

0 = none
1 = small amount (size of 10p piece)
2 = moderate amount (diameter of base of cup)
3 = considerable amount (twice diameter of base of cup)

Similar ratings can be used for the *amount of food eaten* $(0, \frac{1}{4}, \frac{1}{2}, \frac{3}{4}$ full meal).

Latency Measures. In some cases the patient may perform the behaviour very well, but may take a long time to do so. Measuring how long someone takes to eat a meal from the time he sits down at the table may help us appreciate more clearly the extent of his 'obsessional slowness'. How long he takes to get up after being called; to dress or shave or walk to the occupational therapy department are similar examples. In many cases these measures may be indirect measures of the extent to which the patient is pre-occupied, if we assume that such cognitive problems interfere with his daily routine.

Sampling Methods. Where a behaviour occurs at random intervals throughout the day a 'time-sampling' method may be indicated. Incontinence provides a good example. Since it is not possible to predict exactly when the behaviour will occur, observations may be taken at intervals during the day or night. These 'samples' (every 30 minutes) check for signs of the product of incontinence: a wet patch which might be rated in terms of size. However, this observation format may be confounded if the patient changes himself between 'samples'.

Comment

The striking feature of all these methods is their potential for 'inhumanity'. They remind me of the kind of army life which sends a shiver up my spine, or the 'body inspection' procedure of POW camps. However, there is no need for such observations to degrade the patient, providing that some sensitivity and creativity are shown. These observational methods are a necessary evil: they are akin to many medical diagnostic procedures, which are equally uncomfortable for the patient. Many of the observations can be made discreetly, without disrupting the patient. Where contact is necessary, a tactful and sincere explanation of the purpose of the check should avoid any embarrassment.

Social Behaviour

The patient's social behaviour presents us with a much bigger challenge, in terms of the range of behaviour and the technical problems of measurement. Here we would include general social behaviour and the specifics of inter-personal interaction. Inter-personal behaviour has been defined as 'greeting staff, answering awareness questions, and participating in group discussions'.[11] Other studies, however, describe much simpler patterns of behaviour. Some report any utterance the patient makes, whereas others demand sentence construction. In this section I shall not attempt to offer a definition. Instead I shall simply discuss ways of collecting different sorts of measures.

General Interaction

Where the patient is severely limited in social skills a frequency count of the number of times he speaks each day may be a highly valuable measure. Staff might interact with him for a short period at intervals throughout the day, saying (e.g.) 'How are you, John?' or 'What are you going to do now?' The patient's responses might be recorded simply as 'response — no response'. Alternatively a rating might be used:

0 = no response
1 = mumbled — unintelligible
2 = single word — audible
3 = short sentence

The kind of rating required is determined by the nature of the problem. For a delusional patient the rating might cover the degree of 'rational speech present'. In the case of an agitated or hypomanic patient the level of 'excitability' or 'pressure of speech' might be assessed. Such ratings may be taken at random times during the day, to rule out the influence of certain time periods.

Random Observations. If observations are to be taken every 30 minutes a random time schedule might be planned as follows. All the times between 9.00 a.m. and 9.00 p.m. would be plotted on a piece of paper. A time between 9.00 and 9.30 would be selected — for example by sticking a pin in the list with eyes closed. Then a time between 9.30 and 10.00 a.m. would be selected by the same method, and so on throughout the day. As a result the observations would be done *on average* every 30 minutes. However the first one might be at 9.06, the second one at 9.52, and the third one at 10.04.

Consequently the patient would not grow accustomed to the timing of the observations, therefore ensuring a more 'natural' observation.[12]

Structured Interviews. Structured questionnaires are favoured where the patient is withdrawn or the content of his speech is bizarre. A withdrawn patient might be questioned about his feelings, activities or hobbies, using the kind of simple rating scale already illustrated. Where such a format is used it is easier to ensure agreement as to 'correct' or 'incorrect' answers. The quality of the response may be rated further by judging the length of the reply or the use of adjectives to describe things.[13]

Group Discussion. An observer may record patients' responses in a group: e.g. answers to questions; initiated contributions; asking questions. Positioning herself just outside the group, she can clock up single behaviours using a tally counter, or tick off various behaviours for each patient as they occur, using a checklist. On a more difficult level she might measure the length of speeches using a stop-watch, or might rate various verbal and non-verbal behaviours using the kind of scale described in the last chapter.

Opinions and Feeling Talk. Since many long-stay patients have difficulty in expressing their emotions, the assessment of feeling talk is an important area.[14] The nurse might record the number of times patients say 'I think' or 'I feel'. Alternatively, patients might be asked specific questions designed to elicit feelings or opinions, e.g. 'How do you feel about the other patients on this ward?' The patient's answers may be rated on the amount of affection, approval or liking of others expressed.[15]

Comment

A range of methods can be used to measure the occurrence of certain patterns of social behaviour. I have discussed only the simpler methods here. In some settings it may be more appropriate to audio- or video-tape record sessions, using this for a more detailed analysis later. Such a record might pick out the number of times the patient said 'Yes' or a rating of the fluency of speech. However, no observation is possible without first specifying clearly the aim of the assessment. Does the patient talk too much? too little? too fast? or with bizarre phraseology? Such goals will have been decided from the global assessment. Some casual observation of the patient will help establish *how* the measure should be taken. Finally, some practice must be done, to ensure that each nurse using the recording format is able to assess the patient reliably. Deciding whether to observe the patient under natural conditions or in a structured setting is usually a technical one. Observation in the 'natural environment' is always best. It is also always the most difficult. Observations taken in a structured setting — like a discussion group or role play — are much easier. However, the patient's behaviour under these conditions may be quite different to the way he functions under natural conditions.

Psychotic Behaviour

We have already discussed how the psychotic patient has a potential for unusual experiences. It is not possible for us to study such experiences directly, due to their covert or private nature. We can, however, observe patterns of behaviour that we can assume are associated with such phenomena.

Delusional Speech

Delusions may be defined as patterns of speech content which are at variance with accepted reality. Since the content of delusional speech can vary enormously from one patient to another, no standard format can be recommended. It may be appropriate simply to make a catalogue of all the delusional statements the patient makes, using this as the basis for a checklist to monitor the frequency of such statements.[16] Delusional speech patterns may vary in length. In such cases the length of time spent in delusional talk would be a more appropriate record. Recording the frequency of delusional speech is much easier than recording duration. Perhaps the easiest method would involve rating short, medium and lengthy 'delusional statements', having defined these clearly in terms of *time*.

Structured Situations. In a classic study Wincze and his colleagues[17] asked nurses to select 15 questions from an original pool of 105. Each question dealt with the patient's known delusional speech content. The nurses spent three minutes with the patient 20 times a day on a random basis, judging his responses as either 'delusional'

Figure 9.2

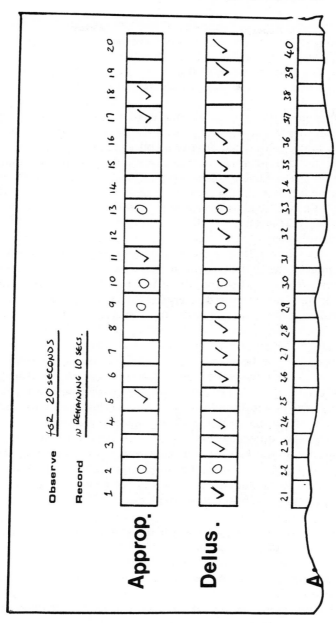

or 'appropriate'. More recently, Myers[18] selected 11 questions from an original pool of 55. The nurses were instructed to interact with the patient, maintaining eye contact after each answer, nodding after each sentence and allowing five seconds' silence after a correct answer, and cutting off lengthy answers after one minute.

Interval Recording. As an alternative to simply counting or rating sentences the nurse who can record the patient's conversation (on audio-tape), or who can observe a colleague talking to the patient, might try this interval recording method. This involves noting whether the patient is silent, speaking appropriately or showing delusional speech during short time intervals. The method may be used 'live' or to analyse a recording. The nurse listens to the patient for exactly 20 seconds. She then judges his speech — silent/appropriate/delusional — and records her judgement in the appropriate box (see Figure 9.2). Ten seconds are allowed for this. She begins listening to the patient again at the start of the next 30-second interval, repeating the procedure. As a result, the whole session is broken up into 30-second intervals: 20 seconds listening and 10 seconds recording the judgement of his speech. During a 10-minute interview 20 such recordings could be made. A fairly accurate estimate of the proportion of time spent in delusional versus appropriate speech can be calculated. We can see that on this record the patient did not speak on four occasions. Of the remaining 16 intervals, he spent 75 per cent of his time in delusional speech and 25 per cent in appropriate conversation. In using this format the nurse must ensure that the patient spends *the majority* of the 20-second period engaged in one form of speech or another. If he spends *more than half* the time interval speaking, this is recorded; *less than half* the interval and he is recorded as 'not speaking'. As a result this format does not provide a direct measure of the duration of delusional speech — only a rough guide.

Latency Measures. It is also possible to record delusional speech by noting how long the patient can hold a 'normal' conversation, *before* introducing material of a delusional nature. This is a fairly simple procedure. The nurse simply starts a stop-watch, preferably in her pocket, at the beginning of the conversation and stops it as soon as the patient begins to speak in delusional terms, noting the duration of normal conversation.

Comment

The measurement of delusional speech is complex because the *quality* of the behaviour is likely to vary from one situation to another. On some occasions the content of the patient's speech will be highly delusional, and on others only a little 'odd'. Sometimes he may say very little of a delusional nature and on other occasions his delusional monologues may run on for many minutes. The assessment of the patient's delusional state must reflect this range of possibilities. As a result, the assessment procedure is likely to be a complex one. Some of the procedures I have described briefly require little effort to apply. Others, like the interval recording method, must be practised to perfection. In general, the key to a 'good' assessment lies in its planning. The patient should be observed in a number of real-life situations, where he is given an opportunity to be rational *or* delusional. By using a wide range of questions — in the manner indicated — the patient's potential to speak 'normally' may be assessed and, by implication, the intrusion of his delusional ideas may also be monitored.

Hallucinatory Behaviour

This presents even more problems than delusional speech, if we are interested in reliable and valid measures. Hallucinatory behaviour has been described, somewhat pedantically, as the presence of verbal, facial and/or gestural responses to an unobservable stimulus. If we are to be the judges of objective reality, we are talking about the patient appearing to respond to something or someone *who is not there*. Hallucinations may take various forms. The only ones we can discuss by direct observation are those of an auditory or visual nature, where the patient appears to be reacting to something, usually indicated by his speech. For other kinds of hallucinations, we must try to recruit the assistance of the patient, to 'self-monitor' his own experiences. Of course, this is possible with only a small number of patients.

Observing the Patient. If the patient is observed alone — such as in a viewing room, or on closed circuit television — this makes identification of such behaviour easier. If no one else is present, there will be no one to make 'normal' responses to. Usually, this is not feasible. Instead, it may be necessary to study the patient closely for a short period, perhaps over a few days, noting the sorts of things he says and does which might be illustrative of a hallucinated state. This list might then form guidelines for observation.

The Structured Setting. To solve the problem of having to observe the patient continuously, some structured setting might be arranged. The patient might be observed during meals, at his workplace or in social interaction: all situations where hallucinatory behaviour might be unacceptable. In theory, there is no reason why someone should not hallucinate when no one else is around. Bob Liberman counted the number of times a patient showed any one of a number of clearly defined behaviours, during structured conversations.[19] Other studies have used a simple rating scale to estimate the amount of hallucinatory behaviour present during set periods, such as mealtimes.[20] Using a similar interval recording format to the one previously described, the presence or absence of hallucinatory behaviour during short time intervals can be studied. If a nurse spends 10 minutes talking to a patient, another nurse can monitor the presence or absence of hallucinatory behaviour by breaking the total period down into (e.g.) 60×10-second intervals. She then merely ticks the presence or absence of hallucinatory behaviour within each 10-second interval. Again this provides a measure of the proportion of the total time spent showing hallucinatory behaviour.

Self-monitoring. These kinds of methods require the nurse to be highly objective and systematic. The methods are difficult not because of the complexity, but because of the long-term strain of looking/recording; looking/recording. The measure produced is necessarily crude and in no way reflects the reality of the experience. Many patients experience hallucinations but show no obvious sign of this. In such cases it may be necessary to enlist his support, through self-monitoring. The patient might be asked to keep a diary, noting each time he heard or saw something that disturbed him. Or he might be asked to carry a tally counter in his pocket, clocking up every hallucinatory incident as it occurred. This is appropriate only when 'voices' or 'images' appear and disappear quickly. Where the hallucination lasts for a longer period of time the patient may need to learn how to rate the experience. Two of my students showed how easy it is to gain fairly reliable records of such experiences. Mike Aslin[21] asked a patient to record each time she heard voices by immediately informing the staff, who recorded this on a chart in the office. Anne Hume[22] asked a chronically paranoid patient to record each time she heard a 'threatening voice' by clocking this up on a tally counter. This measure was taken during structured interviews with the nurse, because it was assumed that the hallucinations were at least partly a function of interpersonal anxiety.

Comment

Some of the methods I have discussed briefly above might be viewed as simplistic. I would accept this. However, I would maintain that they all have a major head-start on some of the highly biased reporting methods that are used in most clinical settings, where global ratings are done for a daily or even weekly period. Often, no clear definition of 'hallucinated behaviour' is available and each nurse uses her own. Such measures give no indication of severity or fluctuations across situations. Hallucinations are a highly complex phenomenon, involving patterns of observable behaviour, psychological functioning and perhaps also physiological activity. It has been suggested that delusions and hallucinations may be seriously studied only if measures of all three domains are taken: (1) what the patient *says* he thinks or perceives (verbal-cognitive); (2) what he can be seen to be saying or doing (behavioural-motoric); and (3) through measures of physiological or autonomic activity.

Other Patterns of Behaviour

The psychotic patient may show a vast array of other disturbed or disturbing behaviours. We cannot discuss all of them here. Especially in the long-stay population, aggressive, self-injurious, destructive and abusive behaviours are common. These may be related to other kinds of experience, such as hallucinations or delusions. These patterns of behaviour can be recorded simply, using the kind of frequency or duration measures already discussed. Bizarre posturing, hoarding of rubbish or food, persistent questioning or repetitive speech patterns can all be measured providing that the 'target' behaviour is clearly defined. The simple rule is — if the behaviour is short-lived (such as a brief verbal outburst), then a *count* of the frequency is appropriate. If the behaviour lasts for varying amounts of time (such as posturing or speech patterns), a measure of the time spent in the behaviour is more appropriate.

The Nurse as Film Director

I acknowledged at the beginning of this chapter that the assessment of psychotic patients would present us with many problems. Perhaps the reading of the last few pages confirms this. The very nature of the problem causes us major technical difficulties. Much of what we call 'psychosis' is a personal experience. Apart from asking the patient to describe this, which often is not possible, little in the way of direct assessment can be done. As a result, most of my recommended methods focus upon studying what we can see and hear: the patient's observable behaviour. This may, however, be a blessing in disguise. As I shall discuss in Chapter 11, we are still uncertain of what, exactly, we mean when we talk about 'psychosis'. For this reason alone, the collection of *highly objective measures* of the patient's behaviour may help us understand better the meaning of 'psychosis'. In many settings nurses, knowing the patient's diagnosis in advance, fail to see anything other than 'psychotic behaviour'. Not only is their observational format highly suspect, but they may be blind to any display of appropriate behaviour by the patient.

The kinds of measures and strategies described here simply quantify various facets of behaviour or experience associated with what we call a 'psychotic state'. No explanation of why the patient behaves in this way is produced. As I noted in my introduction, this was not my aim. I have discussed the nurse's role as an assessment director. Like a film director, she needs to know what sort of 'scene' she wishes to shoot. Does she want to depict self-care skills or delusional speech? This is her first decision. Then she must decide on the location. Where does she want to shoot the assessment? In a natural setting or in a special 'studio'? This is her second decision. Then she must select a 'cameraman', someone who is expert at taking 'good' pictures, someone who will follow her direction to the letter. Next she must select her 'cast'. Who will be in the film? Nurse and patient? Patient alone? Perhaps a group of patients with a member of staff? The cast list must be defined, and each 'actor' should appear in every shooting. Next, she must write a script: this will describe in detail what the actors are doing and gives specific instructions to the 'cameraman' how she should record the scene. Once all these decisions have been taken the filming may begin. Like all the best movies, a number of takes may be necessary before the scene is captured to the director's satisfaction. For us, this represents some of the trial and error necessary to *develop* a satisfactory method, and to practise using it.

Notes

1. See R. D. Laing, 'The Schizophrenic Experience' in *The Politics of Experience* (Penguin Books, Harmondsworth, 1967), Ch. 5.

2. The following discussion is heavily influenced by the writings of G. Reed, *The Psychology of Anomalous Experience* (Hutchinson, London, 1972).

3. This is a reference to Schneider's 'first-rank symptoms'. See Reed, ibid.

4. In this context we might seriously consider the position of all religious cultures, but especially the 'born-again Christians', many of whom claim to have had a personal communication with God.

5. G. Honigfeld, R. O. Gillis and C. J. Klett, 'NOSIE-30: A Treatment Sensitive Ward Behaviour Scale', *Psychological Reports*, **19** (1966), pp. 180–2.

6. A. E. Phillip, 'Prediction of Successful Rehabilitation by Nurse Rating Scale', *British Journal of Psychiatry*, **134** (1979), pp. 422–6.

7. M. Lorr, J. P. O'Connor and J. W. Stafford, 'The Psychotic Reaction Profile', *Journal of Clinical Psychology*, **16** (1960), pp. 241–5.

8. M. Lorr and N. D. Vestre, *The Psychotic Inpatient Profile* (1968). Published by Western Psychological Services, 12031 Wilshire Boulevard, Los Angeles, California 90025.

9. REHAB is available from Vine Publishing Co., 2a Eden Place, Aberdeen.

10. T. Ayllon and N. H. Azrin, *The Token Economy: A Motivational System for Therapy and Rehabilitation* (Appleton-Century-Crofts, New York, 1968).

11. G. L. Nelson and J. D. Cone, 'Multiple Baseline Analysis of a Token Economy for Psychiatric In-patients', *Journal of Applied Behaviour Analysis*, **12** (1979), pp. 255–71.

12. F. E. Sterling, 'Net Positive Social Approaches of Young Psychiatric In-patients as Influenced by Nurse's Attire', *Journal of Consulting and Clinical Psychology*, **48** (1980), pp. 58–62.

13. J. M. Hall, R. D. Baker and K. Hutchinson, 'A Controlled Evaluation of Token Economy Procedures with Chronic Schizophrenic Patients', *Behaviour Research and Therapy*, **15** (1977), pp. 201–6.

14. S. Page and E. V. Copeland, 'Reinforcement of Conversation Operants in Psychiatric Patients', *Canadian Journal of Behavioural Science*, **4** (1972), pp. 348–57.

15. D. A. Tracey, D. W. Briddell and G. T. Wilson, 'Generalisation of Verbal Conditioning to Verbal and Non-verbal Behaviour: Group Therapy with Chronic Psychiatric Patient Dyads', *Journal of Applied Behaviour Analysis*, **7** (1974), pp. 391–402.

16. R. P. Liberman, C. J. Wallace, J. Teigen and J. R. Davis, 'Interventions with Psychotic Behaviours' in K. S. Calhoun, H. E. Adams and K. M. Mitchell (eds.), *Innovative Treatment Methods in Psychopathology* (John Wiley, New York, 1974).

17. J. P. Wincze, H. Leitenberg and W. S. Agras, 'The Effects of Token Reinforcement and Feedback on Delusional Verbal Behaviour of Chronic Paranoid Schizophrenics', *Journal of Applied Behaviour Analysis*, **5** (1972), pp. 247–62.

18. A. Meyers, M. Mercatoris and A. Sirota, 'Use of Covert Self-instruction for the Elimination of Psychotic Speech', *Journal of Consulting and Clinical Psychology*, **44** (1976), pp. 480–3.

19. Liberman *et al.*, 'Interventions with Psychotic Behaviours'.

20. L. T. Anderson and M. Alpert, 'Operant Analysis of Hallucination Frequency in a Hospitalised Schizophrenic', *Journal of Behaviour Therapy and Experimental Psychiatry*, **5** (1974), pp. 13–19.

21. M. Aslin, 'The Reduction of Hallucinatory Behaviour in a Hospitalised Schizophrenic Patient', unpublished report, Royal Dundee Liff Hospital, 1977.

22. A. Hume, 'The Use of Self-monitoring in the Reduction of Auditory Hallucinations in a Chronic Paranoid Schizophrenic Patient', unpublished report, Royal Dundee Liff Hospital, 1984.

10 A HOME FROM HOME: THE PATIENT AND HIS ENVIRONMENT

Circumstances! I make circumstances. — Napoleon

So far we have talked only about the assessment of the patient and his functioning. I hope that we have assumed that the patient does not live in a vacuum. Much of our behaviour involves reactions to our environment. We respond to traffic lights, bicycle bells, fire alarms or the sight of someone important entering the room. We also act upon the environment: pressing buttons and pulling levers to gain access to cigarettes, fresh air, more or less sunlight. We may also act in a particular way to detain or scare off that dignitary who has just entered the room. We are all tied up, inextricably, with our environment: the world we inhabit. This rule applies equally to the psychiatric patient. Especially where the patient is severely disturbed, it is all too easy to forget that his environment may have played a part in the creation of that disturbance. It has been noted that the psychiatric patient is not wholly absolved from the rules governing normal social behaviour.[1] By implication, we can assume that abnormal social behaviour may have something to do with the unnatural circumstances under which he lives. The rules and regulations of the institution are the bells and buzzers which control his functioning, to a greater or lesser extent. In this chapter I want to take a look at the patient's environment. This might be the long-stay 'back ward', where the patient has lived for many years. Or it might be the home for the elderly, the day hospital, or the hostel in the community, where the patient is a relative newcomer; or where this situation represents only a part of his environmental experience. I shall refer to all of these settings as *institutions*. These environments all 'provide procedures through which human conduct is patterned, or compelled to go, in grooves deemed desirable by society'.[2] Some might resent the use of the term: 'institution' has become a dirty word in this new age of enlightenment in psychiatric care. However, as our discussion develops, it may become apparent that the term has no real 'value' connotations: it can represent the humanitarian as well as the restrictive organisation of a life in care.

I intend to say little about individual patients here. I am more interested in the way in which the environment acts upon the patient, or induces him to act upon his environment in return. Our discussion must focus on the way the environment is organised in an architectural sense. However, most of our interest should lie in the abstract organisation — the schedule of rules and regulation, some pinned to the notice-board, other simply part of the verbal culture, which are potent influences on the behaviour of patients and staff alike. In a sense we are looking, indirectly, at staff behaviour and its effects upon the patient. Architects and planners may give us the environmental shell, but nursing staff are often responsible for constructing and manipulating the 'living environment'. Often they are oblivious of the processes involved. This is especially so in the total institution, those environments which represent the totality of the patient's experience, such as the locked long-stay ward. I hope that I do not patronise them too much when I say that many staff are unaware of their surroundings, content to work through a shift thinking, perhaps, about having a drink or meal after work, or next week's FA cup tie. For them, the environment is temporary. For the patients who will still be there, after the staff have left for the pub or are on the terraces, the environment means something else: it can be a cocoon or a constraint. In understanding something of the effects of the environment upon the patient's behaviour, we should try to establish its general function first. Does it promote the growth of the individual, or does it function as a shelter: a genuine asylum in a storm-tossed world? Does it retard his growth; encourage his dependence; propel him further or faster into chronicity? In addition to these general questions, we need also to consider ways in which we can take some reliable measure of the workings of the environment. I do not intend to take either of the typical views of the role of institutions: while I do not believe that they are totally to blame for the plight of the patient, nor do I see them as entirely blameless. My own position can best be summarised by quoting the words of Thomas à Kempis, who asserted that 'occasions do not make a man either strong or weak, but merely show what he is'. I believe that institutional environments can bring out *either* the best *or* the worst in patients. The major aim of our assessment of the environment should be to discover ways of ensuring that the former always triumphs over the latter.

Man and his Environment

The relationship between the individual and his environment has been compared to the relationship between a record and a record-player. The kind of music played, whether classical or popular, is determined by the record. The quality of the music played depends, however, on the record-player. The same record can sound harsh and squeaky, or smooth and full of tone, depending on the kind of record-player used. The same is true of people. The language they speak, the behaviour they show and the beliefs they hold can all be influenced by their culture: the world they inhabit. However, the quality of their performance depends upon hereditary talents and capabilities, or upon biological functions that may have developed during their lives.[3] Even today, there is still much debate about which is the more important influence on a person's behaviour: his environment or his heredity. The question is rather like asking which is more important to the running of a car — the petrol or the engine? In our consideration of the role of the environment I am willing to accept that the patient's behaviour may have its origins in some dysfunctional biochemical state, or some disorder of psychopathology. I am willing also to accept that the environment that the patient inhabits also plays a part in his 'presentation of self'. As I noted earlier, our institutions provide us with grooves similar to those of a record, and we are required to follow these grooves in order to satisfy certain concepts of appropriate behaviour. The environment of the psychiatric institution provides similar grooves: staff decide what constitutes 'appropriate behaviour' and the patient is required to conform to this pattern in order to stay within the institution. It is interesting to note that 'appropriate behaviour' in a psychiatric hospital is, invariably, unacceptable behaviour on the outside. As soon as patients start to show 'inappropriate' hospital behaviour, it is time for them to leave the institution. In considering the role of the institution, one of the key questions we must ask is, 'To what extent does the environment assist the patient to show "inappropriate" behaviour?'

The Total Institution

Out concept of the total institution is derived mainly from the classic text by Erving Goffman, the American sociologist. Goffman describes how it is normal practice for people to move from one environment to another, to engage in different activities or patterns of behaviour.[4] We sleep, eat, work and play with different people, usually in quite different situations. In the 'total institution' such natural barriers are conspicuously absent. He observed that in many cases all such social, recreational, occupational and self-care activities might take place under the one roof, often with little movement of the residents. In this sense the setting for top-security prisoners and psychiatric patients differs little. Neither have much of a 'life' outside the confines of the institution. Of course not all psychiatric hospitals are total institutions, in this sense. It is more appropriate, perhaps, to distinguish the extent to which an environment approximates to a total institution. To what extent is it restrictive? To what extent does it promote normal living? Why should we ask such questions? For the simple reason that for many years we have known that care environments can be damaging to their residents. The classic text by Russell Barton on institutional neurosis showed how care could lead to a deterioration in the funtioning of individuals.[5] This was more likely to happen where patients wore the same clothes, ate from the same bowls, shared the same public toilet and bathing facilities, and were regimented and corralled by the same set of restrictive institutional practices. The patient, as described by Barton, was stripped of his personality in much the same way that prisoners and refugees are stripped of their individuality. With this loss of their intrinsic self comes the deterioration in physical habits, an increase in apathy and a general loss of interest in life itself. Clearly, we now know what kind of environment would be best for our patients. How often we can put this into practice? In evaluating the quality of care in our total institutions we have to accept that there are limitations upon how 'natural' or therapeutic these environments can become. This acknowledgement should not deter us from asking how far can we push back the boundaries of the restrictive environment? To what extent can we normalise an abnormal situation?

The Half-way House

With the advent of more progressive policies for the psychiatric patient has come the development of a range of alternative institutional settings. Rehabilitation units within the hospital grounds, hostels and group homes in the community now exist to facilitate the transfer of the patient from the 'abnormality' of the locked back ward to the reality of life in the community. All such settings function as stepping stones. They are not closed environments, like the total institution described above. However, we still need to question the extent to which the life enjoyed by the patient is anything like as normal as is often assumed. To what extent is he able to come and go? To what extent is he restricted? Does the environment continue to exert a significant influence upon his behaviour? In what way can this be changed or modified to bring about an increase in his personal development? Although the day hospital is a much more transitory environment, it should not escape a similar kind of analysis. It is true that the patient may spend only a small proportion of his day there, but the content may be more significant than the time of the exposure. Consequently, I would include day hospitals for acute, chronic psychiatric and elderly patients in this category: a further setting that might benefit from detailed analysis.

The Therapeutic Environment

We cannot leave this discussion of 'institutions' without discussing the concept of the therapeutic milieu, or therapeutic community. Most of us like to think that the environment is arranged to suit the patient's needs, and to reduce his distress. The term *therapeutic community*, however, has a very special meaning, and one which is pertinent to our discussion here. In the early 1950s a number of experimental projects tried to offer a different kind of care and treatment to young, mainly anti-social, psychiatric patients. The rehabilitative process used shunned the use of the disciplinarian, custodial practices that were the legacy of the early asylum days and the 'moral treatment' tradition. Instead, emphasis was given to sharing decision-making between staff and patients. Staff no longer had a monopoly over the direction of the environment. Where anti-social behaviour was evident, efforts were made to tolerate it — rather than punish it — in the hope that the individual would assume more responsibility for his actions. The roles of staff were greatly reduced: less attention was paid to rank and status and an atmosphere of informality was cultivated. Finally, the environment concentrated, almost exclusively, on confronting patients with the reality of their own behaviour, usually through psychotherapeutic counselling and feedback, individually or in groups.[6] In one sense such environments tried to achieve an atmosphere of normality, through the appearance of informality and lack of structure. In another sense, however, it was heavily organised and — therefore — institutionalised, through its detailed progamme of daily meetings, discussion groups, debate and decision-making over even the most trivial of matters. Such intensity is hardly to be found in the typical semi-detached sitting-room. In many ways it is sufficiently intense to make even the most custodial traditionalist wince.

Whose Responsibility?

Much of the assessment methodology discussed so far can be used, with discretion, by nurses at any level in the rankings of the hierarchy. The same cannot be said of the decision to study the environment. The *decision* — at least — must be taken by someone in authority. Since some of the observational practices recommended for analysing environments resemble 'time-and-motion' methods, an uninformed work-force may think that their 'working', rather than workings of the environment, is under scrutiny. Such a misconception could sabotage the whole exercise. Consequently, the decision to study the environment should always be taken by someone with the appropriate authority and should always be relayed in detail to the work-force who might be included in the survey. The process of conducting the assessment, however, may be the responsibility of fairly junior members of staff.

An assessment of the patient's environment is usually undertaken for one of the following reasons. In order to:

(1) assess the 'quality of care' in a particular setting. This often involves an analysis of one or more of the following factors: the amount of nurse-patient interaction; levels of disturbed behaviour; levels of appropriate activity for the setting; expressed levels of satisfaction amongst the patient population.
(2) identify the effects of specific changes in the environment: this might involve rearrangement of the furniture; revision of staff rotas or routines; or even the effects of transferring patients from one ward to another.
(3) evaluate the changes in any of the factors mentioned above, across time. Rarely is it sufficient to identify problems and purpose solutions. In any environmental context it is important to monitor these interventions across time: do these solutions last in the medium or long term?

The responsibility for proposing such an analysis will usually lie with the nurse in charge of the ward, hostel, day unit, etc.

Alternatively, the suggestion may come from a visiting psychologist, or from some other individual within the therapeutic team. Although such an analysis is often undertaken to resolve some major problem, or following some external criticism of the environment, ideally this kind of assessment should be routine in all care settings. The assessment of the environment is a kind of 'quality-control' measure. It begs the question, 'Does the environment achieve what it sets out to achieve?' Such a question has as much relevance to the care setting as it does to the production setting, where the ideas of quality control and goal achievement were born.

Some General Considerations

The Design of the Environment

The first issue we should consider is the fabric of the environment. This constitutes the skeleton, or framework, of the ward or unit. Around this framework is draped the social world staff and patients inhabit. I do not wish to go into this in any great detail, for clearly this is a subject in itself. However, in assessing any environment it is clear that we must look at how it is built: does it have small rooms or large, echoing chambers? Are the ceilings twenty feet from the ground, resembling St Pancras Station? Or does the 'day room' resemble a large living-room in a modern semi-detached? In addition to considerations about size and shape, we must also include colour, decoration and function. Is the colour scheme stimulating, drab or psychedelic? How is it furnished? Are there pictures and *objets d'art* appropriate to the age, cultural background and interests of the client group? Does the ward 'living-room' have a pool table in one corner and a Space Invaders machine in the other? Are these common fixtures for the average 'living-room'? Such questions are not simply aesthetic. Many of the attempts to improve institutional environments have involved trying to turn the back ward into a page out of the Habitat catalogue. It never seems to occur to such designers that hessian wall coverings and hi-tech furniture may be just as alien and uninspiring to the residents as the gloss-painted walls and tubular armchairs they replace. The design of an environment is not concerned solely with comfort. Its primary aim is to facilitate the performance of behaviour: that is why a bathroom, a dormitory and a dining-room should differ markedly from each other. It is clear from numerous research reports that many aspects of institutional environments deter, rather than encourage, the performance of behaviour. Take, for example, the typical toilet annexe in a large psychiatric hospital. This was designed to allow large numbers of mobile patients to wash in close proximity to one another. Such places are often noisy — every sound reverberating around the terrazoed walls and floors; cold — the size and absence of double glazing making heating in winter a virtual impossibility; and generally inhospitable. Such factors may well deter old Mrs Smith from rising from her comfortable chair in the day room to 'pay a visit'. Incontinent behaviour is not always a function of loss of sphincter control.

When we are looking at the design of an environment we should ask, 'Does it help or hinder the performance of the activities associated with the setting?' I have suggested above that toilets need to be comfortable, private places, especially for the elderly patient who may have been used to such comfort. Designers of 'normal environments' are at least aware that certain colour schemes are stimulating, while others are restful. The decoration of day rooms, dormitories, toilets and bathrooms should in some way reflect the aims of that particular environment. The arrangement of furniture is by now well accepted as a factor in the promotion, or discouragement of, social interaction. Chairs arranged around the walls, or spread out to allow easy staff movement, or a clear view of the television for everyone, are rarely conducive to confidential conversation. Little wonder that the level of conversation in the typical back-ward day room is so low, and the level of shouting is so high. When we are assessing how much social interaction, recreation, mobility or 'apathy' is taking place we cannot study the patients in isolation. We need to consider the role the environment plays in assisting or stimulating such behaviour. Some people have tried to assess the quality of the patient's environment by comparing it with similar staff facilities. Are the toilet paper, cutlery, menu, levels of privacy (etc.) the same for staff and patients? If not, why not? This is hardly a foolproof system, for someone is bound to comment that 'the patients' needs are different'. However, many of the improvements in institutional environments have come about through staff *sharing* facilities with patients in the manner of the therapeutic communities mentioned earlier. In assessing the quality of the patient's environment it may be worth while considering how long *you* could tolerate the level of privacy, comfort, stimulation and freedom afforded to the patients in your care.

The Staff

The members of staff are as much a part of the environment as the television set and the wallpaper. We have to consider how they appear to the patient. This 'appearance' may have a part in the construction of their behaviour. I have mentioned already the air of informality cherished by the famous therapeutic communities. It would appear that little of their philosophy generalised to the profession as a whole. Instead, the military model of nursing has witnessed something of a rebirth, especially with the boom in psychogeriatric care. Although nurses sprouting badges, epaulettes and a variegation of bands and stripes are diminishing in some areas, in many others they are proliferating. I use the term 'military model' since it is clear that the profession that found its feet in the mud and bullets of the Crimea has persistently used the machinery of rank, status and discipline to try to establish itself further as a profession in its own right. In psychiatry there is much debate about the role of uniform. To the sociologist there is no such dilemma. Uniforms function to place a barrier between one person and another. The various grades of uniform, and the ranks which accompany them, function as further barriers between those wearing uniforms. The uniform, therefore, encourages social distance. The same is true of titles and forms of address. Titles such as 'Sister', 'Doctor', 'Mister', even plain 'Nurse' help create social distance. First-name terms, on the other hand, signify friendship, trust or a level of intimacy. Of course, the use of such forms of address can be classed as 'over-familiarity'. In such contexts it would be necessary, perhaps, to assess why a member of staff felt threatened by this invasion of her professional territory. The use of nicknames involves a similar concern. These are commonly used on long-stay wards and in many a geriatric area. Calling James 'Jacko' may be a form of endearment. It can also be patronising. In many cases the nickname is highly inappropriate: calling an elderly spinster 'Granny' or a man with one eye 'Gunner' are typical examples. When assessing the role of staff in the patient's environment we must begin with their raw status as staff. To what extent do staff deploy uniforms, titles, medals, pet names, etc. as mechanisms of control? Such information may tell us much about the social psychology of the institution. Since I have stressed the 'interpersonal context' of psychiatric nursing throughout this book, it is important that we gauge the extent to which staff are able to relate to patients, and vice versa. We also need to know the extent to which the encumbrances of authority and professional*ism* may obstruct them from doing so.

The Organisation of the Environment

The operation of the environment is determined by two classes of instruction. The first involves 'abstract' rules and regulations. These are enforced often as though they were written on tablets of stone. When these rules are questioned, often no record can be found: they represent the verbal culture of the ward. The second is the formal organisation of the interaction of staff and patients: the 'routine'. This is usually well documented on a notice-board if not on a tablet of stone. When we consider the role of rules and regulations — of either variety — we need to evaluate their effect on patients. Does the environment dictate the same rule for everyone: when to get up; when to go to bed; when to have a bath or wash his hair; where he can smoke; whether or not he can drink alcohol; have a girlfriend in his room; or change the décor of the wall above his bed? Some kind of order is necessary where a large number of people live under one roof. But is the environment overly restrictive? Some people would say, 'Of course the patient can't decide when to have a bath, or paint his wall . . . he's in hospital after all!' Again we are back to our original dilemma. What is the hospital for? Can its traditional face and function be adapted and modified to suit 'new needs'? I am not making recommendations one way or the other. I am simply acknowledging that the way our environment is organised has an effect upon us: sometimes it encourages us to conform, and we follow the grooves in the record. In other instances we rebel, either publicly or deviously. Especially in those settings where patients appear to be 'bucking the system', we need to consider whether or not the environment needs changing, rather than the patient.

I have drawn a thread of person-centred care throughout this book. This might be wholly impractical in many settings, especially where staff are required to provide a shepherding function. Yet even in situations where staffing levels are low, or the organisation of staffing is less than efficient, it is all too easy to blame the disorder on the 'chronicity' or 'dementia' of the patients. In looking at the organisation of activities throughout the day we need to evaluate whether the organisation encourages or discourages the performance of the desired behaviour. Does the routine include specifications about the arrangement of privacy at bathtimes? Do the staff and patients eat at the same tables? Does the nurse work alongside the patient at occupational therapy? Do patients spend a lot of time 'waiting': on food, drugs, the toilet or other forms of staff attention? In many closed institutions the patient's day is ordered beyond the level necessary for avoiding cold dinners or congestion in the toilet area. Our assessment needs to ask: is such a level of organisation and control therapeutic or restrictive?

The Orientation of the Institution

Richard Lovelace, the English poet, was the first to remark that 'stone walls do not a prison make, nor iron bars a cage'. The quotation is particularly apposite when we consider the *function* of institutions, as distinct from their appearance. Many a care setting may appear comfortable, airy and potentially therapeutic. We need to analyse its function to decide whether such a promise is realised. Most analyses of the function of environments, from Goffman to the present day, have involved asking the question, 'For whose benefit is the institution run?' Numerous studies have suggested that the answer is not always 'the patients''.

In the early 1970s Raynes and King conducted a number of studies of the 'quality of care' of handicapped children in residential settings. Local authority homes, voluntary homes and hospitals were studied in order to detect any significant differences.[7] Although they focused on the care of the mentally handicapped, it is now well recognised that their findings have relevance for other patient populations in other residential situations. These authors developed a scale to measure the quality of care. This measured:

(1) Rigidity of Routine. The degree to which management practices were flexible — viz. to what extent did staff accommodate 'individual differences' among residents; did routines vary according to the day of the week, time of year, occasion, etc.?

(2) Block Treatment. The degree to which the residents were treated as individuals or merely as members of a group — viz. did the residents bathe, use the toilet, have meals, etc. according to individual need, or was this determined by a group practice policy?

(3) Depersonalisation. The degree to which the residents had the opportunity to aquire and maintain personal possessions; enjoy privacy; use their initiative; make decisions, etc.

(4) Social Distance. The degree to which the residents engaged in 'normal' interaction with staff — viz. did the residents dine with staff, play and talk with staff on an individual basis? Were the residents bathed, dressed, fed, etc. by one member of staff, or were they *processed* by several?

Raynes and King found that although there were major differences between the different residential units studied, these differences were *not* explained by the *overall* size of the institution, the *actual* size of the care units or *differences* in staff-patient ratios. Instead the differences in *role orientation* served to distinguish one setting from another. Raynes and King argued that there was a direct relationship between the orientation of staff and the pattern of care they ultimately offered. In short, they found that those staff who had been trained in large institutions to work with 'mentally handicapped people' were more task-oriented, and spent little time engaging in close interaction with the residents. Those staff who had been trained in child care were more orientated towards the individual child, displaying this orientation through higher levels of individual contact. In similar studies it has been shown that even where the fabric and structure of the environment are changed, to allow increased individualisation of care, the negative features of the total institution highlighted by Raynes and King will survive if the person running the unit retains a custodial philosophy.[8]

The features highlighted in the Raynes and King study are echoes of some of the considerations already mentioned. Barton highlighted the 'inflexibility' of routines in his study, and this was one of the key elements in Goffman's research. Many other researchers have pointed out that institutions deprive patients of an opportunity to engage in complete cycles of activity, e.g. shopping, preparing and cooking food, eating the meal and then doing the washing up. Instead they are consistently catered for, often like guests in a second-rate hotel. Staff attitudes play a large part in influencing block treatment or the process of personality stripping. Traditionally we have distinguished between 'custodial' and 'therapeutic' staff. I am not sure that such a distinction is always clearcut. However, it is clear that any analysis of the patient's environment must take account of the prevailing attitudes of the staff. It has been noted that nurses who tend to view patients as 'people', similar to themselves, will tend to be more patient-oriented, whereas those who are task-oriented tend to be dominated by the use of diagnostic categories or sub-types in their experience of the patient.[9] The authoritarian tradition of nursing is of obvious relevance here. It relates strongly also to the issue of social distance, as we have already discussed. In theory, psychiatric nursing is based upon the establishment of open, trusting, therapeutic relationships between staff and patient. In assessing the patient *for* treatment or help-giving, we must consider whether or not it will be possible to offer help. The question can only be answered by an analysis of the climate of care, as expressed through the attitudes of staff and the patterns of care they project.

The General Assessment of the Environment

The considerations I have listed above are a rather anarchic grouping. How can one possibly evaluate the quality of a ward or a day-care setting, covering everything from the architecture and décor of the building to the caring orientation of the staff? The answer is that such a wide-ranging assessment is probably impossible. I include these merely as considerations. An 'assessment' might look only at the fabric of the ward, problems patients meet in moving from A to B, and the ease with which they can turn on and off taps, or unravel the toilet tissue. Another 'assessment' might deal exclusively with the daily timetable: does it accommodate the celebration of birthdays, having a lie-in on Sundays, or having a sandwich in front of the television, instead of the regulation 'high tea'? Other assessments might try to evaluate the function of staff attitudes — towards certain kinds of patients, towards routines, individualised care or the wearing of uniforms. In suggesting that we might focus our assessment of the environment on specific facets, I am aware that many nurses have taken the complete 'environment' as their canvas and have lived to tell the tale.

Specific Considerations

In the second part of this chapter I want to consider ways of assessing specific aspects of the patient's environment. The methods I shall discuss are examples of standardised measures, methods that have been developed through research to yield fairly firm data regarding what is happening within the environment. Since these are specific methods, they tell a very incomplete story. However, these methods may be further examples of the kind of 'thermometers' mentioned earlier: they may help us to take the temperature of the ward or day unit from a variety of angles.

The Ward Atmosphere Scale

When we talk about the atmosphere in a ward or unit we do not mean the air pressure or the various gases circulating around us. Instead we are referring to another 'invisible' feature of the environment that is equally influential — the various attitudes, relationships, rules and regulations and other organisational factors that go to make up the 'social environment'. We have considered many of these items already. But how do we assess the 'social environment', especially when we cannot see it? In 1972 Moos[10] developed a scale, designed for use with staff and patients, that tried to assess the perception of the ward atmosphere. The format has seen a number of revisions and developments with perhaps the best-known being the 100-item questionnaire, which required the staff member or patient to circle 'true' or 'false' against each item. Typical statements are:

11. Patients never know when a doctor will ask to see them.
30. The patients are proud of this ward.
82. Patients are encouraged to show their feelings.

The various items on the scale represent ten discrete dimensions that can be grouped under factors involving *relationships* (1–4); the *treatment programme* (5–7); and the *administrative structure* (8–10). The ten dimensions analyse the atmosphere as follows:

(1) *Involvement* assesses the extent to which the patients take an active part in the routine running of the ward.
(2) *Support* assesses the amount of help and understanding available from members of the staff and from fellow patients.
(3) *Spontaneity* assesses the extent to which patients are encouraged to express their feelings openly towards staff or other patients.
(4) *Anger and aggression* assess the extent to which these emotions are tolerated or encouraged by way of therapeutic expression.
(5) *Autonomy and self-direction* assess the extent to which patients

are encouraged to take responsibility for their own affairs or relationships with others.

(6) *Practical orientation* measures how much preparation the patient is given for his discharge back into the community.

(7) *Personal problems* assess the amount of help given to patients to identify and understand their problems and emotions.

(8) *Activity planning* and *organisation* assess the importance of routine and order and their relationship to the planning of schedules and activities.

(9) *Programme clarity* assess the extent to which the patient understands the rules and regulations of the ward and the various procedures involved.

(10) *Staff control* assesses the amount of restriction imposed upon patients through rules and regulations and other controlling measures.

A vast amount of research has been done to standardise this scale: initially 160 psychiatric wards were used in the development of the scale and a number of outcome studies have been reported.[11] The scale was revised slightly in 1972 for use in community treatment progammes, such as half-way houses, hostels, rehabilitation centres and day hospitals. This revision was retitled COPES — the community oriented environment scale — and carries 102 items which are scored 'true' or 'false'.[12] These are summarised using the same ten dimensions on the original Ward Atmosphere Scale. Both these measures have shown marked differences between environments that are manifestly 'therapeutic' or 'custodial'. In an early ward-based experiment it was found that patients who were involved in a token economy programme reported greater levels of involvement and general 'satisfaction' than patients in three standard settings.[13] Similar findings were reported later for the COPES format.[14]

Although the WAS and the COPES scales are very simple to use, the value of the information they produce should not be underestimated. The picture of the environment offered by both scales is relevant to any institutional setting. This is obviously most true of the *relationships* and *administrative* dimensions, which are part and parcel of any institution: school, hospital or prison. The scores on the *treatment programme* dimensions, which involve personal development, would be expected to differ across different environments. Moos has found that this scale tells us a great deal about the patients' perception of their environment. On some parts of the scale staff and patients are in complete agreement, for example regarding the levels of organisation. However, patients often rate 'staff control' higher than staff. Moos' research has also shown that where there are large numbers of patients and few staff the levels of 'support' and 'spontaneity' are low and the amount of 'staff control' is high. Finally, where the environment is more 'open', with fewer restrictions on patients and less of an 'institutional' atmosphere, this is reflected in high scores for 'spontaneity; autonomy and self-direction; personal problems and anger and aggression'.

The cynic might well argue, 'Well, we knew that already.' And in some settings she could be right. Some environments are obviously open, supportive and therapeutic. Others are obviously confining, restrictive and custodial. Between these two extremes there exists a vast grey area where we are uncertain of the extent to which the environment is a positive or a negative force. The Ward Atmosphere Scale and its community-oriented derivative may help resolve some of our doubts. However, even where we are certain of the status of the environment, surely there is no harm in 'taking the temperature' of the ward or day unit. By using a standardised scale we can assess exactly how custodial or therapeutic the setting is. We can also identify in which areas (or dimensions) the setting is rich or deficient. Of supreme importance is the fact that, by using such a scale, we can evaluate how the environment changes — or remains the same — across time. Earlier in the book I drew an analogy between psychiatric assessment and taking the patient's temperature. The analogy is apposite in this context. Although we *know* (i.e. believe) that the patient is feverish, we still take his temperature, using a standardised instrument. If we know (i.e. believe) that our environment is therapeutic, shouldn't we adopt the same objective evaluation?

The Assessment of Activity

The WAS and COPES formats focus attention on the perception of the environment, by staff or patient. These scales pay no attention to the 'effectiveness' or 'workings' of the environment. Clearly, these are difficult concepts to define, far less measure in any direct fashion. A number of attempts have been made to assess the effectiveness of environments by studying the behaviour of the residents. These studies have taken the view that if an activity or pattern of behaviour can be identified as *appropriate* for the setting, then a measure of the extent to which people engage in that activity might be one measure of the success — or effectiveness — of the environment. If most people are 'eating' in a dining-room, 'relaxing' in a lounge, or 'studying' in a library, then we might assume that the organisation and planning of these environments had come to fruition. People are doing what they are supposed to be doing. The environment 'works'. In psychiatric hospitals even casual observation reveals that many patients do not perform behaviour that is appropriate for the environment they are in. Indeed, in a sense this may be part of the reason they are in hospital. Patients withdraw into themselves in the lounge, and pace back and forth in the dining area. Although we may assume that such patterns of behaviour are symptomatic of the patient's mental disorder, we need to ask, 'To what extent does the environment serve to promote or reduce the performance of such behaviour?' In evaluating the effectiveness of psychiatric wards or other departments, we are asking the same question as we would if we were evaluating the effectiveness of a public house ('Do the people drink, laugh and talk a lot?') or a gymnasium ('Do the people puff, pant and exercise a lot?'). In any environment appropriate behaviour could be retitled 'planned activities': the environment was planned, or designed, in order to encourage certain kinds of behaviour. In the early 1970s Todd Risley and his colleagues developed an observational system which they called the Planned Activity Check (PLA-CHECK). Although much of their research involved children and the mentally handicapped, the system is appropriate for any environment.[15] In recent years a version of the system has been used to analyse the effectiveness of various environments for the elderly.[16]

PLA-CHECK. Risley's method was remarkably simple. Because the amount of *time* spent engaged in an activity seems to be more important than the number of times the person smokes, eats, looks at television or lifts a newspaper, a 'time-sampling' method was used as the basis for the observations. Time-sampling simply means that the observations were taken at set intervals during the day, rather than for any continuous period of time. Much of the early work was done in school classrooms and the method was designed to suit observers who had little experience of formal assessment procedures.[17]

Procedure. The first step in the PLA-CHECK involves defining the 'planned-activity'. This will vary according to the area in which the observation takes place. In a lounge this might be 'socialising'; in a games room it would be 'recreation'. To ensure that each observer takes note of the same behaviour patterns these broad categories will be defined further. A list of activities representing 'socialising' or 'recreation' would be drawn up. Usually these are defined in very specific terms, to avoid any confusion over what is, or is not, the 'planned-activity'. The list for 'socialising' might include:

Talking to another person
Laughing in the company of other(s)
Listening to someone else speaking
Singing and/or clapping hands, tapping feet in time to music with other(s)
Showing object (e.g. newspaper, photograph) to other(s)

If the patient performs any of the activities on the list he is deemed to be 'participating'. If he is engaging in *any other behaviour* he is deemed to be a non-participant in the planned activity. He might, for example, be waiting: for lunch to be served; for a nurse to take him for a bath; or for the television to be switched on. Such waiting behaviour, if it is not on the list, would be discounted. So would other behaviours that might be appropriate in other settings: e.g. playing cards at the dining table, or pacing around the television room. These are not discounted because they are 'disruptive' or 'deviant', but simply because they are not the planned activities for the area. Of course, any anti-social behaviour, e.g. shouting, throwing furniture, undressing in public, would also be classed as failing to meet the criteria of the planned-activity.

In Figure 10.1 an example of a typical PLA-CHECK recording is illustrated. The place where the observations are conducted is noted along with the name of the observer, the date and the time observations began. The observations are made every 5 minutes — noting how many people are present — or available in the area (in column A); and how many of the group are participating in an appropriate activity (in column P). In the illustrated section 'Jessica' began her observation at 8.30 a.m. in the breakfast area. Twenty people were present when she took her first 'sample'. However, only 4 of the group were participating in appropriate 'breakfast' behaviour. In the next observation cell 2 of the group left the table and went

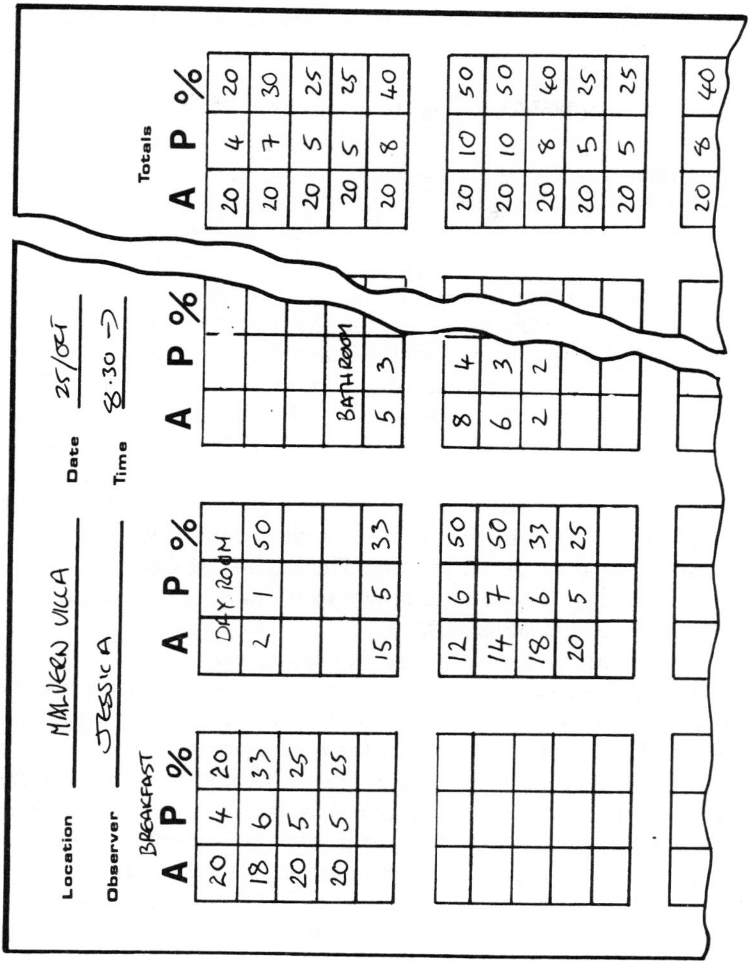

Figure 10.1

| Location | MALVERN VILLA | Date | 25/OCT |
| Observer | JESSICA A | Time | 8·30 → |

BREAKFAST

A	P	%
20	4	20
18	6	33
20	5	25
20	5	25

DAY ROOM

A	P	%
2	1	50
15	5	33
12	6	50
14	7	50
18	6	33
20	5	25

BATH ROOM

A	P	%
5	3	
8	4	
6	3	
2	2	

Totals

A	P	%
20	4	20
20	7	30
20	5	25
20	5	25
20	8	40
20	10	50
20	10	50
20	8	40
20	5	25
20	5	25
20	8	40

into the adjoining day room. After Jessica had sampled the 18 people at the breakfast table, she moved into the day room and noted the behaviour of the 2 people in this area. The record sheet shows that by the next observation cell these 2 people had rejoined the rest of the group at the breakfast table. After about 20 minutes the whole group left the breakfast area: some went to the day room; others to the bathroom. The observations continued, every 5 minutes, in these two areas — showing how many people were present, and how many were participating in appropriate behaviour *for that area*. At the end of the series of observations rough percentages can be calculated, showing the proportion of people who were participating in appropriate behaviour. These proportions can be worked out for each situation — e.g. breakfast, day room, bathroom; and as combined totals for each 5-minute cell. This very simple recording format allows 'Jessica' and her colleagues to calculate the percentage of appropriate behaviour shown at breakfast, in the day room, bathroom, etc. She could also note any fluctuations that occurred in the levels of appropriate behaviour, across situations, or throughout the day. The PLA-CHECK manual gives highly practical advice regarding the training and assessment of 'reliability' of the observers.

Once the observations have been completed the information can be graphed in the manner shown in Figure 10.2. This shows the extent to which patients 'participated' in various activities programmed as appropriate for a long-term ward. The dotted line shows how many patients were present during the observations: this fluctuates due to departures and arrivals of patients during the day. The full line shows how many patients were participating in the planned activities at each observation. As the figure shows, the level of 'participation' in the planned-activities also fluctuates. However, only twice are there more than half the patients involved in appropriate behaviour. The level of 'social behaviour' rose sharply during the conversation group when a dog was brought in as a conversation piece. The graph also shows clearly the number of patients who were 'non-participants', which is represented by the gap between those in 'attendance' and those 'participating'. This kind of information can be helpful in deciding whether or not an environment needs restructuring in some way. New activities might be introduced gradually, their value (or effect) judged by evaluating any change in levels of participation. Alternatively, the general organisation of the environment might be revised: the radio

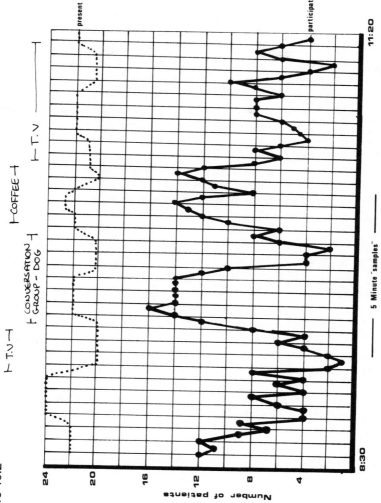

Figure 10.2

which plays all day, every day, might be turned off; the arrangement of the seating might be changed; or the amount of space between beds might be increased.[18] The effect of these aspects of the environment could be evaluated by assessing any change in the level of participation in the planned activity. In one of their early experiments with PLA-CHECK Risley and his colleagues studied levels of interaction and participation in games or craftwork in a home for the elderly.[19] By introducing new pieces of equipment and apparatus and by increasing the use of prizes and awards, they were able to change levels of attendance at bingo, art and reading classes. By rearranging the furniture they found that levels of social interaction improved. These experiments answered many of the questions we have posed already about the environment's role as an influence on the patient's behaviour. Of even greater importance was the demonstration of PLA-CHECK's value as a simple yet reliable way of assessing this influence.

Engagement — One Step Beyond

The original PLA-CHECK format was developed further in the UK by the Health Care Evaluation Research Team based at Winchester. Led by Albert Kushlick, this team extended Risley's format, preferring the term 'engagement' to 'participation'. Their approach had similar aims. They wanted to assess the proportion of patients who were engaged in some positive, productive behaviour. Any patients who were performing some *neutral* activity, like waiting, sleeping, or sitting, or some negative or anti-social behaviour were designated as 'disengaged'. Instead of defining 'planned-activities' for every new situation, they developed a simple classification of four categories of 'appropriate' or positive behaviour, viz.:

(1) *Social activity*: talking or listening to another or a group; participating in a sing-song, playing bingo, etc;
(2) *Daily living activity*: handling cutlery at the dinner table, making a bed, drying face with towel, climbing into the bath, etc.
(3) *Recreational activity*: looking at or handling books, newspapers, writing materials, gardening, or looking at television.
(4) *Mobility*: propelling wheelchair, walking with frame, getting up or down with aid of Jacob's ladder, etc.

If the patient was involved in any of these activities — which were more specifically defined in their manual[20] — he was classed as 'engaged'. Kushlick's team recommended a slight revision of Risley's procedure for conducting the observations. The observer was advised to observe each person *for one second* from left to right, around the area, judging whether or not he was 'engaged', before moving on to the next person. The observer kept a running count in her head of the number of 'engaged' patients as she conducted the observation, noting down the final number as shown in Figure 10.3. *Then*, she would record the total number of patients present. The observer also noted the predominant activity going on at the time of the observation. As with the PLA-CHECK format, these observations are usually repeated at 1-, 3- or 5-minute intervals.

The 'engagement' method appears even simpler than PLA-CHECK, but here again I would emphasise the need for nurses to acquire the skill through careful practice. It is not enough to pick up a scrap of paper and begin counting. To ensure that any nurse is able to judge engagement *reliably*, comparisons between different nurses during practice are necessary, using the kind of format described in their manual. In my own experience I have found that staff at various levels can use this approach to good effect. The major advantage of the 'engagement' system is that four classes of appropriate behaviour are defined which can be used as guidelines across a range of social, recreational or daily living settings. This allows the observations to be a little more flexible than the PLA-CHECK, which may be best suited to classroom and nurseries, where planned-activities are more fixed.

The Ward Activity and Socialisation Profile (WASP)

Some years ago Jim McGlynn, a former colleague of mine in Dundee, was studying 'life in a psychogeriatric ward'. He had been asked for advice about individual patients and decided that the most appropriate assessment would be of the environment, rather than single patients. We collaborated on a number of observational exercises, which attempted to study the social behaviour of the patients and their interactions with staff. Due largely to limitations on our time and the staffing of the unit, we concentrated our energies on studying the behaviour of the patients outwith the routine 'care periods' — when they were being bathed, dressed, fed, etc. Since the majority of the population were frail, and

Figure 10.3

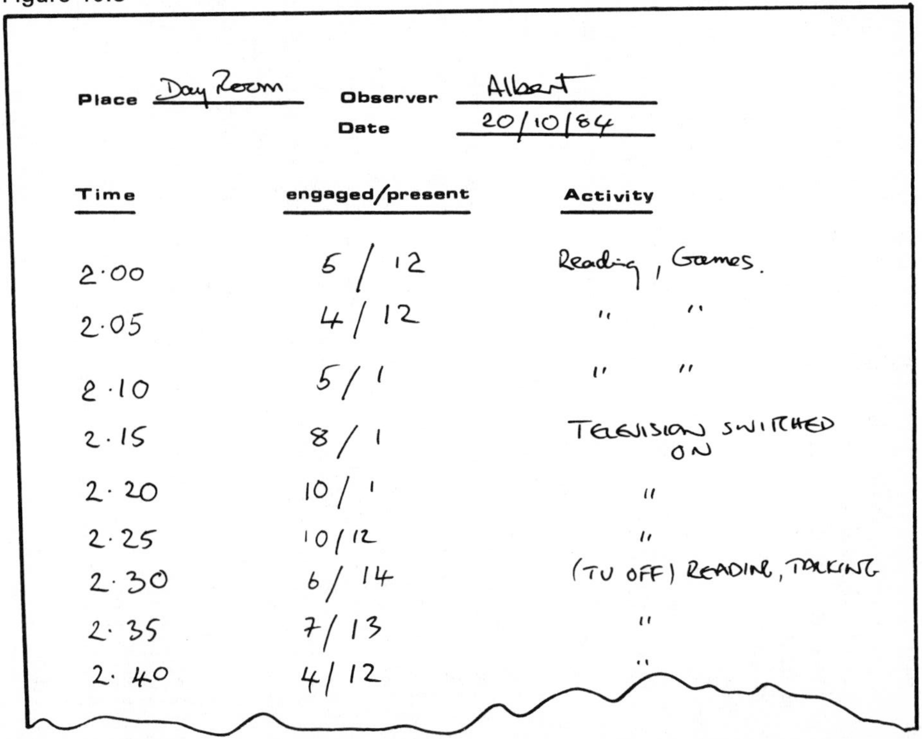

Place Day Room	Observer Albert	
	Date 20/10/84	
Time	engaged/present	Activity
2:00	6 / 12	Reading, Games.
2:05	4 / 12	"
2:10	5 / 1	" "
2:15	8 / 1	TELEVISION SWITCHED ON
2:20	10 / 1	"
2:25	10 / 12	"
2:30	6 / 14	(TV OFF) READING, TALKING
2:35	7 / 13	"
2:40	4 / 12	"

Figure 10.4

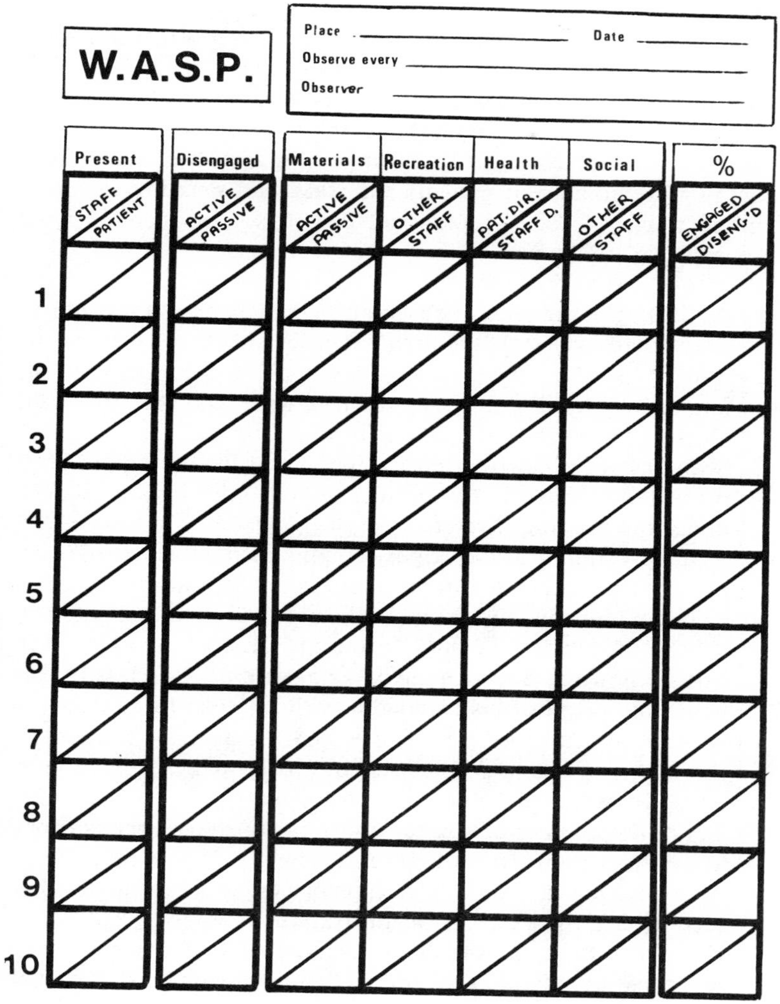

W.A.S.P.

Place ______________ Date ______________
Observe every ______________
Observer ______________

	Present	Disengaged	Materials	Recreation	Health	Social	%
	STAFF / PATIENT	ACTIVE / PASSIVE	ACTIVE / PASSIVE	OTHER / STAFF	PAT. DIR. / STAFF D.	OTHER / STAFF	ENGAGED / DISENG'D
1							
2							
3							
4							
5							
6							
7							
8							
9							
10							

physically handicapped in some way, we decided to focus on socio-recreational activity: hence the title, 'Ward Activity and Socialisation Profile' — WASP for short. Because we hoped to study the effect of environmental changes on specific patterns of behaviour, the 'engagement' format yielded insufficient detail for our purposes. Since the staff were few in number, but key components of the environment, we thought that their presence should also be noted. The final format — shown in Figure 10.4 — involved counting the number of patients and staff who were involved in a limited range of socio-recreational activities. The recommended procedure is as follows:

(1) At the beginning of each observation take up a position with an unrestricted view of 'the area': this should be defined as 'the lounge' or the 'day room'. Only staff and patients in the *immediate vicinity* of this defined area will be observed. Outside this area is 'off limits' to the observer.

(2) Scanning the area from left to right count the number of staff present and record the number in the appropriate triangle under the heading 'Present'.

(3) Again, scanning left to right, count the number of patients present and record the number in the appropriate triangle.

(4) Look up immediately and begin the observation of the patients' behaviour. Scanning from left to right, observe each patient in turn, allowing approximately *one second* to classify his behaviour. Record his behaviour with a stroke ('|') under the appropriate category (see Figure 10.5 for details). Proceed to the next patient, and so on, until all the patients have been observed and their behaviour categorised.

(5) Count the number of strokes under each behavioural category and enter a total score within each triangle. Where no patients were engaged in a particular category enter a zero under that section. See Figure 10.5 for illustration.

(6) Calculate the approximate percentage of patients who were 'engaged' or 'disengaged'. Enter these percentages in the final column. This completes the observation.

Definitions of Engagement and Disengagement. Examples of the definitions of appropriate and inappropriate behaviour are given below. Due to the more extensive range of behavioural categories more practice is required to achieve satisfactory degrees of

Figure 10.5

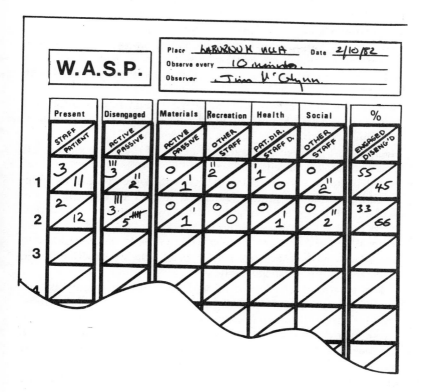

'reliability' between observers. The method has, however, been taught successfully to untrained nurses and nurses in training, as well as more sophisticated nurse observers.

Disengaged (active): any *disruptive* or antisocial behaviour — e.g. shouting, banging on window, tearing up newspapers, mannerisms.

Disengaged (passive): any *neutral* activity — e.g. sitting or standing (only), lying on floor, sleeping, 'waiting'.

Materials (active): any active manipulation of some material object(s) — e.g. smoking a pipe, knitting, reading a book, doing a jigsaw.

Materials (passive): any passive engagement with a material object
— e.g. watching television, sitting under a hairdrier, watching a
goldfish in a fish tank.
Recreation (other): any collaboration in an activity with other
patients — e.g. playing dominoes, cards, etc., or doing a jigsaw,
building a collage, etc. with others.
Recreation (staff): engagement in any of the above activities with
staff.
Health (patient directed): any engagement in an activity important
to health, which is performed unaided — e.g. drinking, eating,
taking medication, putting on hand cream.
Health (staff directed): engagement in any of the above where staff
assistance is required.
Social (other): any social interaction with other patients — e.g.
talking, laughing, smiling, listening, singing along with.
Social (staff): any engagement in the above activities with staff.

Note: Where patients are engaged with materials *or* in recreation *or*
health activities *and* are interacting socially their behaviour should
be classified under 'social' only.

The length of any observation is determined mainly by the
number of patients in the area, and the amount of activity going
on. Our studies have shown that with 12−15 patients in a day area
the average observation takes about 90 seconds. Where this method
has been used with larger populations — especially those who are
more active — it has proved less reliable. Where patients move very
quickly from one part of the area to another, possibly changing
their activity in the process, this can cause some confusion for the
observer. Erring perhaps on the side of caution, I would recommend the WASP for small groups of patients (up to twelve) who
are not overly active, such as the elderly.

Summary

In this chapter I have tried to address some of the issues involved in
looking at the patient's *circumstances*, and the effect this has upon
his functioning. Circumstances is a rather outdated expression but
one which neatly summarises our concerns here. The patient's
circumstances are the particular elements that directly affect him. It
might be difficult to prove, unequivocally, that the general
organisation of the patient's environment directly affects the way
he functions. However, the evidence does point in that general

direction. I have noted that a wide range of factors might be having an invisible effect upon him. It is not only the obvious restraints of the physical settings but also the social order of the environment that matter: the rules and regulations, not to mention expressed attitudes of a whole host of staff. Our single most erroneous belief in the history of psychiatry was that the patient's 'mental illness' existed entirely within him. We are now aware that the patient is not interpersonally isolated. He is very much a part of his environment and we need to be aware of his relationship with it. I have made some suggestions about how we might study that relationship more closely. We might have several reasons for wanting to do this, from gaining a simple understanding of how the living area 'works' to obtaining detailed measures of the patients' behaviour under various environmental conditions. By concluding the chapter with some methods for studying the *patient population* — rather than the ward — I have restated my belief that the patients are to a large extent, like the rest of us, a function of their environment.

Notes

1. K. T. Erikson, 'Patient Role and Social Uncertainty: a Dilemma of the Mentally Ill', *Psychiatry*, **20** (1967), pp. 263–74.

2. P. L. Berger, *Invitation to Sociology: A Humanistic Perspective* (Penguin Books, Harmondsworth, 1966).

3. R. Bierstedt, *The Social Order: An Introduction to Sociology* (McGraw-Hill, New York, 1963).

4. E. Goffman, *Asylums: Essays on the Social Situations of Mental Patients and Other Inmates* (Doubleday, New York, 1961).

5. R. Barton, *Institutional Neurosis,* 2nd edn (Wright, Bristol, 1966).

6. M. Jones, *Maturation of the Therapeutic Community: an Organic Approach to Mental Health* (Human Sciences Press, New York, 1976).

7. N. V. Raynes and R. D. King, 'Residential Care for the Mentally Retarded' in D. M. Boswell and J. M. Wingrove (eds.), *The Handicapped Person in the Community* (Tavistock, London, 1974).

8. J. Tizard, I. Sinclair and G. Clarke, *Varieties of Residential Experience* (Routledge and Kegan Paul, London, 1975).

9. V. Turner, 'How the Nurse can Help Preserve the Patient's Individuality', *Nursing Mirror*, 20 and 27 Jan. 1977.

10. R. Moos, 'The Assessment of the Social Atmosphere of Psychiatric Wards', *Journal of Abnormal Psychology*, **73** (1968), pp. 595–64.

11. R. Moos, *Evaluating Treatment Environments: A Social Ecological Approach* (John Wiley, New York, 1974).

12. R. Moos, 'The Assessment of the Psychosocial Environment of Community-oriented Psychiatric Treatment Programs', *Journal of Abnormal Psychology,* **79** (1972), pp. 9–18.

13. R. F. Gripp and P. A. Magaro, 'A Token Economy Program Evaluation with Untreated Ward Comparisons', *Behaviour Research and Therapy*, **9** (1971), pp. 137–49.

14. J. B. Milby, P.E. Pendergrass and C. J. Clarke, 'Token Economy versus Control Ward: A Comparison of Staff and Patient Attitudes towards Ward Environment', *Behaviour Therapy*, **6** (1975), pp. 22–30.

15. K. LeLaurin and T. R. Risley, 'The Organization of Day Care Environments: Zone versus Man-to-man Staff Assignments', *Journal of Applied Behaviour Analysis*, **5** (1972), pp. 36–43.

16. J. Jenkins, D. Felce, E. Powell and B. Lunt, 'Measuring Client Engagement in Residential Settings for the Elderly', Research Report (1977), Health Care Evaluation Research Team, University of Southampton, Southampton SO9 5NV.

17. Copies of the PLA-CHECK manual, along with reports on the development and testing of these materials, may be obtained by writing to T. R. Risley, Center for Applied Behaviour Analysis, AA 313 Bristol Terrace, Lawrence, Kansas 66044, USA.

18. S. M. Hereford, C. C. Cleland and M. Fellner, 'Territoriality and Scent-marking: A Study of Profoundly Retarded Enuretics and Encopretics', *American Journal of Mental Deficiency*, **77**(4) (1973), pp. 426–30.

19. L. E. McClannahan and T. R. Risley, 'The Organisation of Group Care Environments: Living Environments for Nursing Home Residents', paper presented at the American Psychological Association, 1972.

20. Copies of the 'Handbook for Observers' for measuring client engagement are obtainable from the Health Care Evaluation Research Team (see note 16).

11 ISSUES AND DILEMMAS

> All colours when placed in the shade appear of an equal
> degree of darkness among themselves. Placed in the light
> they never vary from their true and essential hue. —
> Leonardo da Vinci

In this book I have tried to discuss ways of looking at patients;
ways of helping patients to look at themselves; and a few of the
issues which are involved in the whole practice of assessment. We
have talked about some of the problems of making observations on
the nature of people's lives, and difficulties involved in making
judgements or pronouncements based upon these observations.
There are also a few other problems which might be classified as
philosophical, moral or ethical in nature. No matter how alien such
'intellectual' pursuits might appear to us, we dare not avoid our
duty to confront the issues which such questions might raise. We
have, during the course of this book, considered our right to judge
and comment upon the lives of those we call 'patients'. We need
now to consider our attitudes towards the patient body in more
general terms. We need to bring into sharper focus the philosophical and ideological base upon which we stand in order to gain a
clearer view of the patient.

Who do you See when you See me?

It is an inescapable fact that we are obliged to judge patients. The
kind of clear-cut signs and symptoms of disorder that are evident in
many physical disorders are not so evident in the so-called mental
illnesses. We have to make subjective judgements about what we
see, or even what we think we see. Much emphasis of this book has
been devoted to methods of trying to ensure that we have indeed
seen (or heard) or otherwise witnessed something. In the first part
of this chapter I want to extend our efforts to gain a more objective
picture of the patient by considering the problem of seeing things
that may not be there at all! I am not suggesting that nurses might
be hallucinated or deluded. However, in some situations we may be
so blinded by a stereotyped perception of the patient that we may
fail to see the 'real' person who is there. We witness only our
stereotyped image of the person. Such stereotyped images can be a

problem to all of us in our everyday interactions with friends and family. I remember some years ago a colleague entering my office one morning and asking me for a light for his cigarette. I told him several times that I had no matches, but he appeared to doubt my word, appealing to me to check my pockets and desk drawers for an odd match. Finally he asked me what I was using to light my pipe. I had by then been a non-smoker for more than two years. My colleague clearly had retained the old 'image' of me with pipe perpetually in hand or mouth. His perception of me, in that one respect, was stereotyped.

The Position of Patients

Standard medical diagnosis is concerned with evaluating some deviation of physical or physiological functioning. This may be one of degree — when a person has high blood pressure; or of nature — when a patient has a gastric ulcer. The diagnosis is based upon knowledge of normal physiological functioning. The doctor does not diagnose a condition within a person. Instead he identifies a disorder within one of his physiological systems. As a result patients are described as *having* a certain condition: he has emphysema or congestive cardiac failure. We do not refer to these patients as though they were synonymous with their condition. The patient is not called an emphysemic. We adopt this convention only when we view the problem as a chronic, or perhaps incurable, one. For instance we refer to diabetics, spastics or asthmatics. In this context it may well be that the long-standing nature of the patient's condition encourages others to see the patient and his condition as inseparable.[1]

It is common practice for nurses to want to know what is wrong with a patient before they begin to work with him. Student nurses, especially, are often anxious to establish the patient's diagnosis so that they will know how to treat him. In one sense this is something to be encouraged. This way we might assume that the patient will receive the correct care and attention. In another sense the diagnostic label may merely stereotype the person: squeezing him into a diagnostic pigeon-hole which only crudely summarises the nature of his problems, and says even less about 'him'. The patient might well be excused for thinking, 'I am not a real person, I'm a schizophrenic [or whatever].' Often the labels we apply to patients are assumed to represent their total identity, but one which is very much a spoiled identity.[2] I shall return to this point again in a moment.

The importance of this point is that in medical diagnosis (such as diabetes) we do not assume that disorders in one area of functioning always bring about disorder or dysfunction in other areas. Indeed a patient may have several disorders at the same time, but this does not mean that they all originate from the same cause. Moreover, the individual can retain his personal identity throughout his various trials and tribulations. He *has* a number of complaints or ailments. He has not been taken over by them.

The All-Embracing Disorder. In psychiatry the position is quite different. Although we use the same kind of labelling process and the same kind of descriptive terminology, the principles of classification have a wholly different rationale and effect. As we shall discuss later, in many cases our assertion that the patient suffers from a certain mental disorder is more of an assumption than a proven fact. Although no one can offer me unequivocal proof of the existence of the majority of the mental disorders patients I work with are assumed to suffer from, I must accept that such disorders exist. If I did not, there would be no point in me writing this book, or in your reading it. However, we should not pretend that the disorders we are talking about are in any way similar to gastroenteritis or cancer of the colon. Not only is there disagreement as to the constitution of many psychiatric disorders, but even where such conditions are clearly defined, difficulties are met in establishing a reliable diagnosis. When we say that a diagnostic criterion exists, we mean that anyone should be able to identify the presence or absence of the condition, providing that they use the same assessment process. A number of studies have shown that many categories of psychiatric disorder use 'overlapping criteria' or are poorly defined.[3] Patients showing much the same symptoms may be assigned to quite different diagnostic categories. The key feature here is that the diagnostic label reveals so little about the person and the way he functions. Other studies have shown that the patient's behaviour (or symptoms) are not greatly related to his diagnosis. For instance, a diagnosis like schizophrenia is more common in the USA than in many other Western countries. The chances of being labelled schizophrenic vary, however, from one state to another, and even from one ward to another. The best predictor of whether or not a patient will be so labelled is *where* the psychiatrist was trained and the therapeuric model that guides his practice.[4] The same accusation could be levelled at nurses. Not only do nurses tend to look at patients in the same way as their ward consultant,[5] but their application of labels like 'hostile' or 'hyperactive' depends more on their background training than any obvious pattern of patient behaviour. In a recent study involving the use of the term 'confused', massive discrepancies were found amongst nurses and doctors. Some used the term to refer to simple disorientation, whereas others meant the kind of disturbed state characteristic of severe dementia or hallucinosis.[6] The use of diagnostic labelling is a convention with obvious positive qualities. It serves as a means of communicating simply about the patient among professionals, and may also help identify treatment goals and methods. It is apparent, however, that the label may not only be irrelevant at times, but may be highly inaccurate. A label conveying so little information about the person merely 'typecasts' him. More importantly, it may be very difficult for the patient to escape from such a stereotype.

The Self-fulfilling Prophecy. Diagnostic classifications must surely distinguish patients with psychiatric disorders from so-called normal people. If they do not fulfil this criterion, then they are of little value. In a classic, and still controversial, experiment, Rosenhahn showed that it can be difficult to distinguish normal people from the psychiatrically disturbed. He arranged for eight research assistants to gain admission to twelve different mental hospitals in the USA by simply telling the admitting doctor that they heard the sounds 'thud' and 'crunch'. They showed no other problems. Once in hospital they stopped reporting these sounds and behaved 'normally'. It took an average of two weeks before these patients were discharged as 'schizophrenia in remission', having previously been labelled 'schizophrenic'. Rosenhahn noted with interest that nowhere in the vast literature on schizophrenia was hearing the sounds 'thud' and 'crunch' listed as a symptom of the disorder. His conclusion that the existing criteria, which have since been amended, were not adequate to differentiate the 'sane' from the 'insane', were reinforced by the observation that other patients became suspicious of the pseudopatients about two or three days after their admission. He also commented that once people are labelled as schizophrenic, staff attitudes towards the 'patient' change. The normal behaviour of the patient may be overlooked or profoundly misinterpreted. The psychiatric label appears to have a life and influence all of its own.

This paper caused a storm of outrage in the American psychiatric establishment. Rosenhahn was clearly challenging the value of the classification system and the competence of psychiatrists to use it appropriately. My aim in recalling this experiment is quite different. As I have noted repeatedly, nurses are not required to diagnose patients. This issue, therefore, is of largely academic interest. However, once a patient has been classified, we must be beware of stereotyping him. We must guard against assuming that the patient is no more than the diagnostic label suggests. Once a patient has been diagnosed we may expect him to behave in a particular way, to fulfil our expectations. If he behaves in a different manner we may interpret this as further signs of his problems or 'disease state'. We may begin to create, albeit unwittingly, an environment which may be hell-bent upon ensuring that he fulfils the criteria of the label which has been applied to him. This is the self-fulfilling prophecy in action.

The Position of Women

Our gender determines our lives from the minute we are born. In the early days there are no differences between the sexes, except for their genitalia. However, they are treated differently. Females are seen as being more fragile and are encouraged to be dependent and passive. Males are seen as hardy and are encouraged to pursue a path of aggressive self-reliance. As children the sexes are prompted to think, act and even feel differently. Studies have shown that even in the case of hermaphrodites the child reared as a female will become a woman, while an identical child reared as a boy will become imbued with male interests and acquire male privileges.

Women are reared to be passive, accepting, unquestioning, beautiful, supportive and co-operative. Young girls are restricted from an early age from enjoying the freedom and adventure that boys enjoy. They are restrained most specifically in their cumbersome dresses, which restrict their movements and which should never be sullied. They carry this symbolic restraint throughout their lives until as adult women they teeter precipitately on stiletto heels, or are partially handicapped by elongated painted talons, which serve no functional purpose. These kind of erotic exaggerations are designed, transparently, to meet the needs of the voyeuristic male. Where women stray from this path they may be conveniently labelled as 'tomboys' or in the best Hollywood tradition characterised as 'dowdy'. The social training of women is designed to meet their limited roles as mothers, housemaids, male assistants or sex-objects.

Sexist Psychology. I am generalising of course, but no more than I would be if I called men strong, self-reliant leaders and providers. I merely wish to acknowledge that it is little wonder that the sexes grow up differently. Traditional reasons given to explain such differences — biology and personality — are now largely discredited. The reality is that in a male-dominated society women are judged by male standards. Joanna Rohrbaugh comments wryly upon the 'female catch 22'. She notes that women can never win when they are defined and evaluated by male standards. In aptitude tests where men score higher on mathematical or spatial ability, these tasks are assumed to be of supreme importance. Where women display an advantage, as in verbal ability, they are classed as different, rather than better.[8] Psychology has been a male-dominated science throughout its long history. When Freud tried to translate it into even more scientific terms he set the seal on its sexist status with his idiosyncratic view that women were creatures who were mourning the loss of the penis. Countless studies have continued to perpetuate his myths about sex differences. The clue to all of this, as Rohrbaugh points out, is power: penis envy may be a curious translation of power envy.

So what is the relevance of all this to psychiatric assessment? Without wishing to project a closet feminist line, it seems apparent that women have been the victims of massive prejudice in the mental health field, as well as within wider society. Many of women's problems reflect male prejudice. This is true even where women perpetuate the myth. Any woman who refuses to toe the feminine line is seen as competing with men and may be classed as 'aggressive' or 'butch' or with some other complex or chip on her shoulder. Where she acts out the feminine role to the full she may be described as neurotic, frigid or hysterical.

Female Disorders. The prevalence of certain mental disorders in women has often been explained by reference to their unique biological system. Hysteria was first proposed by Hippocrates, who thought that female psychological disorders were hidden signs that the woman's body was pining for a child: thus we gain the concept of the 'wandering womb', from the Greek *husterikos*. Although professionally we now recognise the foolishness of this idea, we retain the notion that hysteria is peculiar to women. In certain sections of the male population the idea that vigorous sexual intercourse will provide the solution to any female problem is a cherished fantasy which still carries considerable street credibility. However, even today some professionals still retain the notion that only women are afflicted by any *neurotic* disorder. A nurse told me recently that she worked in a 'neurosis unit for women'. When I asked if there was an equivalent for men she replied, 'Our consultant says there is no such thing as a male neurosis.'

Depression in its various forms appears to affect women more consistently and seriously than men. Some female writers have argued that this is because women are in a continual state of mourning — mourning the freedom and privilege they have never had, or have sampled all too briefly.[9] Arieti has noted that women are depressed more often than men because we still live in a patriarchal society, in which women are raised to be dependent upon another person.[10] Returning to the notion of penis envy, Arieti and Bemporad noted somewhat dryly that

it is easier to affirm that depressed women are more likely to mourn not for the castration of their penis, which would be pure fantasy on their part, but because they really have been castrated — in a metaphorical sense. The symbolic penis of which they have been deprived is the male role in the world, including all the opportunities and privileges connected with that role.[11]

They go on further to comment that women in operas are typically depicted as (e.g.) sick, frail, exploited, loose and promiscuous, mechanical, beautiful when young but with a youth of short duration. 'We can conclude that either a woman's life is made miserable by men and therefore she has a right to be depressed; or she is regarded by men in such a negative way as to justify being in a state of despondency.'[12]

Anorexia nervosa — the so-called 'slimmer's disease' — and bulimarexia — where starving, gorging and purging routines are intermingled — are two other problems strongly associated with women. Traditionally these have been depicted as sexual disorders. The analyst argues that these women refuse to eat because they fear impregnation: they gorge themselves from time to time as unconscious desires to become pregnant break through. This sounds curiously like a latter-day Hippocrates at work. Feminist analyses of these problems take a different view with both feet planted on empirical soil. A large study of bulimarexic women noted that nearly all reported a perceived or actual male rejection incident prior to the beginning of their diet. Their discontinuation of relationships with men was not concerned with pregnancy fears, but a fear of performing inadequately and being rejected again.[13] Not surprisingly, the women in this study reported an extreme concern with their weight and appearance, and concerns that they were unattractive to men. This feminist analysis is not entirely at odds with the analytic tradition. It is accepted that such eating disorders are an expression of sexual conflict. However, whereas the Freudians emphasise the fear of impregnation and the underlying rejection of femininity, the feminists emphasises the fear of rejection and the underlying eagerness to be feminine.

Disorders of Living. It is not my intention here to present a feminist critique of traditional psychiatric attitudes towards women. I simply wish to emphasise, if such emphasis is necessary, that in some areas women have greater and more persistent problems than men: certain anxiety states, depression, some habit disorders and aspects of social relationships figure strongly in this respect. In many cases this appears to be more a function of their social upbringing and position within society than a function of any biological or personality sex differences. As Rohrbaugh has pointedly commented:

> in a frantic attempt to please others, some of these women become conventional, martyred caretakers, who are then vulnerable to the depression that accompanies the empty-nest syndrome. Some become depressed trying to conform to the expectations of the Dominant Other. Some women starve themselves in demands for autonomy or in a vain attempt to attain a distorted image of physical beauty they see as the path to happiness and fulfilment through male attentions.[14] Still other women rely upon superficial social charm and emotional appeals to manipulate the men in their lives.[15]

In our attempts to assess the nature of any problem of a psychological nature in women we should be aware that some, if not many, of these problems may be bound up in the experience of being female. Although, as Rohrbaugh notes, millions of women are already re-evaluating their assumptions, attitudes and value systems, the questioning of established values should not be exclusive to women. As a member of the opposite side, I wish to emphasise my own willingness to come to grips with some of my own prejudices, dysfunctional attitudes and distorted value-systems. I have made a point of emphasising the role of women throughout this book as the 'therapeutic agency', where the patient is mostly referred to in the male gender. Here, I have attempted to reverse the traditional procedure of depicting the weak and dependent person as a woman, and the person who invariably comes to her rescue as a dashing 'father-figure'.

Although female consciousness made a remarkable flourish over the last two decades, I fear that it is being battered into submission by powerful market forces, if not also the political rear-guard in many countries which desires a return to some of the older values. In our own society hoardings, newspapers, television and the cinema are intent upon pressuring women to conform to the male fantasy of the sexual object or the male reality of the homemaker and child-rearer. Certainly many more women are able to assert a more honest kind of sexuality, which is equal and different to men's. But the indications are that the pressures upon women to project a 'female stereotype' are being subtly reinforced by the pressures on males to project the male — or *macho* — stereotype. American cinema is most notable in this particular campaign, as they resurrect the idea of the screen hero (cf. Indiana Jones). Even ageing American presidents try to project their abilities for leadership through demonstrations of (alleged) physical fitness and a fine head of hair, not to mention their capacity for arm-wrestling other presidential candidates into submission.[16] I believe that these issues are not merely sociological curiosities. There is an implicit tragedy for men here as well as for women. For instance, it is well known that many psychological *and physical* disorders in men are a function of the massive restraint they exercise over their emotions, and their desperate efforts to attain the physical or professional ideals which may be wholly beyond them. In the assessment of people who either are in the process of becoming patients, or who are well established in their careers, there is a desperate need for us to penetrate the veneer of the sexual stereotype that most, if not all, of us erect around ourselves. Our assessment should attempt to understand the effects that sexual stereotyping may have upon the patient as well as the effects it may have upon our perception of the patient. Although I will accept that this need is pressing also for men, especially the extremist *macho* male, I believe that psychiatry has a major task in hand in attempting to repair the disservice done to women.

The Position of the Disabled

Within any psychiatric population we may find a number of patients who are physically as well as psychologically disabled. This disablement, which we refer to conveniently as *handicap*, can be wholly physical, as in spasticity or choreo athetosis, or mental, where a range of levels of intellectual impairment may prevail. In recent years we have popularised the notion that the physically handicapped person may be normal in all other respects. This seems to be more a vain hope than a reality. Certainly, this new liberal philosophy has yet to extend itself with any credibility to the person with a mental handicap. At present society discriminates to varying extents against handicapped people; but discriminate against all of them it does with impressive consistency. In the assessment of people with psychiatric disorder who may also be suffering from some accompanying physical or mental handicap we need to consider the extent to which our views of the person are coloured by the handicapped label which is applied.

What's in a Name? In one of the truly valuable and readable contributions to our understanding of the effects of disablement Miller and Gwynne make the important observation that although the word 'cripple' is seen as offensive, the synonyms are hardly an advancement in humanitarian terms. Popular alternatives such as the *in*firm, the *dis*abled, the *in*valid or the *de*formed all carry negative prefixes, expressing the absence of socially desirable attributes.[17] In more primitive societies, or I should say less bureaucratic and competitive societies, the crippled person is better accepted. Although he may be denied the privilege of high office, he is usually given a role which is commensurate with his abilities. In such societies the disability is seen more as a natural phenomenon that might happen to anyone. As a result cripples suffer less discrimination. In the West our tradition of discrimination has a long history. The Bible, Greek myths, drama and literature since the Renaissance, and contemporary comics and children's fairy stories are filled with crippled villians or 'bogeymen'. The Bible gives clear guidelines for excluding cripples, or virtually anyone with a physical affliction or blemish, from entering the priesthood.[18] This tradition has stood the test of time. In the Eastern religions it is common for such crippling afflictions to be seen as a punishment for misdeeds in previous lives. It is hardly surprising that the cripple is poorly catered for in such a climate of retribution. In short, our labelling of the 'crippled' person is not merely descriptive; it serves a function. It is designed to locate him somewhere at a distance from the rest of us. This symbolic distancing was, of course, fulfilled geographically in the establishment of colonies and institutions for the handicapped.

The classic discriminatory statement made against the handicapped person can be heard on an outing to a local restaurant where the waitress turns to his obviously 'normal' carer and asks, 'Does he take sugar in his tea?' This form of blindness is not exclusive to the layperson. I have heard high-ranking medical staff proclaim that mentally handicapped people never suffer from psychiatric disorders: 'They aren't bright enough!' On a more vigorously ignorant level, a parent told me how she had asked her general practitioner why her mentally handicapped son seemed to follow his father's instructions, but paid little attention to her. 'They're like dogs, you see. They only obey one master' was the authoritative reply. I fear that the doctor knew as little about the canine fraternity as he did about his human patient. In such examples we have clear illustrations of people who cannot see past the handicap. Or rather, they have a vivid impression of a stereotype that blinds them. A handicapped person, writing about D. H. Lawrence's depiction of Lady Chatterly's enfeebled husband, wrote:

> However one rates the human species, a man must be considered as a whole. His body is an incredibly wonderful piece of fully automated engineering, but in itself it is not a man. His mind, soul, spirit, is an even more wonderful and complex thing, but in itself it still does not constitute a man . . . He is much more than the sum of these parts, but a deficiency in one means a deficiency in the whole. Lawrence's view that after Sir Clifford became a cripple he was no longer a man is extreme, but it contains more truth than we like to admit. A cripple is still a man, but, as it were, on a smaller scale. His totality is diminished, his image distorted. He is not a whole.[19]

The writer affirms with impressive candour that although

handicapped people may be accepted to a limited extent, their sexuality presents major problems for the lay public, and often more so for those caring for them. Surprisingly, the blind, who are deficient in a crucial sense, are not discriminated against in the same way. As the writer notes, some kind of Jungian complex may be at play here. Blindness does not have the same sinister connotations that a physical abnormality has in the collective unconsious. Instead, as history demonstrates, blindness is often seen as an asset: e.g. in poetry or the exercise of philosophical wisdom.

Discrimination. The stereotyped disabled person in the psychiatric hospital can take various forms. In those settings where the mentally handicapped are still integrated with psychiatric patients, the intellectually impaired person may be seen as less complex and more of a one-dimensional man, the key dimension being intelligence. Where staff are anxious to exercise their skills on the stronger meat of ego-defence mechanisms or ephemeral group processes, the mentally handicapped person may be viewed as *just* a 'mental defective', a 'subnormal' or 'a bit simple'. In a conversation with staff on a long-stay ward a man was described to me as a mental defective. I asked what this meant. 'Well, he's got very simple needs, a very simple guy.' How did he know? I enquired. 'Because he doesn't appreciate things.' So why didn't he help him to appreciate things? 'Because he wouldn't understand. He's too simple.' This is the kind of self-fulfilling prophecy, uttered with complete conviction, that used to be the prerogative of the American white discussing the Negro, or the British describing the Indian at the height of the Raj. 'Why is the Negro inferior?' 'Because he is ignorant.' 'Then why don't you educate him?' 'Because he can't learn. He's inferior.' George Bernard Shaw once remarked that in America 'they force the Negro to shine their shoes for them, and then look down upon him because he is a bootblack'.

In all institutions set up to deal with dependent people there is a danger that the residents will become an equivalent of the victim of racial prejudice. Because *some* of the patients are highly dependent, requiring total care and attention, everyone is perceived in this way. In many geriatric settings the patients are reduced to the lowest common denominator, that of physical incapacity. As a result, other needs may be discounted or rarely considered. Where they are acknowledged, they may be seen as secondary or subsidiary concerns. The patient may be viewed as more sick, frail, helpless, or incapacitated than he really is. This perception is maintained by the fact that the philosophy of care is orientated towards physical care. As Goffman has shown, this is another example of the self-fulfilling prophecy.[20] The patient's needs are seen as largely physical in nature. Consequently, this is the only kind of care on offer. As a result, the patients' demands are largely of a physical nature. (They can only request what is on the 'menu'.) These demands in turn reinforce the staff view that the patient's needs are purely physical in nature.

The Creation of the Stereotype. Why do staff develop a stereotype of the disabled patient as being dependent, helpless and childlike? It seems clear that this idea is fuelled by the amount of time the staff spend working closely with *some* patients who indeed fulfil this stereotype. Highly dependent patients consume vast proportions of staff time. This tends to colour their attitude towards 'working in a disabled area'. There is a tendency to over-generalise, suggesting that all disabled people behave in the same way as the high-dependency group. The psychogeriatric ward is an obvious example. Here there are a number of patients who are very frail, extremely disoriented, and perhaps reduced to a basic level of functioning. However, every patient — by the law of averages — cannot be similarly disabled. If we are willing to remove our blinkers we will find varying residues of cognitive functioning, healthy emotions and differing levels of motor and social behaviour.

It has been widely reported in institutions for the physically disabled that where patients do not fit the stereotype, they are branded as trouble-makers or disruptive elements. Increasingly, my colleagues and I have been asked to offer advice and guidance to nurses in geriatric or chronic sick areas where patients are allegedly 'disturbed' or perhaps even 'mentally ill'. On closer examination, these patients have invariably turned out to be more competent than their peer group, both mentally and physically. Their 'problems' often involved their desire to exercise what independence they had left. Where the care system is routine and rigid, such independence is not catered for, and naturally disruption will take place. Where such patients were viewed, and often treated, like difficult children, the patient's reaction was often one of natural resentment or anger. Often this merely added fuel to the fire and provided further evidence that the patient must be 'mad'.

Conformity to the stereotype of the passive, pathetic and ever-lastingly grateful patient is the criterion by which we often judge the 'good patient'.

Clearing the Air

These few comments about some of the problems with stereotypes that we might meet during the course of assessment are not meant to be in any way exhaustive. I offer these comments merely as stimulus for further deliberations. Although I have talked exclusively about patients, it is clear that we tend to sterotype ourselves — the carers — in the same way. Where interpersonal conflicts crop up on a ward, these may be attributed to the emotional reactions of the female staff; the extreme old age or youth of various members; or the fact that someone's stupidity is causing frustrations or tension. Age-ism, sex-ism, and intellectual-ism are three of the commonest stereotyping devices used by staff on each other. They correlate highly with the use of similar strategies in common use with patients. I have been encouraged by the new syllabus for psychiatric nurse training,[21] which begins with assisting student nurses to see themselves: their attitudes, beliefs, prejudices, etc. Only once this period of learning is over will they be encouraged to look at patients. In this sense my comments in the last few pages are already unnecessary. Where nurses are being pre-pared to appreciate their own prejudiced perceptual set, they will require less prompting to un-blinker their vision of the patient in their care. Such self-awareness will clear the air: clearing a way to a truly objective, impartial assessment of the patient.

What is Wrong with this Patient?

One of the questions I have refrained from asking during the preceding chapters is, 'Does the patient really have a problem?' We should not take it for granted that simply because a patient carries a certain label, or has been referred for assessment with a certain complaint, that this is any proof of the existence of real problems. We would do well to remember the moral of Rosenhahn's story in this respect. I am not saying that we should be in perpetual doubt. I merely advise against taking too much for granted. Many nurses believe that it is not their job to challenge the authority of the psychiatrist. I would agree. Reporting information that appears to weaken the diagnosis, and suggests a different interpretation of the patient's state, is, however, simply 'good nursing'. It is not a challenge to anyone's authority. The nurse has a responsibility to remain as impartial as possible, whilst offering the patient support and advocacy.[22] Many, if not all, psychiatrists in a hospital setting rely upon the reports of nurses to arrive at their final diagnosis. The nurse cannot afford to hide her opinions or judgements without risking endangering the patient in the process.

It is a truism that many patients suffer psychiatric treatment because of the problems of their families or even society itself. At least one commentator has questioned our responsibility to make people 'fit into' a mad society. Perhaps it is our responsibility to reshape society to make it less distressing for its inhabitants.[23] On a more domestic note it is clear that our perceptions of mental disorder can be grossly misleading. The apocryphal tale of the man who saw a unicorn in his garden, by James Thurber,[24] is a wry reminder that sloppy labelling can be not only offensive, but might also work against us. The man told his wife that he had seen a unicorn in the garden one morning. 'You are a booby, and I'm going to have you put in the booby hatch,' she replied. The man, who had never liked the words 'booby' or 'booby hatch', thought for a moment and then said, 'We'll see about that.' His wife telephoned the police and a psychiatrist and when they arrived she proceeded to tell them about her husband's sighting of the unicorn. They began to believe that she was the insane one. When her husband arrived on the scene he failed to confirm her story, so off she went to the 'booby hatch'.

We might do well to remember that sometimes, when we are studying crazy behaviour, we might be better employed in looking at the conditions that give rise to these apparently crazy phenomena. In another sense we might ask ourselves, what exactly do we think we mean when we say that someone is mentally ill? The concept of mental illness is little more than a comfortable convention. Like an old overcoat, we dare not investigate it too closely in case it starts to fall apart.

Mental Illness and Mental Health

Throughout this book I have mixed the use of technical terms like 'psychotic' or 'anxiety' with the concept of problems of living. I have tried to avoid talking about psychiatric nursing as a mere subsidiary of the diagnosis of mental disorder. From this viewpoint nurses are, at least in theory, involved in collecting a much wider body of information about the patient's functioning than is necessary for the formation of a diagnosis. We cannot leave the discussion of nursing assessment without considering some of the dilemmas inherent in psychiatric diagnosis, since these dilemmas might represent further reasons why we should be attempting to extend our own assessment expertise and technology.

It would be foolish to assume that assessment is not influenced by the ideological orientation of the assessor: her 'school of thought'. So what sorts of things do nurses believe about their patients? I find the answer an elusive one. There appears to be no central theoretical model of psychiatric disorder that might help unite nurses in the way they look at patients. In the UK at least nurses tend to follow their leader. They adopt the theoretical model of the consultant-in-charge, accepting his notions of mental illness in the best-behaved tradition of the handmaiden.[25] So if nurses do not have a central philosophy or science, what kinds of models do their mentors follow? Models of mental disorder range from traditional psychoanalysis to contemporary anti-psychiatry. In between there are various convictions about what is wrong with the patient. These are influenced by medical viewpoints (the biophysical school); psychodynamic or intrapsychic beliefs and sociological viewpoints (social psychiatry). In some countries (e.g. Italy and the USSR) the school of thought may be heavily influenced by political standpoints.

A Change of Heart. Nurses are encouraged from their first introduction to their craft to accept the idea that mental illness exists. By implication it is assumed that mental health can be similarly defined. In recent years, the disruptive effects of writers like Szasz, Laing and a number of sociologists have led us to question our rather concrete view of mental illness. Here I want to comment upon only some of the more notable problems involved in trying to understand what is wrong with the patient. I proffer no solutions. I am merely sharing some of my doubts and anxieties with you. I believe that we are in a position which is analogous to riding the horns of a rather hyperactive dilemma. We need to learn how to position ourselves on this dilemma to afford ourselves as much comfort as we can. I see no sign of the dilemma disappearing, or in us having an opportunity to dismount.

There has been a growing trend among a number of health care workers to acknowledge that the traditional distinctions between one disease category and another hinder us from understanding fully the meaning of *health* and its numerous irregularities. The medical tradition has encouraged all of us — doctors, nurses and laypersons — to think of illness in terms of pathology: the functional or structural changes caused by disease. However, it is clear that not all human disease follows the rules laid down in the textbooks. Selye's research into the role of stress in health and disease concluded that people react to stress in a variety of ways.[26] It may be more important to try to understand how people become 'sick' than simply to catalogue the variety of disorders that they might suffer from.

The 'holistic' model of health care which is gaining favour reflects an ecological view of man. Everything here is interconnected. This is in stark contrast to the medical model, which explodes the patient in order to study disease in one part of his functioning. We are now beginning to experience a change of heart. Instead of viewing patients as some sort of billiard balls responding passively to the forces exerted upon and through them, we are beginning to see illness and health as more dynamic features of the person's total functioning and interaction with his world.

The Roots of Psychiatry. I have observed already that many of the mental disorders that our patients suffer from say very little about the people to whom these labels are applied. In an incisive analysis of the diagnostic approach Mathew Dumont highlights what he calls the 'nonspecificity of mental illness'.[27] Taking schizophrenia as an example, he reminds us that Bleuler, who first coined the term, described a number of 'primary symptoms': associative looseness, affective disturbance, autism and ambivalence. These were all prefixed with the letter 'A' to make them easier for medical students to learn. Delusions and hallucinations were classed as 'secondary symptoms'. Bleuler did not suggest how often the four As occurred together, nor did he indicate how often these 'symptoms' occurred in the non-schizophrenic population. However, the idea of the disease of schizophrenia was born thus in 1911. The picture has cleared little today. Despite the massive body of evidence from research, we are no clearer as to the meaning or origins of the disorder. Everyone is aware that something is there, but no one knows exactly what. The illusion that there are natural boundaries to the thing we call schizophrenia has been maintained for generations.

This assumption has allowed various researchers to draw meaningful inferences from statistical trends which, like the edges of a moving cloud, tend to fulfil the fantasies of the beholders. If we remove the labelling process, with all its classist, racist, sexist underpinnings, what we are left with is a diffuse population of socially disturbed people who are in no specific or characteristic way neurologically damaged. And it may be that a major reason for the clustering of major mental illnesses among the lower socio-economic classes is the whirlpool of teratogenic influences to which the poor are subjected.[28]

How do we Function?

In Chapter 1, I suggested that we function on a range of levels. One of the major problems in trying to understand mental illness is that traditionally we have tended to split people up into compartments. As we noted earlier in this chapter, a mental disorder is often seen as taking over the person. Much of the debate of the last hundred years has focused upon the dualism between mind and body: are they separate or are they the same? Dumont has tried to solve the problem by comparing the way we function to the formation of ice on a lake. In order for the drop in temperature to lead to the formation of ice, a complex chain of actions and interactions must take place. These involve, mainly, the electromagnetic forces around individual molecules of water. This leads to the formation of crystals which congregate to form what we call ice. Dumont compares the formation of patterns of behaviour to this complex process of action and interaction. When we reach out to save a child from falling (a single behaviour) this action is derived from a template which connects memory, intelligence, imagination, emotion, perception and numerous other individual functions, by a network of gossamer threads. The net result is a template which resembles a hologram. Like a hologram it may appear in one form but function in another, quite different, dimension. This model of behaviour seems to reflect contemporary science and technology in much the same way that Freud was influenced by ideas about the combustion engine, which led to his concepts of drives, energy and catharsis. Dumont argues that in the light of this hologram analogy the idea that a gene — a very small cluster of amino acids — can *cause* the structure of a huge, amorphous mass of behaviour like schizophrenia is like assuming that the structure of H_2O can explain the outline of a cloud. It is an error of scale of such magnitude as to be something of a thought disorder itself.[29]

Whatever mental illness is, it will not be ameliorated by use of a process of classification as the basis for different treatment interventions. Instead the patient's problems must be seen in ecological terms, connected to and continuous with other functions of our biological, cultural and social existence. Dumont's ideas might seem a little radical to many nurses reared upon a simple diet of diseases and syndromes. Perhaps they might be forgiven for thinking that he is denying the very existence of mental illness. Nothing could be further from the truth. He acknowledges that people suffer disturbance and distress. However, these must be seen as problems that are a function of their total experience as people projecting through their own biological space to interact with their social and cultural world, and ultimately with the influences of the environment, whether, natural or man-made.

Health? Clearly all of us accept the notion of health and sickness as concrete things, if only for simplicity's sake. When we come to analyse what we mean by such terms we start to feel the horns of the dilemma even more sharply. Yet we might do well to question the idea of illness, in order to appreciate better the meaning of health. Peter Sedgwick has made the highly provocative assertion that there are no illnesses or diseases in nature.[30] Illness is something man defines. He selects out certain states that he *chooses* to call illness. These are the natural causes which lead to the death or loss of function of a limited range of species: people, pets, domestic livestock and the plants we cultivate for gain or pleasure. All of these may be classed as disease-ridden or illness-prone. We do not normally talk about spiders, lizards or desert grass as sick or diseased. These are of little importance to us. Sedgwick argues that the labelling of disease or illness is a social value system. Illness simply does not exist: it is a social construction. We have grown to believe that illness is defined by our medical wizardry. This also is mythical. Concepts of illness were in use centuries before man even understood the circulation of the blood. Even today different cultures interpret sickness or disease differently, either as a disturbance of the body or the spirit, and occasionally both.

Illness as Deviancy. So what does all this mean? Is Sedgwick saying that we simply believe in illness and make it happen? No. Merely that our perceptions of illness are heavily influenced by concerns that have little to do with pathology. In my introduction I suggested that illness might be seen as deviancy: the ill person is different from other people; he differs from the established norm of biological or psychological functioning. However, when we are talking about 'the norm', do we mean healthy? Massive variations regarding the meaning of healthy occur within, as well as across, cultures. Sedgwick again notes that in 1911 it was found that hookworm was seen as part of normal health in parts of North Africa. In one South American tribe the disease of dyschronic spirochetosis, which is marked by coloured spots on the skin, is so normal that anyone without the condition is disqualified from marriage. Social and cultural norms clearly influence our perceptions of normality and pathology. In Western society the doctor has traditionally held the exalted status equivalent to the witch doctor or priest in more primitive societies. Doctors are, as a result, called upon to comment upon not only obvious physical problems, but also matters such as contraception, sexual relationships, child-rearing practices and emotional management. In the world of psychiatry Freud popularised the notion that no one was free of neurosis. A psychotherapeutic growth industry has developed, despite any evidence of its value, which encourages people to seek solace or repair for what may well be 'natural emotions'. In the wake of an upsurge of iatrogenic disorders doctors are now urging people to recognise that problems of living cannot be remedied by taking tranquillisers or antidepressants *ad nauseam*. These are some of the problems of living that are the responsibility of the world, its politicians and ultimately its individuals. We must solve such problems by our own moral actions. We have done many a human being a disservice by *medicalising* his natural suffering: by applying a label to something that should be seen as a function of that person's distress as a result of his interaction with his own world.[31]

The reader might be forgiven for thinking that I have been attempting to confuse her over the past few pages. I have questioned the logic by which we arrive at definitions of psychiatric disorder. I have questioned the philosophical and sociological bases upon which we construct our models of health or sickness. I have caused this confusion simply to deter nurses from assuming that the understanding of health, illness or what is wrong with this person can ever be a simple business. The evidence for the existence of *specific* psychiatric disorders is slight, and I leave it to other, more articulate commentators to argue the subtleties of this debate with you. However, it seems clear to me that the 'conditions' we call 'schizophrenia', 'manic depressive psychosis' or the various psychoneurotic states are rather fluid by comparison with disorders of a physical nature. More importantly, there may be a distinct disadvantage in trying to look for conditions that inhabit a private world. We may miss the important relationship which exists between the patient's biological state and his environment. The *process* of this relationship should be the true focus of our attention in any assessment. Nurses should be more interested in studying how people function in an ecological sense, rather than assuming that the patient inhabits a vacuum.

Some Ethical Concerns

Ethics does not relate only to treatment. Ethics is the discipline concerned with the moral guidelines governing the nurse's actions towards the patient, *under any condition*. This must begin with assessment. If nurses are not ethical — i.e. right and just — at this stage, how can they ever redeem themselves later on?

The Nurse as an Agent of Treatment

Nurses might be excused for thinking that they fulfil only a minor role in the successful treatment of psychiatric patients. Largely, this is a function of the confusion between the terms 'care' and 'treatment'. Shirlee Passau-Buck comments:

> the hospital family consists of mothers (nurses); fathers (physicians) and children (patients) and is based upon the patriarchal family system of western society . . . the subordinate position of nursing is reinforced by the care/cure myth that values caring, the traditional female nursing role, less than curing, the male medical role . . . [this is] further emphasised by the fact that doctors are well paid for curing, but not so nurses for caring.[32]

The gentle irony of this situation is that although curing and caring are different, both are essential. *Healing* in its fullest sense involves both care and cure. It has been observed repeatedly that nurses often do both in practice. For this reason nurses can never afford to take their relationships with the patient lightly. Society, and indeed the patient, may assume that other staff are more important, for whatever reason. This does not absolve nurses from their responsibility to be aware of their own importance. Nursing assessment should never be assumed to be inferior to medical diagnosis: it is merely different.

Asking Questions

Does the nurse have the right to ask the patient questions about any aspect of his life? Perhaps this question should read, 'Does the nurse have a right to ask the patient any questions?' The patient need not answer any questions, or participate in any part of the assessment process, if he does not wish to. In a legal setting the person has a right to 'remain silent'. This should extend to psychiatric assessment. The importance of this issue is that nurses should be aware that the patient might feel threatened by an interview or some other form of assessment. In some situations the *content* of the assessment questions may be more threatening than the form they take. We should respect the patient's concern on this issue and should try to make life easier by modifying the questions, or trying to put him more at ease. However, if the patient is unwilling to answer certain, or any, questions, what right have we to coerce him further? Apart from the absence of any such right, such an action will merely prejudice further relations with the individual.

The Role of Prejudice

It is commonly assumed that nurses are angels in disguise. Although I am a great believer in the humanitarian potential of everyone, I must also accept that, by the law of averages, nursing — like any other professional group, must have its quota of bigots. I doubt very much whether even a library full of ethical essays would change their attitudes. Even if we see ourselves as liberal and free-thinking, we should not forget our potential for prejudice. I have already covered three areas where our stereotyped notions of people may obscure our ability to see them clearly. In other areas we may be blinkered by moral or religious standards. Wife or child battering, sexual deviations and even the use of foul language are areas where our own moral philosophy might bring us into conflict with the patient. Even political prejudice might be involved if we are confronted by someone with radically oppositional views to our own. These problems are not such a problem with the seriously disturbed patient, where we can attribute his behaviour to the 'ravings of a madman'. In less severe cases conflicts might be experienced if the nurse interprets his behaviour as meaningful. She must guard against such conflicts influencing her judgement.

The Use of the Assessment

The assessor cannot separate herself from the use to which her information will be put. I am taking the view that assessment in nursing is rarely for statistical purposes. I have already emphasised the need to identify problems that are problems *for the patient* rather than any other person. Our role is to act as the patient's advocate, acting on his behalf wherever necessary, even to the extent of helping ensure that the assessment goals are in his best interest. In this context it is important that the nurse does not let herself be used to 'trick' the patient into confiding material he might previously have been unwilling to disclose. If the nurse has established a good relationship with a patient, he may make such disclosures because he trusts her. If the nurse wishes to pass on such information, she should seek his approval. Otherwise she will risk breaking a confidence and prejudicing the relationship.

It is worth while telling the patient at the very outset *exactly* why the nurse wants to ask certain questions, and what she intends to do with the information. By stating the aims and objectives of the assessment the nurse is keeping an *open agenda*: there are no hidden motives or uses to which the information will be put. This openness will do much to strengthen the relationship.

Records and Notes

I have stated a number of times already my conviction that we should try wherever possible to confine ourselves to stating the facts. When we comment upon a patient we should strive to report verbatim what he said and did; what he thought and felt about what he did. We should leave it at that. There is no need for interpretation.

I worked recently with a young man who spent most of our first meeting discussing the records I was keeping, which were lying closed in their folder on the desk. He also talked a lot about the sorts of things he knew other people were saying about him. He had asked a number of people (GP, social worker and psychiatrist) whether he could see the records they were keeping, asking whether they could be destroyed after he had ended his contact with the service. He reported that he had lost a number of jobs 'on account of my health record'. I was intrigued to find a reference in his notes to this young man's 'pathologically suspicious and paranoid behaviour'.

On the surface this man did appear to be making unreasonable demands. It would be all too easy to lose patience with him. However, he had a valid point. The records that were kept by the psychiatric service were concrete documents. They cannot be handed over to the patient. He cannot even view them. And there is no question of their contents being destroyed once he ends his contact with the service. Vernon Coleman, a general practitioner, has suggested that if patients were able to keep their own health records this would rule out much of the danger of breaches of confidentiality.[33] This, however, would be only a partial solution for my patient. He was concerned about the factual basis of what was being put into the records. Such fears are well grounded and certainly are not paranoid. Each time a patient meets a new health care professional, the sketch of him already in his record will colour the perceptions of his new contact. I tend to avoid reading case notes before meeting a patient for the first time in order to limit the development of preconceived ideas, shaped perhaps by the pen of the previous contact. There are occasions when staff are required to commit their beliefs to paper: when they believe a patient is dangerous or suicidal. These statements should always reflect their dubious status and the decision to record such information should not be taken lightly. The patient will carry this record idefinitely.

Confidentiality

There are undoubtedly many pressures put upon nurses to report the content of confidential discussions held with patients. It is important that we are aware of the limitations of the relationship and the conditions under which this confidence may be breached.

It is a good idea to tell the patient what the aim of the assessment is. Then he is in no doubt about the purpose to which his comments might be put. If the nurse tells the patient that she wants to find out how he feels so that she can plan some programme of care for him with the rest of the team, then it is implicit that anything she says may be reported back to the rest of the team. If he asks for clarification on this point, honesty must prevail. If the nurse takes rough notes, which may later be transcribed into a case file, the nurse can read these notes back to check that her observations were correct. If the patient asks to see what she is going to write about him, she may let him see the rough notes. Once the notes are written up, *formally*, they become a legal record. These notes no longer belong to the patient or the nurse, but to the Secretary of State. It is for this reason that the patient is disbarred from witnessing his own notes. Although I have suggested that nurses may allow the patient to read their 'rough notes', on no account can they allow the patient to read other people's comments, without their approval. This would involve breaking a professional confidence.

In this context it need hardly be emphasised that nurses should not discuss with patients comments alleged to have been made by some other nurse or other professional. The patient may be annoyed or worried about something someone has said. He may wish to discuss this with his 'favourite nurse'. She may invite comments from him and further details, questioning him as to how he feels and what he thinks about what has been said. However, it is not appropriate for her to pass any opinion on such matters. This should be stated with some clarity.

Breaking a Confidence. Are there any situations in which a confidence may be broken? Muyskens[34] lists three situations in which the nurse might feel obliged to breach confidentiality with the patient. The first example is where the patient is in a temporary fit of depression or anger and discloses his intention to harm or kill himself, which would clearly prejudice or destroy his prospects for leading a full, autonomous life. The nurse's decision here is clearly a paternalistic one. She makes a judgement over the head of the patient, in much the same way as parents do over children. Although the information may have been imparted in confidence, the nurse believes that the patient's best interests will be served by breaking this confidence. In the second example the rights of some third party might be threatened. He quotes the example of a mother who threw her child down a flight of steps, afterwards claiming that it was an accident. Later, in a state of depression, she confessed to a nurse, imploring her to remain silent. What is the nurse's moral duty? Muyskens notes that in most states a legal responsibility would exist to report the incident. Is the moral requirement any different? He acknowledges that, since the risk of further damage to the child cannot be predicted, the decision is a difficult one. He decides, however, that the protection of confidentiality does not extend to situations where the rights of a third party are at risk, no matter how small. In the third example he states that confidentiality may be breached where there is some danger to the general public. A patient who talks about his resentment against society, and his ambition to 'get even', may simply be talking. However, he may be a threat to the lives of innocent people. His ambitions must be publicly acknowledged.

It has not been my intention here to review all the possible ethical dilemmas that might confront the nurse in her assessment of the patient. I have selected only those which appear most common concerns, or are fairly regular obstacles to the development of ethical assessment. The requirement to protect the freedom and dignity of the patient does not begin and end in treatment: it is sketched in the assessment and often becomes the blueprint for ethical practice thereafter.

Conclusion

In this chapter I have tried to share some of my concerns and anxieties relating to the business of assessment. I have expressed my concern that even when we try to be 'patient-centred' one stereotype or another may hinder us from ever becoming truly person-centred. I have expressed my doubts also about the value of the beast we call 'mental illness'. Traditional practice tends to guide all of us — nurses, doctors, psychologists alike — towards thinking that the complex mish-mash of human misery can be reduced to identifiable organic or psychological states, with identifiable causes and outcomes. This seems by all accounts to be a delusional system. The more we know about mental illness, the less we appear to understand. I have offered no ready solutions: just encouragement to avoid being simple-minded. Finally, I have discussed a few of the key issues involved in the practice of ethical assessment. The issues I have addressed are of a fairly concrete consistency and should pose no problems for the nurse who is uneasy with philosophical debate. I have made a few suggestions as to how the planning of ethical assessment can provide the framework for the subsequent ethical care of the patient. Taken together, these three facets represent my sole contribution to the philosophy of assessment. I hope that in the future we will find the need to say more about such philosophical issues. Perhaps by then we will feel more comfortable with the mechanics of the practice.

Notes

1. H. E. Adams, J. A. Doster and K. S. Calhoun, 'A Psychologically Based System of Response Classification' in A. R. Ciminero, K. S. Calhoun and H. E. Adams (eds.), *Handbook of Behavioural Assessment* (John Wiley, New York, 1977).

2. E. Goffman, *Stigma: Notes on the Management of Spoiled Identity* (Prentice-Hall, Englewood Cliffs, NJ, 1963).

3. E. Zigler and L. Phillips, 'Psychiatric Diagnosis: A Critique', *Journal of Abnormal and Social Psychology*, 63 (1961), pp. 607–18.

4. National Institute of Mental Health, *Schizophrenia Bulletin Issue 11* Government Printing Office, Washington, DC, 1974).

5. D. F. S. Cormack, *Psychiatric Nursing Observed. A Descriptive Study of the Work of the Charge Nurse in Acute Admission Wards of Psychiatric Hospitals* (Royal College of Nursing, London, 1976).

6. C. J. Simpson, 'Doctors and Nurses' Use of the Word Confused', *British Journal of Psychiatry*, 145 (1984), pp. 441–3.

7. T. Rosenhahn, 'On Being Sane in Insane Places', *Science*, 179 (1973), pp. 250–8.

8. J. B. Rohrbaugh, *Women: Psychology's Puzzle* (Harvester Press, Hassocks, Sussex, 1980).

9. P. Chessler, 'Patient and Patriarch: Women in the Psychotherapeutic Relationship' in V. Gornick and B. K. Moran (eds.), *Women in Sexist Society* (Basic Books, New York, 1971).

10. S. Arieti, 'Roots of Depression: The Power of the Dominent Other', *Psychology Today*, 12 (1979), pp. 54–92.

11. S. Arieti and J. Bemporad, *Severe and Mild Depression: The Psychotherapeutic Approach* (Basic Books, New York, 1978).

12. Ibid.

13. M. Boskind-Lodahl and J. Sirlin, 'The Gorging-purging Syndrome', *Psychology Today*, 10(2) (1977), pp. 50–2, 82–5.

14. Judith Bat-Ada comments caustically: 'All the special glitter that this male society produces for women — the makeup, the high heeled shoes, the tight little dresses — single us out as women as effectively as did the yellow stars on the coats of the Jews,' and more specifically on the influence of soft pornography: 'women hate themselves for not being like the magazine models they see men panting after. We don't measure up to the measurements touted by the magazines, and we know it. We despair, but because there is nowhere to go with that despair, it turns inward and becomes self-hatred' pp. 118–20 in L. Lederer (ed.), *Take Back the Night: Women on Pornography* (Bantam Books, New York, 1982). (I am indebted to my daughter, Charley, for extending my understanding of the female state.)

15. This quotation is taken from Rohrbaugh, *Women*.

16. C. Beck has suggested that prejudice against the elderly and the stereotyped view of old people is influenced by the following factors: (1) an emphasis upon the importance of youth; (2) an emphasis upon work, activity and efficiency; (3) a denial of death and suffering; (4) increasing secularisation; (5) a romanticised view of mental health. See C. Beck, 'Mental Health and the Aged: A Values Analysis', *Advances in Nursing Science*, 1(3) (1979), pp. 79–87. It would appear that many old people also 'buy' such prejudiced views, like the aforementioned American president.

17. E. J. Miller and G. V. Gwynne, *A Life Apart* (Tavistock, London, 1972).

18. Leviticus 21: 17–23. Quoted by Miller and Gwynne (ibid.).

19. Quoted in P. Hunt (ed.), *Stigma: The Experience of Disability* (Geoffrey

Chapman, London, 1966).

20. E. Goffman, *Asylums* (Doubleday, New York, 1961).

21. *Training Syllabus: Register of Nurses Mental Nursing*, published by the General Nursing Council for England and Wales, 23 Portland Place, London, 1982.

22. Schrock has suggested that nurses need to fulfil such a role in order to co-ordinate the activities of the various groups of professionals involved in the delivery of care. R. A. Schrock, 'Planning Nursing Care for the Mentally Ill', *Nursing Times*, 17 April 1980.

23. Laing has commented: 'Psychiatry could be, and some psychiatrists are, on the side of transcendence, of genuine freedom, and of true human growth. But psychiatry can so easily be a technique of brainwashing, of inducing behaviour that is adjusted, by (preferably) non-injurious torture. . . . I would wish to emphasise that our "normal" adjusted state is too often the abdication of ecstasy, the betrayal of our true potentialities, that many of us are only too successful in acquiring a false self to adapt to false realities.' R. D. Laing, *The Divided Self* (Penguin Books, Harmondsworth, 1965), p. 12.

24. Taken from *The Thurber Carnival* (Penguin Books, Harmondsworth, 1953).

25. Cormack, *Psychiatric Nursing Observed*.

26. H. Selye, *Stress in Health and Disease* (Butterworth, Boston, 1976).

27. M. P. Dumont, 'The Nonspecificity of Mental Illness', *American Journal of Orthopsychiatry*, **54**(2) (1984), pp. 326–34.

28. Ibid.

29. Ibid.

30. P. Sedgwick, *Psycho Politics* (Harper and Row, New York, 1982), pp. 28–42.

31. Taken from 'More Wealth, Less Health — An Interview with Ivan Illich', *Psychology Today*, **2**(6) (1976).

32. S. Passau-Buck, 'Caring versus Curing: The Politics of Health Care' in J. Muff (ed.), *Socialisation, Sexism and Stereotyping* (C. V. Mosby, St Louis, Mo., 1982).

33. V. Coleman, 'Why Patients should Keep their Own Records', *Journal of Medical Ethics*, **1** (1984), pp. 27–8.

34. J. L. Muyskens, *Moral Problems in Nursing* (Rowman Littlefield, Tottowa, NJ, 1982).

12 SOME AFTERTHOUGHTS

We know accurately only when we know little;
with knowledge doubt increases. — Goethe

When I was a boy I used to learn to draw at my grandfather's knee. On Saturday afternoons I would look over the park and draw the trees bordering the road on the hill as it climbed out of the village. Later, my grandfather would often 'shape up' my drawing, abstracting faces, animals and people from my fumbling sketches of the trees. At first I was angry, and for a long time afterwards. At times I dreaded the lesson. Later he said, 'Draw what is there, not what you *think* is there.' As time passed I too began to see the people and animals that were *hidden* in my trees. As time passed I grew to doubt more and more the 'truth' of what I saw. Paradoxically, I grew to know better the things I was drawing. My sketches of the trees became more honest, less ambiguous. Although my grandfather is long gone, the lesson goes on. In this book I have indulged something of my experience as a doubtful 'seer', sharing my own doubtful vision of the patient with you.

I have discussed two kinds of assessment. In one, we have an approach which can tell us *something* about virtually anyone. These are the general assessment strategies that help us to identify (e.g.) the presence or absence of a certain skill or the level of 'assertiveness' in an individual. These methods, which are usually rigorously tested, have 'high generalisability'. They tell us something about everyone, but very little about one person. The second kind is the method which focuses attention on one person, often providing us with a mountain of information that we find difficult to handle. These methods are 'person-centred' and, as a result, tell us nothing about other people. Although they are quite different, these two approaches both reflect a 'scientific' attempt at assessment. They are quite, quite different from the 'seat-of-the-pants' awareness which often guides nurses' judgement of patients. If I was asked to single out one single moral from the whole of this book it would be this: *intuition can be dangerous*.

I have always believed that 'life' is the great teacher. The passage of even the most tedious of days provides a plentiful supply of learning situations. Often, however, we can become complacent

361

and may forget that we know, as yet, very little. When one is cast in the role of an expert — such as being asked to write a book like this — it is altogether too easy to forget how little one has really experienced or how blunted one may have become to the experience of life. Recently, I had the good fortune to supervise a student who was working with a man with a forty-year history of depression and anxiety. 'Jackie' presented with agitation, sleep disruption and a pervasive anxiety which fuelled a range of 'obsessional checking' rituals. These problems stemmed from experiences in a Japanese prisoner-of-war camp towards the end of the war. Through careful questioning we were able to piece together the horrific background to his contemporary nightmare: a picture which had been wholly ignored during the series of repeated attempts to quell his disturbance through drugs and ECT. Jackie made a number of startling comments early on in the interviews which I found to be rather outstanding. Perhaps they are not all that remarkable, and may only reflect my own limited experience. As he grew to trust his interviewer more, he began to relate a little of the horror of his experience. The story had a seductive quality, even for those who believe that they do not have a morbid temperament. As he recounted his story Jackie turned and in a rather desperate voice said, 'I'm not looking for sympathy. I don't want anyone to feel sorry for me.' What I found remarkable about this little incident is simply this. Although I feel that I have led a fairly rich life, with its share of ups and downs, the story that Jackie unfolded made me feel exceedingly humble. At the same time I felt honoured that he should be willing to share it with my colleague and myself. A stock 'empathic' phrase, which too easily trips off my tongue, is 'I know how you feel' or 'I understand how you are feeling.' Some patients are quick to point out that we do not know how they feel. Jackie never made a particular emphasis of this point. However, he serves as a perpetual reminder that, only rarely, can I ever know how the patient feels. In this context it may well be that 'humility is strength'.

In this book I have tried to explore some of the avenues of assessment that have been chartered by some important figures. Much of what I have discussed represents the culmination of significant research work and a powerful tradition of human enquiry. Much of what I have described represents 'a way' of charting unknown territory. It is certainly not '*the* way' — in the sense of representing any significant truths. It is undeniably not the 'only way'. I have attempted to portray a simple, practical approach to understanding some of the vagaries of the human condition. Of necessity, I have done it my way, and that is often a clumsy one. Often the emphasis upon structure, systems, methods and standardisation serves only to blinker our 'natural vision'. In a sense, however, that is the challenge of assessment. Each time we complete an assessment to our satisfaction we need to remind ourselves that the picture we have drawn is, despite all our efforts to the contrary, no more than a caricature, a crude representation of a uniquely indefinable entity. I make this rather emotive plea for the simple reason that I regularly forget this fact: I assume that I am alone in this respect.

The message I have conveyed in this book has been brought to you through the medium of my clumsy usage of what can, in the right hands, be a wonderfully communicative language. This may explain my repeated recourse to the 'wordsmiths' to help express what I instinctively feel about various aspects of assessment. I have suggested on a number of occasions that our concept of mental disorder is primarily an idea, something we explore through the medium of language. Often that language is pitifully impotent to describe the complexity of what we witness or what the patient reports. I believe that we need to remind ourselves that our use of the language can become corrupt. We can become complacent in our communications about the people we call patients. Often we do not say what we mean: or (I hope) we do not mean what we say. It has often been said that we have become insensitive, or sceptical, about the language to which we are exposed. The main culprit appears to be the steady bombardment we receive in the form of slick, loquacious mass media communication and advertising. Advertising, which deals almost exclusively in superlatives, has succeeded in devaluing our language to a point where it is now well accepted that most of the words displayed on billboards, in magazines or within the jingles of the TV commercial are *completely meaningless*. A yawning gulf has opened between language and reality. Writers have persistently bemoaned this gulf, especially where it exists in the form of jargon: here I am thinking not only in terms of psychiatric jargon but how we are assailed by jargon in everyday life. When we use jargon we are talking about people in a language that is divorced from reality; consequently it is easy to lose sight of the 'real person' who is the subject of our discussion. The dramatist Ionesco has written that 'our knowledge becomes separated from life, our culture no longer contains ourselves (or only an insignificant part of ourselves) for it forms a social "context" into which we are not integrated'. He goes on to argue that to bring our lives back into contact with our multiple realities we may need to 'kill our respect for what is written down in black-and-white, to push human beings again towards seeing themselves as they really are'.

This is a subtle and complex concept, and one which I have advocated *ad nauseam* throughout this book. We should try to use our language sensitively, carefully and creatively, to *build up* a picture of the complexity of the human state. We should avoid, wherever possible, categorising, simplifying, caricaturing and ultimately distancing ourselves from the reality of the patient's experience of us — and our experience of him. I recognise that, at least according to my own standards, I have failed to do this in the text.

The assessment process I have described attempts to study the patient as scientifically as possible. This approach is based on the clear understanding that people cannot be analysed in the same way as geological formations. A substantial part of our assessment involves our interaction with the patient, who may influence our perception of him in ways which the rock, the plant or even the lower-order species animals never could. Assessment in psychiatric nursing is not a one-way traffic. In the introductions to the various chapters I have tried to indicate that our assessment practice is influenced by a wide range of schools of thought: medical, psychological, sociological, artistic, literary, anthropological and even political. The net result is that psychiatric nursing assessment relies heavily upon *judgements* — judgements we make about the patient's behaviour, based upon our earlier judgements of the various influential schools of thought. As a result our assessment is not so much based upon 'fact' as upon our translation or interpretation of the facts. These are the views which we, the care-givers, hold about the person who is called 'patient'.

In this book I have tried to communicate a little of what I believe to be the substance of psychiatric nursing assessment. Many will challenge the value and the validity of much of what has appeared in this book. Many will challenge the relevance any of this has to psychiatric nursing. This is only right and fitting. For only by such disagreements will we clarify, to our greater satisfaction, the meaning of the term 'psychiatric nursing assessment'.

INDEX